Mindfulness in Behavioral Health

Series Editor

Nirbhay N. Singh
Medical College of Georgia
Augusta University
Augusta, GA, USA

More information about this series at http://www.springer.com/series/8678

Lynette M. Monteiro • Jane F. Compson
Frank Musten

Editors

Practitioner's Guide to Ethics and Mindfulness-Based Interventions

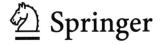 Springer

Editors
Lynette M. Monteiro
Ottawa Mindfulness Clinic
Ottawa, ON, Canada

Jane F. Compson
University of Washington
Tacoma, WA, USA

Frank Musten
Ottawa Mindfulness Clinic
Ottawa, ON, Canada

ISSN 2195-9579   ISSN 2195-9587   (electronic)
Mindfulness in Behavioral Health
ISBN 978-3-319-64923-8   ISBN 978-3-319-64924-5   (eBook)
DOI 10.1007/978-3-319-64924-5

Library of Congress Control Number: 2017956123

Printed on acid-free paper

This Springer imprint is published by Springer Nature
The registered company is Springer International Publishing AG
The registered company address is: Gewerbestrasse 11, 6330 Cham, Switzerland

To all my teachers, friends, and family who bring clarity to the complex joys of values, morals, ethics, and their purpose as the emergence of love: the teachers and participants at the Ottawa Mindfulness Clinic whose trust make this work a joy; Jane Compson, Anne Schlieper, Cary Kogan, Mu Soeng, and Pierre Ritchie for their continuous support and embodied ethics. To Alexandra Monteiro Musten and Mike Valiquette for their love and dearest Amelia who fills us with hope. To Frank, for everything.

Lynette M. Monteiro

To my friends and teachers in the secular and Buddhist mindfulness communities. To Jay Schneller for tirelessly supporting me, and to Lynette Monteiro for making all this happen and being a wonderful model and guide in so many ways. To my wonderful colleagues at UW Tacoma who offer support, humor, and inspiration. To my lovely family (and other animals) who keep my feet on the ground.

Jane F. Compson

To the teachers at the Ottawa Mindfulness Clinic whose collaboration in designing and teaching our courses has enriched my awareness of the ethical space we create when we teach: to Marie-Andree Papineau and Caroline Douglas, my partners in bringing ethically based mindfulness programs into organizations; Alexandra who inspires me with her dedication to caring for those who live in the margins of society, her partner Mike whose imagination is a constant source of wonder, to Amelia whose constant smile can brighten any day, and to Lynette who is constantly striving to encourage the good in all of us. As always, thank you for being my North Star.

Frank Musten

Contents

Contributors

David G. Addiss, MD, MPH Task Force for Global Health, Decatur, GA, USA

Eck Institute for Global Health, University of Notre Dame, Notre Dame, IN, USA

Center for Compassion and Global Health, Atlanta, GA, USA

Ruth Baer, PhD Department of Psychology, University of Kentucky, Lexington, KY, USA

Shalini Bahl, PhD The Reminding Project and Downtown Mindfulness in Amherst, Amherst, MA, USA

Isenberg School of Management, UMass, Amherst, MA, USA

Sean Bruyea, MA Independent freelancer, Nepean, Canada

Bruno A. Cayoun, DPsych Mindfulness-integrated Cognitive Behavior Therapy Institute, Hobart, Tasmania, Australia

Jane F. Compson, PhD University of Washington, Tacoma, WA, USA

Anthony A. DeMauro, PhD CISE Department, Curry School of Education, University of Virginia, Charlottesville, VA, USA

James R. Doty, MD The Center for Compassion and Altruism Research and Education, Stanford University, Stanford, CA, USA

Christopher Germer, PhD Cambridge, MA, USA

Candy Gunther Brown, PhD Department of Religious Studies, Indiana University, Bloomington, IN, USA

Patricia A. Jennings, PhD CISE Department, Curry School of Education, University of Virginia, Charlottesville, VA, USA

James N. Kirby, PhD The University of Queensland, St Lucia, QLA, Australia

The Center for Compassion and Altruism Research and Education, Stanford University, Stanford, CA, USA

Michael Krasner, MD Olsan Medical Group, Rochester, NY, USA

Donald McCown, PhD, MAMS, MSS, LSW Center for Contemplative Studies, West Chester University of Pennsylvania, West Chester, PA, USA

Laura M. Nagy, PhD Department of Psychology, University of Kentucky, Lexington, KY, USA

Patricia Lück, MD, MA Olsan Medical Group, Rochester, NY, USA

Pittman McGehee University of Texas, Austin, TX, USA

Lynette M. Monteiro, PhD Ottawa Mindfulness Clinic, Ottawa, ON, Canada

Frank Musten, PhD Ottawa Mindfulness Clinic, Ottawa, ON, Canada

Kristin Neff, PhD University of Texas, Austin, TX, USA

Stanley R. Steindl, PhD The University of Queensland, St Lucia, QLD, Australia

About the Editors

Lynette M. Monteiro, PhD is a clinical psychologist and Director of Training at the Ottawa Mindfulness Clinic. She is trained in CBT, Cognitive Processing Therapy for veterans and active military personnel, several mindfulness-based interventions, and Buddhist chaplaincy. Her primary treatment interest is exploring the development of values through mindfulness programs; she also serves as a personnel selection psychologist for police and military units. As Clinical Professor at the University of Ottawa, she trains PhD clinical psychology candidates in Mindfulness-Based Symptom Management. She is coauthor of *Mindfulness Starts Here*, contributor to *Buddhist Foundations of Mindfulness*, and several articles and presentations on contemporary mindfulness, ethics, and treatment issues.

Jane F. Compson, PhD is an assistant professor in Interdisciplinary Arts and Sciences at the University of Washington, Tacoma. Her PhD is in comparative religion, and she has training in MBSR and Buddhist chaplaincy. She teaches in the topics of comparative religion and applied ethics and is a member of a clinical ethics committee. Her research interests are in the application of contemplative practices, particularly those associated with Buddhist traditions, to contemporary contexts. She has published articles in the journals *Contemporary Buddhism*, *Mindfulness*, *Journal of Nursing Education and Practice* and *Interdisciplinary Environmental Review*.

Frank Musten, PhD is a clinical psychologist and co-founder of the Ottawa Mindfulness Clinic. In private practice, he treats persons managing stress-related disorders and relationship issues. In the Ottawa Mindfulness Clinic, he has developed a Burnout Resilience program for executives, police, and military personnel and conducted mindfulness programs with various military units. Working with military and police services since 1970, he has developed various programs for dealing with stress and currently is involved with clinical and pre-deployment assessment and post-deployment treatment of military members, including using mindfulness-informed treatments to manage PTSD. He also trains and supervises health care professionals in developing ethics-based mindfulness for clinical treatment.

About the Authors

David G. Addiss, MD, MPH is a public health physician whose work has focused on the prevention and treatment of neglected tropical diseases—causes of immense suffering and disability. He has worked as a general medical practitioner in migrant health, an epidemiologist at the US Centers for Disease Control and Prevention, and a program director at the Task Force for Global Health. David completed the lay chaplaincy training program at Upaya Zen Center. He teaches global health ethics at the Eck Institute for Global Health, University of Notre Dame. His current interests include global health ethics and compassion in global health.

Ruth Baer, PhD is Professor of Psychology at the University of Kentucky, a licensed clinical psychologist, and an Associate of the Oxford Mindfulness Centre at the University of Oxford. She conducts research on mindfulness and teaches and supervises several mindfulness-based interventions. Her interests include assessment and conceptualization of mindfulness and compassion, effects of mindfulness-based programs, mechanisms of change, and professional training and ethics in the mindfulness field.

Shalini Bahl, PhD is an advocate of mindfulness in business, education, and society. She is committed to integrating the transformative potential of mindfulness in marketing, business, and policy to enhance consumer, employee, and societal well-being. Her research on self-awareness and mindfulness has been published in premier marketing and public policy journals. Through her organization, The Reminding Project, she designs and delivers mindfulness-based solutions that address workplace challenges. In her studio, Downtown Mindfulness, she is co-reating a community to promote mindful living. She has received professional training with the Center for Mindfulness at UMass Medical School and the Search Inside Yourself Leadership Institute.

Sean Bruyea, MA graduated from the Royal Military College in 1986. He served as an intelligence Officer in the Gulf War (1990–91) where he suffered disabling physical and psychological injuries. Since retiring from the military, Sean has devoted himself to investigating, presenting, and writing extensively about injured serving and retired military. He has also been a frequent commentator in both Canadian and international media. In 2010, the Canadian government issued a rare official apology to Sean for widespread violations of his privacy carried out as a reprisal for his advocacy on behalf of disabled veterans. In 2016, Sean completed his Master's in Public Ethics focusing upon the obligations governments have to their military veterans.

Bruno A. Cayoun, DPsych is a clinical psychologist in private practice and principal developer of Mindfulness-integrated Cognitive Behaviour Therapy (MiCBT). He is Director of the MiCBT Institute, a leading provider of MiCBT training to mental health services since 2003. Dr. Cayoun co-supervises mindfulness research in collaboration with various universities. He has practiced mindfulness meditation and attended intensive training in the Burmese Vipassana tradition of S. N. Goenka in France, Nepal, India, and Australia since 1989. He is the author of three books, including *Mindfulness-integrated CBT: Principles and Practice* (Wiley, 2011) and *Mindfulness-integrated CBT for Well-Being and Personal Growth* (Wiley, 2015).

Jane F. Compson, PhD is Assistant Professor in the School of Interdisciplinary Arts and Sciences at the University of Washington, Tacoma, where she teaches religious studies and philosophy. She studies the application of contemplative techniques in contemporary secular contexts and has authored articles in journals including *Mindfulness, Contemporary Buddhism, Journal of Nursing Education and Practice, Interdisciplinary Environmental Review,* and in the books *Contemplative Approaches to Sustainability in Higher Education: Theory and Practice* (Eaton, Hughes and MacGregor, 2017) and *Meditation and the Classroom* (Simmer-Brown et al., 2011).

Anthony A. DeMauro, MS is a doctoral candidate at the University of Virginia's Curry School of Education in the Curriculum, Instruction, and Special Education Department. Anthony's research focuses on how teachers' personal mindfulness practice influences their professional teaching practice such as their abilities to build relationships with students, respond to students' needs, and manage their classrooms. He also works with pre-service teachers as an instructor for classroom management and in-service teachers as a CARE for Teachers training facilitator. Anthony previously worked as a Behavioral Specialist Consultant.

James R. Doty, MD is a professor of neurosurgery at Stanford University and the founder and director of the Stanford Center for Compassion and Altruism Research and Education. He works with scientists from a variety of disciplines examining the neural bases of compassion and altruism. His work also examines how being compassionate with intention affects peripheral physiology in regard to health, wellness, and longevity. He is the *New York Times* bestselling author of *Into the Magic Shop: A Neurosurgeon's Quest to Discover the Mysteries of the Brain and the Secrets of the Heart* now translated into 30 languages and is the senior editor of the *Oxford Handbook of Compassion Science*.

Christopher Germer, PhD is a clinical psychologist and lecturer on psychiatry (part-time) at Harvard Medical School. He is a co-developer of the *Mindful Self-Compassion (MSC)* program, author of *The Mindful Path to Self-Compassion*, and co-editor of *Mindfulness and Psychotherapy,* and *Wisdom and Compassion in Psychotherapy.* Dr. Germer is a founding faculty member of the Institute for Meditation and Psychotherapy as well as the Center for Mindfulness and Compassion, Cambridge Health Alliance, Harvard Medical School. He teaches and leads workshops internationally on mindfulness and compassion and has a private practice in Arlington, Massachusetts, USA, specializing in mindfulness and compassion-based psychotherapy.

Candy Gunther Brown, PhD (Harvard University, 2000) is Professor of Religious Studies at Indiana University. Brown is author of *The Word in the World: Evangelical Writing, Publishing, and Reading in America, 1789–1880* (University of North Carolina Press, 2004); *Testing Prayer: Science and Healing* (Harvard University Press, 2012); and *The Healing Gods: Complementary and Alternative Medicine in Christian America* (Oxford University Press, 2013). She is editor of Global Pentecostal and Charismatic Healing (Oxford University Press, 2011) and co-editor (with Mark Silk) of *The Future of Evangelicalism in America* (Columbia University Press, 2016). Her current book project is tentatively titled: "Secular AND Religious: Yoga and Mindfulness in Public Schools, and the Re-Establishment of Religion in America."

Patricia A. (Tish) Jennings, MEd, PhD is an Associate Professor of Education at the Curry School of Education at the University of Virginia. She is an internationally recognized leader in the fields of social and emotional learning and mindfulness in education. Dr. Jennings led the team that developed CARE for Teachers, a mindfulness-based professional development program shown to significantly improve teacher well-being, emotional supportiveness, and sensitivity and classroom productivity in the largest randomized controlled trial of a mindfulness-based intervention designed specifically to address teacher occupational stress. She is the author of *Mindfulness for Teachers: Simple Skills for Peace and Productivity in the Classroom.*

James N. Kirby, PhD is a Lecturer at the School of Psychology at the University of Queensland. James is a practicing compassion-focused therapist and evaluates the impact of compassion-based interventions. He has published over 30 peer-reviewed journal articles and has presented at international conferences on his compassion research. James worked at the Center for Compassion and Altruism Research and Education at Stanford University as a Research Fellow to Dr. James R. Doty. He is also the co-founder of the Compassionate Initiative at the University of Queensland.

Michael Krasner, MD, FACP is a Professor of Clinical Medicine at the University of Rochester School of Medicine and Dentistry, practices internal medicine, and has taught mindfulness-based interventions to patients, medical students, and health professionals for over 16 years, with over 2200 participants and 800 health professionals. He is engaged in several research projects including investigations of mindfulness on the immune system in the elderly, chronic psoriasis, and medical student stress and well-being. He was the project director of *Mindful Communication: Bringing Intention, Attention, and Reflection to Clinical Practice*, sponsored by New York Chapter of ACP and reported in *JAMA* in September, 2009.

Patricia Lück, MD, MA is a Palliative Care Physician, Certified MBSR Teacher, and Medical Educator. She worked for many years in palliative medicine in South Africa before moving to London, UK. She is a faculty member for the Mindfulness Certificate Program at the University of Stellenbosch Medical School, South Africa, as well as the Mindful Practice program in the Division of Medical Humanities at the University of Rochester School of Medicine. Her interest is in growing clinician capacity, a necessary component of heartfulness and deep listening within medicine in order to be present to the diversity of human suffering within a variety of complex settings.

Donald McCown, PhD is Associate Professor of Health and Co-Director of the Center for Contemplative Studies at West Chester University. Over the past two decades, he has taught mindfulness-based programs at Thomas Jefferson University, Won Institute of Graduate Studies, and in the postgraduate program in Family Therapy at Council for Relationships. He is primary author of *Teaching Mindfulness: A practical guide for clinicians and educators* and *New World Mindfulness: From the Founding Fathers, Emerson, and Thoreau to Your Personal Practice*; author of *The Ethical Space of the Mindfulness-Based Interventions*, and primary editor of *Resources for Teaching Mindfulness: An International Handbook*.

Pittman McGehee, PhD is a licensed psychologist in private practice in Austin, Texas. He received his doctorate from the University of Texas, Austin, focusing his research on the connection between psychological health and the concepts of mindfulness and self-compassion. In addition to his private practice, Dr. McGehee is a certified Mindful Self-Compassion teacher and teacher-trainer, is currently adjunct faculty at Seton Cove Spirituality Center, Austin, Texas, as well as teaching faculty in the Department of Educational Psychology at the University of Texas, Austin.

Lynette M. Monteiro, PhD is a psychologist, Clinical Professor (University of Ottawa), and co-founder of the Ottawa Mindfulness Clinic. Co-developer of Mindfulness-Based Symptom Management, she facilitates pain management and military-focused Operational Stress Injury programs. She coauthored the book, *Mindfulness Starts Here* (Friesen Press, 2013), journal articles in *Mindfulness* and *International Journal of Psychotherapy* on ethics in traditional and contemporary mindfulness, and contributed a chapter to *Buddhist Foundations of Mindfulness* (Springer, 2015). In private practice, she treats military and veterans experiencing PTSD and conducts personnel selection for police and military services. She is Director of Training at the Ottawa Mindfulness Clinic.

Frank Musten, PhD is a clinical psychologist in private practice and Director of Programs at the Ottawa Mindfulness Clinic. His work in applied organizational behavioral research began with the Canadian Armed Forces and then with the Royal Canadian Mounted Police at the Canadian Police College. His private practice primarily focusses on work stress and person-organization fit. In 2003, he co-founded the Ottawa Mindfulness Clinic where he and other clinic teachers have developed mindfulness-based interventions designed to foster burnout resilience as well as promote well-being among engaged high performers in various organizational contexts. He is the coauthor of *Mindfulness Starts Here* (Friesen Press, 2013) and several articles in the popular press and peer-reviewed journals.

Laura M. Nagy is a PhD candidate in clinical psychology at the University of Kentucky. Her research interests include mindfulness, borderline personality disorder, self-criticism, and rumination and her clinical work focuses on using mindfulness-based interventions.

Kristin Neff, PhD is currently an Associate Professor of Educational Psychology at the University of Texas at Austin. She is a pioneer in the field of self-compassion research, conducting the first empirical studies on self-compassion over a decade ago. In addition to writing numerous academic articles and book chapters on the topic, she is the author of the book "*Self-Compassion: The Proven Power of Being Kind to Yourself*," released by William Morrow. In conjunction with her colleague Dr. Chris Germer, she has developed an empirically supported eight-week training program called Mindful Self-Compassion, and offers workshops on self-compassion worldwide.

Stanley R. Steindl, PhD is a clinical psychologist in private practice at Psychology Consultants Pty Ltd, Brisbane, Australia, as well as an adjunct associate professor at the School of Psychology, the University of Queensland, Brisbane, Australia. He is a researcher and teacher in compassion and compassion-based interventions, and in 2014 he established the UQ Compassion Symposium, an annual conference aimed at promoting compassion in society.

Chapter 1
Introduction: A New Hope

Donald McCown

How Shall I Begin?

This chapter starts in the first person, so that I am assuming responsibility for all nuances of expression. It starts from a question that is not merely academic, but also engages the well-being of the community of mindfulness-based practitioners. And it starts at the very beginning of ethical thought in the West, with Aristotle as a foundation of science and poetics—and the tension between them.

I'm writing here to satisfy my own curiosity, in hope that readers, particularly members of the mindfulness-based practitioner community, are curious, as well. In 2010, I became interested in the ethics of mindfulness-based programs (MBPs), and determined to make it the subject of my dissertation (McCown, 2013). When I spoke with colleagues then, I was mostly met with puzzled reactions, such as "Why are you thinking about that?" or some variant of "That's inherent in what we do." The implication was always that there were more pressing theoretical challenges, such as coming to clarity on a definition of mindfulness or ensuring quality in teacher training.

The mindfulness-based programs community seemed insulated against if not isolated from direct confrontation with ethical critiques, as year to year the empirical evidence mounted, and interest in and adoption of mindfulness continued to blossom, both inside and outside the therapeutic intervention context, and both with and without informed understanding (that definition problem!). By January of 2014, *Time* magazine's cover was announcing the "Mindfulness Revolution." The illustration on the cover was reflective of the less-informed manifestations in the culture, rather than of the MBPs on the ground. Not coincidentally, a backlash was

D. McCown, PhD, MAMS, MSS, LSW (✉)
Center for Contemplative Studies, West Chester University of Pennsylvania,
Sturzebecker Health Sciences Center, #312, West Chester, PA 19383, USA
e-mail: DMcCown@wcupa.edu

© Springer International Publishing AG 2017   1
L.M. Monteiro et al. (eds.), *Practitioner's Guide to Ethics and Mindfulness-Based Interventions*, Mindfulness in Behavioral Health,
DOI 10.1007/978-3-319-64924-5_1

taking hold in parallel to this growth in popularity. The neologism "McMindfulness" for the often less-informed approaches to mindfulness, particularly in the corporate world, rapidly achieved currency through a *Huffington Post* blog entry (Purser & Loy, 2013).

This line of critique arose mostly within the Western Buddhist community, focused on a fear that mindfulness, presented as a "secularized" version of a Buddhist practice, is thereby unmoored from its ethical anchors in traditional and religious context, and available for exploitative and unethical applications. A central, politically tinged argument is that mindfulness training may be aimed to make corporate employees both more productive and more docile, while the image of the "mindful sniper" is a potent rhetorical device for incongruent applications of what may be considered an originally spiritual practice. The tone and temper of this criticism has ranged from sincere to withering, with Anne Harrington and John Dunne noting that, "The scorn evident in some of the criticisms is quite stunning" (2015, p. 662). A mere 4 years later, we can view this counter-blossoming of mindfulness through the lens of popular opinion by returning to *Time* magazine and the headline, "How we ruined mindfulness," introducing an article replete with sniper fears (Krznaric, 2017).

Certainly, this 4-year slice of the popular history of mindfulness offers range for broad political, sociological, and other forms of interpretation. This is not my interest here. I am concerned with the much smaller community of the mindfulness-based programs, where critique also arose—in *Mindfulness*, its "journal of record"—beginning with a chapter by the editors of this volume (Monteiro, Musten, & Compson, 2015) and including, for example, contending views from Theravada Buddhist clergy (Amaro, 2015), academic and clinical psychology (Baer, 2015; Grossman, 2015), religious studies (Lindahl, 2015), and management (as well as Zen clergy) (Purser, 2015).

This was a rich and varied colloquy, opening avenues to be pursued further. The present volume begins this pursuit, bringing together theoretical and practical considerations of the ethics *of* and ethics *in* mindfulness—to use the convenient distinction employed by Lynette Monteiro (2017). In the *of* category, the questions surrounding the tensions of secular versus spiritual framings of mindfulness loom large, including the appropriateness of applying mindfulness—as a spiritually derived practice—with secular populations. I recommend to the reader Jane Compson's insightful and inspiring Chap. 2 for grounding, and the succeeding chapters in Part One for valuable meditations on such issues from different disciplines. The *in* category ultimately reflects the strength and flexibility of the mindfulness-based practitioners who work from the community resources of scientific evidence, curriculum offerings, and pedagogical insights that have been shared within the MBPs across four decades. The questions here surround the place of ethics in the development and delivery of mindfulness-based programs—questions sensitively elaborated in Lynette Monteiro's Chap. 6 and Frank Musten's Chap. 13. The further chapters reflect the often-hidden glory of the MBP community—that is, the creativity and care taken in theory, curriculum, and pedagogy for programs that meet an ever-expanding range of participants where they are.

Toward a Productive Question

Conditions in the MBP community when the current ethical dialogue arose were perhaps different than in the broader culture, and motivations and intentions of the ethical critique might be seen as different, as well. It is the specific situation of the community in this "ethical moment," and its response, that interest me in this essay. The question that I began to form was: Why this sudden eruption of ethical debate? Yes, of course, there was critique outside the community, but this was not directly targeted toward clinical applications, and, after all, leaders of the MBP community drew strong distinctions—for example, Jon Kabat-Zinn announced directly in an interview, "This is not McMindfulness by any stretch of the imagination" (Shonin 2016)—and held to the line that the MBPs have always had a strong implicit and embodied ethic (Crane, Brewer, et al., 2016).

It was not as if the MBP community had been rocked by financial or sexual scandals and needed to concentrate its thinking and resources on ethical reform in order to recover. This actually was the case in many American Buddhist and Hindu practice communities in the 1980s. Consider three high-profile cases:

1. Richard Baker Roshi inherited the leadership of the San Francisco Zen Center and its associated businesses from Suzuki Roshi at the latter's death in 1971. In an austere community, Baker spent hundreds of thousands of dollars on personal expenses, and, among many other infidelities, had carried on a brazen affair with a student—the wife of a close friend and major donor. Finally, in 1983, the board pressed him to take an extended (ultimately infinite) leave of absence (Downing, 2001). Perhaps most distressing in trying to understand the situation is that even 10 years later Baker was both unreflective and unrepentant, stating "It is as hard to say what I have learned as it is to say what happened" (Bell, 2002, p. 236).
2. Osel Tenzin, Vajra Regent of the Shambhala organization and successor to its founder Chogyam Trungpa, was revealed in 1988 to be HIV-positive, and, although aware of his condition, to have continued his long practice of unprotected sex with male and female members of the organization. It further came to light that board members had been aware of his HIV status and had kept silent. On the advice of a senior Tibetan teacher, Tenzin went into retreat, and died soon after (Bell, 2002).
3. Asian Theravada teacher, Anagarika Munindra, teaching an Insight Meditation Society retreat, had sex with a participant—a woman who had been psychologically troubled, and now was further traumatized. While IMS guiding teachers were divided on approach, Kornfield pushed for complete disclosure and an immediate confronting of Munindra, noting, "If parts of one's life are quite unexamined—which was true for all of us—and something like this comes up about a revered teacher, it throws everything you've been doing for years into doubt. It's threatening to the whole scene" (Schwartz, 1995, p. 334).

These are simply examples. By 1988, Kornfield would write, "Already upheavals over teacher behavior and abuse have occurred at dozens (if not the majority) of the major Buddhist and Hindu centers in America" (quoted in Bell, 2002). As the communities, directly affected and otherwise, coped with the aftermath of the scandals, they came to a new maturity—backing away from charismatic leadership into more distributed and democratic models, and adopting formal ethics statements and policies.

As these scandals arose and faded, MBSR was establishing itself. It is interesting to me that any mention of this time period or such incidents is missing from the detailed recounting of the history of the clinical application of meditation through which Harrington and Dunne (2015) attempt to understand the current arising of the "ethics" debate for the MBP community. Yet, there was certainly impetus and opportunity for the MBSR community to think through questions of ethics of this kind.

So, in considering my question, there is no current moral stain on the escutcheon of the MBPs to parallel the narratives above. As drivers for ethical thinking, any historical issues have been lost to memory, suppressed, or ignored. Still, a debate goes on inside the MBP community, under the banner of ethics. My question begins to sharpen: Why choose ethics as the category of critical thought? The questions about ethics *of* mindfulness might be included in the long-standing quandary about the definition of mindfulness and its relationship to secular or sacred derivations and framings (e.g., Brown, Ryan, Loverich, Biegel, & West, 2011; Grossman, 2011; Hölzel et al., 2011; Sauer, Lynch, Walach, & Kohls, 2011). The *in* questions, likewise, already have a pride of place in the community's dialogues, particularly around ensuring quality in curriculum development and teacher training (e.g., Crane, Soulsby, Kuyken, Williams, & Eames, 2016; Cullen, 2011; Grossman, 2010; Kabat-Zinn, 2011; Santorelli, Goddard, Kabat-Zinn, Kesper-Grossman, & Reibel, 2011).

Why not maintain the continuity of these ongoing dialogues? Why hang a new banner if there is room under the old ones? In fact, the definition debate has been the site of a rare opening beyond the insularity of the science-driven MBPs, inviting voices from outside the community and beyond scientific disciplines (Williams & Kabat-Zinn, 2011, and the entire special issue of *Contemporary Buddhism* they introduce). Another case in point is the distinction now being made between "second-generation" mindfulness-based interventions, which explicitly reference Buddhist forms of mindfulness and worldview in their curriculum and pedagogy, and the first-generation, which is presented as secular (Van Gordon, Shonin, & Griffiths, 2015; Crane, Brewer et al., 2016). This distinction is made within the dialogues both on the definition of mindfulness and assurance of quality in curricula and teachers, rather than being framed in ethical terms. Even the strong charges by Candy Gunther Brown in Chap. 3 about the ethical ramifications of the duplicity of the (first-generation) MBPs showing a secular face to participants while heavily relying on Buddhist thought and practice behind the scenes might as easily be located within these already established dialogues. No thinker's answers or positions are concrete or correct; all of these questions should be open for further exploration.

I am puzzled yet again, although my question is very much sharper: What *else* is going on in the choice of ethics as the banner for dissent? Yes, that's it, precisely. I'd like to suggest that ethics is a repository for disappointment and frustration within the MBP community. Or, perhaps it's a yearning to have more intellectual space in which to explore, with different kinds of attention. Ultimately, it may be that the dialogue around ethics is a forum in which to keep the MBPs together—if not exactly unified—in a time of dramatic growth, transition, and potential fragmentation. To make this sensible, however, may require a different starting point.

Shall I Begin Again?

Let's run all the way back, past even Aristotle and *ethics*, to the *Iliad* and a metaphor employing the Greek root *ethos*. Describing Paris running through the halls of Troy to join his brother Hector in battle against the Greeks, Homer likens him to a stallion freed from the stable and racing toward his herd in the pasture, using for that destination the word *ethos*, meaning the place where an animal belongs with others and will thrive (Baracchi, 2008). For Aristotle,[1] when thinking about the ethical, place and time come together in a particular situation where the individual and community might flourish, if the appropriate actions are taken. The ethical is what a community disposed toward the good does in a specific space and time—a present moment (Baracchi, 2008). Perhaps there is something here for our shared (I hope!) curiosity.

Following Aristotle's conception, ethics as a category of philosophy is by necessity extremely imprecise. John D. Caputo (2003) notes that "Ethics stands alone among the sciences or disciplines by announcing right at the start that it is not possible as a science or, if you prefer, that its possibility is co-constituted by a certain impossibility" (pp. 169–170). This is because the ethical investigation is focused on the fullness of a situation among people gathered in community. Its subject is what is emerging within a web of relationships in the present moment. Aristotle uses the term *poiesis* in his descriptions, so we must understand the moment as a situation emerging through a process of artful creation (Baracchi, 2008). That is, the ethical situation emerges differently in each moment and is difficult to comprehend completely.

When people of virtuous character are gathered in the emerging moment, we may hope that what they are doing—what they create—is beautiful and just. For these ethical constructions, Aristotle favors the metaphor of the products of arts and

---

[1] The fact that the MBPs are often presented as derived from Buddhist thought and practice suggests to many that we may look there for ethical discussions. However, the distinction of the moral versus the ethical complicates such an undertaking. Denotation of both words centers on appropriate behavior; however, the moral bears connotations of action in the workaday world, while the ethical connotes philosophical description and analysis of those actions. Western thinkers such as Plato and Aristotle write extensively about ethics, politics, and justice, yet scholars have not found Buddhist equivalents to the *Republic* or the *Nicomachean Ethics*. While Buddhism is one of the most moral of all the world's religions, technically, it may be described as lacking an ethics. The historical Buddha solved the fundamental problem of defining the good life and how to live it, and in his teachings detailed the "how to" of such a life. His followers simply had to live it, not reflect on it. Buddhism's essential pragmatism may account for the mismatch of categories with Western philosophy (Keown 1992, 2006). Mindful of this fact, my discussion proceeds with Western ethical conceptions.

crafts, which are handmade and never repeatable, yet each is bearing the potential to shine out with beauty (and justice) for all. This includes the idea that our understanding of a situation is an artifact in which we have captured something of the moment, and that can be saved for later—it is an artwork or, maybe better, a text, that can be reflected upon and shared in other times and places (Baracchi, 2008). It becomes possible, then, to see how the value of developing one's character, of coming to possess the virtues, does not ultimately lie in individual improvement, but, rather, in the flourishing of the *polis*—the community.

In this very brief description of the beginning of ethical thinking, I trust that I am making available some useful ideas for our current situation within the community of the MBPs. Now, as the main burden of this chapter begins to unfold, I'll be drawing on the essential *im*precision of ethical thought as motivating and shaping the present discourse from which this entire volume springs. I'll be considering virtues and their cultivation from the perspective of their potential within a community, rather than their isolated value to an individual. And I'll center my own descriptions and conjectures in the *poiesis*, the formation, the making, indeed, the poetics of situations in particular places and times—pointing specifically to the MBP classroom, wherever it is to be found.

How Can the MBPs Go On?

As I've suggested, it is certainly possible to locate the bulk of the internal critique of the MBPs within longstanding categories of dialogue, such as the definition of mindfulness, and assurance of quality for curricula and teacher development. However, these critiques are quite often being engaged under the more provocative banner of ethics. To understand why, I believe we must particularly consider the imprecision, the poetic ambiguity of ethical investigation. It stands in direct opposition to the entire trajectory of the MBPs toward the current height of their popularity within health care and mental health care.

Inarguably, the nearly four-decade-long project of amassing an empirical evidence base for the MBPs has been central to their dramatic growth. Inevitably, the nature of the research conducted has recursively shaped the interventions, focused as it is on individual outcomes as measured by self-reported quantitative psychological tests, physiological measurements, and neuroscience imaging. Such an approach locates any pathology and any potential relief inside the patient's mind (or even more intense, the patient's brain). Individualistic and reductionistic assumptions are rampant. The typical becomes a substitute for the actual, and fails to add thickness to our understanding of the embodied experience of the intervention. The vast bulk of the data generated in the MBPs has therefore not been useful in ongoing development of the pedagogy, which relies on complex, poetic (to use our new designation) understandings of the moment of teaching in the community of the classroom. Rather, tending to the requirements of randomized controlled trials has tended to calcify curricula and restrict the options of the teacher in the service of ever more "reliable" data. Although there may be the beginning of a trend toward the use of mixed methods to include qualitative data in larger studies, any such shift is concurrent with the ethical critique, and, in fact, might be interpreted as a response to it.

Opposition to the constriction of certain lines of thought and practice may be, then, what is behind the raising of ethics as the banner for critique. After all, ethics, as Aristotle describes it, is the most imprecise of the sciences, the least amenable to typical means of empirical investigation. Invoking it is a symbolic and concrete protest. As the disappointments of the hegemony of the scientific disciplines become more difficult for some MBP community members to bear, the new possibilities of ethical discourse offer consolation—and new opportunities. Ethics directs attention to the actions of the gathered community in the present moment, where we are better served by a poetic, as compared to a scientific, approach. Here, teachers and researchers can find more "elbow room" for their work; indeed, with the ethical critique, they might be seen as "elbowing a way in" to a space perceived to be closing down.

Ethical critique within the milieu of the MBPs opens new avenues of investigation—from wider theoretical reflections using resources as diverse as Buddhist conceptions of compassion and contemporary feminist care ethics, to creative adaptations of mindfulness-based curricula and pedagogy that accommodate revised views of the relationships and values vital to working successfully with an expanding range of participants. The present volume is representative of this poetic direction and the creative energy behind it. Many of the chapters are approached with sensitivity to the particular situation that is being engaged, such as the needs of medical practitioners in Chap. 5, business professionals in Chap. 14, or military personnel in Chap. 15. Many chapters go further, engaging the creative tasks of actually writing the poems, so to speak—specifying curricula and pedagogical approaches to mindfulness in health care and mental health care, such as Mindfulness-integrated Cognitive Behavior Therapy in Chap. 7, Mindfulness-Based Symptom Management in Chap. 8, and Mindful Self-Compassion in Chap. 11, as well as the CARE program for teachers in Chap. 9, culminating in explorations of compassion (Chap. 10) and self-compassion (Chap. 11).

Within these chapters—further, within the creative actions of MBP participants and teachers in their places in the moment in classes the world over—we may find a way forward that offers countermoves to individualism and reductionism. We may even find that the critical chorus singing under the banner of ethics offers a promise to keep the whole community of the MBPs together.

Pedagogical Discourse of the MBPs

Although their discourse has been subordinated to the overarching scientific discourse of the MBPs over the decades, teachers have a contrasting way of talking about what happens in the classroom with the participants, which colleagues and I have remarked upon and elaborated over many years (McCown, 2013, 2016; McCown, Reibel, & Micozzi, 2010; McCown & Wiley, 2008, 2009). With not too much reflection, it becomes evident that the MBPs, as group-based interventions, are complex situations in which networks of relationships develop from session to session as the course progresses, in both the long stretches of silence and the interactive events of the curriculum.

With colleagues, I have also suggested that the discourse of MBP pedagogy fits very well with a social constructionist approach that reflects a radical interdependence of participants and teachers (Gergen, 2009, 2015; McCown et al., 2010). This approach differs in intensity from the relational understandings applied by others involved in pedagogical theory (Crane, Kuyken, Hastings, Rothwell, & Williams, 2010; Crane, Brewer, et al., 2016). These thinkers maintain the received individualistic view of participants, and grant the teacher a superior position from which to act on the class. More radically, our thinking proceeds from a view of the class as a "confluence" (Gergen, 2009) in which actions of participants are not structured by cause and effect, but rather are continually self-defining. That is, we do not posit a group of discrete participants and teachers who take actions based on directives (however gentle), but rather we see a confluence that continually co-creates its actions and dispositions from moment to moment. This is much like the creative actions of the community of Aristotle's description—drawing us toward a poetics of the MBPs, and, with an expanded attention, perhaps toward a poetics of the MBP community itself. Monteiro and Musten, in the present volume, describe this poetics quite clearly in the context of their "second-generation" MBP, Mindfulness-Based Symptom Management (MBSM):

> …MBSM is far from—and likely never will become—an intervention that is fixed and manualized. The essential truth is that nothing is permanent and everything is in constant state of change; it is both a spiritual claim of Buddhism and of physical science. But there is also a more immediate reason for the constant state of change: every program we offer is new simply because all those who come together are doing so for the very first time. In the space that each program is conducted, everything is happening for the first time. Even as teachers who have walked into that room hundreds of times over the years, we too are new because the relationship with everyone there creates us anew (p. XX).

The focus on ethics as a category of thought may be moving our thinking around or pushing it past the unreflective individualism and reductionism of the scientific focus of the MBPs. Therefore, it may be valuable to sketch—poetically, and with ample room for revisions—what the opposites of individualism and reductionism may look like in practice. In what follows, I am suggesting that on the other side of individualism we will find a healthy community that has been there all along, and that on the other side of reductionism we'll find a rich diversity of participants and their contributions to the moment-to-moment life of the community. It may even happen that, just as Aristotle, I cannot resist proposing some very *un*certain principles that may be of general use in our ethical thinking.

Community, Strong and Weak

An MBP class is a confluence dedicated to the pedagogy of mindfulness. The community is learning and changing as it moves from formal meditation practices to mindful dialogue about the practice to structured engagement with material in specific curricular modules. Participants (I use the word because we don't really have the language to describe persons as *integrated parts* of a confluence) partake of the pedagogy actively or passively, by participating or observing, by speaking to others or remaining silent—they are all affected. Humans are sensitive creatures that "cannot not respond" to the activity around them (Shotter, 2011). In whatever mode they choose for participation, they are connected within the confluence—the ongoing dialogue is part of them as they are part of it. Gergen (2009) notes that what we call thinking may be recast as "unfinished dialogue," so even our "inner self" can be seen as part of the outer confluence. Here we might come back to the idea mentioned above of experience as forming artworks or texts, where such texts—acknowledged in words or actions—become available to all and are generative of further texts, finished or unfinished, that nurture the confluence (McCown & Billington, under review).

An MBP class is, thus, a small community that develops a capacity to generate mindfulness, and to know how to go on together from moment to moment. It has a poetics, and, in fact, it has an ethics as well. Gergen (2009, 2011) describes that the shared meanings and values established through the actions of the confluence define the "good" for the group's life. When such a "first order morality" is present—even if it has never come into direct speech—it governs the sense-making of the group. To transgress it would place one outside the bounds of shared meaning. A simple example is that a participant would be extremely unlikely to sing (out loud!) during a silent sitting meditation—because it would make no sense to do so.

With such thinking, we move away from individualism, in which each participant is a self-contained agent who consults knowledge located "inside" him- or herself to decide how to go on in the group. Rather, within a confluence, knowledge of how to go on together is more sensibly seen as located in the group itself—it is community knowledge. We are certainly relational creatures, and are capable of being in different and possibly even competing confluences. Gergen's description (2009) is that we are "multi-beings" made up of ways of going on that have been instilled by experiences in many different confluences. That which has been instilled is available to us in not only within the originating confluences, but also in others as it is appropriate.

Seemingly, then, holding a confluence together requires bonding of the group, so that incongruous ways of going on do not arise and introduce "nonsense." It may be that a strong community is what is needed to accomplish what seems to be tight control. The first-order morality of an organized crime family, for example, will be powerful, and deviation will be dramatically discouraged. This example also suggests that such a strong community may also choose to impose its will on others that are outside its bounds of sense-making. Clearly, a strong community may be a danger to dissenters within and anyone outside. Nevertheless, bringing a community together can have significant value, as suggested by our example of the MBP classroom.

Is it possible to bond a class tightly into a *weak* community? Is it possible to be both close and safe? Let's consider the actions that bond groups of any type, and then compare and contrast with the pedagogical actions of the MBPs.

For Gergen (2009), three mechanisms are involved in the bonding of any confluence—negotiation, narrative, and enchantment. In the context of the MBPs, all are important, and all must be seen in a particular view—as in a poetics.

Negotiation is the "co-creation of shared realities, and the comfort, reliability, and trust that accompany them" (Gergen, 2009, p. 175). This idea moves straightforwardly into MBP pedagogical thinking. In learning to produce moments of mindfulness together, participants find out how they can turn toward their experience in the present moment and find a way to be both with and in it in a nonjudgmental, or, better, a friendly way. Within the setting and actions of the confluence, they are offered freedom to choose how they will respond in each moment. They are impressed with the need for confidentiality, which offers a feeling of safety in the confluence. There is also a high likelihood of positive physiological reinforcement through the early practices; consider the body scan and the relaxation (or sleep!) that often arrives as a side effect of doing it. Through actions of the pedagogy, participants quickly find that they share a common purpose, often feel more relaxed than when outside the class, and know that the actions in the classroom will unfold sensibly.

Narrative, the second mechanism of bonding, is specifically related to changing a story about "me" into a story of "we." In an ongoing relationship, the individual is invited to soften self-boundaries and instead identify with, or become, the relationship. To say, for example, "in our school we do it this way," or "on our team we always…" involves this kind of narrative. There are, of course, stories that are told within particular confluences to illustrate its special characteristics; Gergen refers to these as "unification myths" (2009, p. 177). The telling of such stories actually prompts actions that are congruent, and that bring the myths into reality. In the MBPs this happens through another kind of text—not a story but a lyric poem, a song, as it were. Through mindfulness pedagogy, participants actually step out of their stories and into the experience of the present moment. Thus, the confluence generates texts of present moment experiences that they share; there is not a storyline, but instead a collection of poems: "Songs from Our Group." This is the burden of the practice of the pedagogy.

While Gergen's description of narrative as a mechanism of bonding highlights the duration of being together—the longer the time, the better the bonding—the MBP view highlights individual moments. We might even see this through the ancient Greek distinction of *chronos*, for sequential, horizontal time, and *kairos*, for vertical time—the moment of opportunity, of significance. So, the group experience of *kairos* in abundance, as it were, may promote bonding, as a lyrical substitute for the long togetherness of a story.

Enchantment is Gergen's third, critical mechanism (2009), through which the confluence takes on a "sense of transcendent importance" (p. 179). The sense is generated especially strongly through language, ritual, and emotion. Let's look at each, within a typical group such as a team, and then see how it might also be applied to descriptions of MBP pedagogy.

Shared words that are performed as oaths, songs, or cheers, or are treated with gravitas, as in founding documents or ongoing records, bring any group together. In an MBP class, which spends much time in silence, we might weight non-verbal expression heavily in lieu of language. How participants hold themselves—posture, attitude, expression, maybe even eye contact—particularly in the moments after practice or while witnessing a moving inquiry dialogue between a classmate and the teacher truly speaks volumes. Messages about group cohesion, caring, and support come through.

Likewise, rituals reinforce the group's meaning to its members—for any group, think of anniversaries, commemorations, even happy hours. In an MBP class, think of meditation practice to start and end, maybe with a ringing bell—participants are called together as a "we" assembled in time. It happens in space as well, when the class is scattered to dyads or small groups for an activity, and then all are called back. Enacted again and again, the meaning arises that we can't go on until we are gathered together.

Emotional expressions at transitions—from simple moments of meeting and parting, to emergent moments of welcoming the new and mourning losses—are displays of commitment to group life and, perhaps, to something beyond. In the MBPs, these socially constructed forms of emotion may certainly take place, yet there is also something more subtle, a feeling tone that seems generated by the facts of being together. Although Gergen eschews physiological description, Steven Porges's (2011) polyvagal theory nevertheless may help in understanding the subtlety here. Porges's theory is based on the evolution of the autonomic nervous system in mammals—particularly the vagus nerves. Mammals adapt to life-threatening situations by "freezing," to challenging situations with "fight or flight," and (here's the new idea) to situations of safety with what Porges calls *social engagement*. In a situation in which others are calm and regulated (as in a class after meditation) and we feel safe, the new vagus nerve slows our heart rate, inhibits fight or flight, and prepares us for optimal sharing with others. Our eyes open wider, inner ears tune to the human voice, face and neck muscles gain tone to make subtle expressions and gestures, and muscles of speech gain tone for better articulation. Perhaps a key to the subtle emotion here is the associated release of oxytocin—the bonding hormone. Maybe the feeling is like coming home.

For a fuller understanding, Robert Frost provides two definitions of "home" through two different characters in his poem, "The Death of a Hired Man." For full effect and understanding, the reader must hold both definitions simultaneously—one follows quickly on the other. First definition: "Home is the place where, when you have to go there, / They have to take you in." The second does not correct this, but adds to it: "I should have called it/Something you somehow haven't to deserve."

So, as we allow the critical discourse of ethics to call attention to the poetics of the MBPs, the individualistic view of the science begins to fade, and what comes into focus is a bonded community. The community created through the pedagogy of the MBPs holds a healthy tension. Its bonding is strong enough to offer the sense of home, yet weak enough not to threaten those who dissent from inside—or who live outside.

Virtues in Community

To understand the healthy tension of MBP classroom communities, we need to view the pedagogy in the widest and most generous way possible. In each class, teacher and participants are learning together how it is possible for them to turn toward to be with and in the experience that is arising in the present moment. There are as many routes to this outcome as there are courses given. The actions within every classroom confluence are entirely contingent on its composition and its location. Each is rich and varied. None are alike. All are shaped by what we are calling poetics. In other words, the pedagogical process is not rote or conceptual learning, but rather is a co-creation of the participants in the moment. The "take away" is not information or knowledge. Instead, it is know-how—a capacity of the confluence that when called for is available as part of the "multi-beings" of participants.

The possible responses of the MBP class to actions of the pedagogy are infinite. As Aristotle states, there are no very useful ways of accounting for a specific choice of actions by applying principles or premises. The same is true for the unfolding of emerging classroom situations. Principles would be at best "navigational instruments" to steer the ship away from the rocks, while what truly matters is the disposition or posture of the participants, as a confluence. When the group is disposed toward the good, the response will promote the good. We are talking here about virtues. The reductionist cast of mind (including Aristotle's) would locate virtues inside individuals, but we are critiquing such moves. What will we find if we locate virtues—the dispositions that produce the good—in the confluence? The confluence itself knows how to produce the good, then, and participants who enter into other, different confluences will have those dispositions available as needed.

What then are the virtues of the confluence of an MBP class? I have previously approached this from a different perspective (McCown, 2013), while creating a model of the space that is generated by the confluence when practicing the pedagogy. To take up the perspective of the critical discourse of ethics as it exists now, I am applying insights from that model to describe three important dispositions that are part of the discourse of the MBP community, and to gesture *very generally* toward a *telos*—a goal or end, to be Aristotelian about it—that the larger MBP community might embrace.

I am proposing these dispositions as virtues that are imbued through the pedagogy of the MBPs at its best, regardless of the structure or generation of the curriculum in use. I find it intriguing that what might be called virtues in Buddhist thought are negatively constructed; that is, they are dispositions *away from* rather than toward particular forms of action. According to Richard Gombrich (2009), the Buddha's ethical process was pragmatic—simply to fix what was broken. Given that immoral behavior is driven by the "three poisons," which are greed, hatred, and ignorance (*raga*, *dosa*, and *moha* in Pali), the three "cardinal virtues" then become non-greed, non-hatred, and non-ignorance (*araga*, *adosa*, and *amoha*). Via this same pragmatism, central dispositions of the MBPs have arisen from the perceived inhumanity of the medical and mental health care system with its labeling of pathologies, hierarchical power structure, and instrumental interventions that ignore the whole person. These may then be expressed the non-pathologizing, non-hierarchical, and non-instrumental virtues—not of individuals, but of the confluence.

Non-pathologizing

This virtue is constantly in tension within the MBPs, as many of them have target populations defined by specific medical or diagnoses, yet insist that they see the whole person. It is certainly easiest to maintain a non-pathologizing disposition within a program open to a heterogeneous population, such as mindfulness-based stress reduction, in which participants from all walks of life, with almost any medical and/or psychological diagnosis, or none at all, may come together as a confluence. In considering this disposition of non-pathologizing, Jon Kabat-Zinn (2011) describes how

> it can be felt in the way the instructor relates to the participants and to the entire enterprise. Although our patients all come with various problems, diagnoses, and ailments, we make every effort to apprehend their intrinsic wholeness. We often say that from our perspective, as long as you are breathing, there is more 'right' with you than 'wrong' with you, no matter what is wrong. In this process, we make every effort to treat each participant as a whole human being rather than as a patient, or a diagnosis, or someone having a problem that needs fixing (p. 292).

Although this description comes from a perspective that valorizes the teacher and discounts the other participants, it does clearly suggest that no one needs to carry their specific diagnosis into the class. The nature of the group undercuts the power of diagnostic discourses—whether of medical conditions or psychiatric disorders. As Saki Santorelli suggests:

> Medicine for the past 120 years has really developed tremendous acumen for the differential diagnosis. We give a single diagnosis and then we develop a single treatment modality to meet that diagnostic condition. In the Stress Reduction Clinic, we have done it the other way around. We've said that instead of making the groups homogenous, we will make them heterogeneous. Why? If people participate for the same reason—say heart disease—well, that's what they have in common and where conversation will naturally gravitate. Sometimes this can be very useful, sometimes not. Conversely, if you have people in the room for 25 different reasons, their common ground becomes the work of developing their inner resources in service of whatever ails them. (quoted in Horrigan, 2007, p. 142)

The non-pathologizing disposition re-creates the participants, replacing their limited diagnostic identities with unlimited possibilities. In effect, all participants carry the same diagnosis—the "stress" or suffering of the human condition that everyone shares. They do not attend class with the intention to remove something unwanted from their experiences, but rather are there to learn to live their lives, as they are, to the fullest.

Also, non-pathologizing counters the tendency of participants to put themselves under surveillance—to subjectify themselves to their diagnosis, as Foucault (1995) would put it. That is, a discipline, such as psychiatry or clinical psychology, establishes power through its discourse, its system of knowledge, which in science means a system of classifications. The categories of the Diagnostic and Statistical Manual (DSM) illustrate this well. The use of the DSM as expert knowledge exerts power over your life and identity. When you allow experts to observe, examine, and classify you, you are labeled nearly indelibly. You are made a subject of the power of a discipline—you are subjectified. It is difficult to escape such power. You don't have the power of expertise or social position to reject or overturn your diagnosis—it can follow you forever. Once depressed, for example, once you've been diagnosed as depressed, you are "a depressive" even when you are laughing, even when you've been happy for years. You live under surveillance: How's the depression? It seems like it's lifted, but it may come back. You are never free. And you are the source of much of that surveillance, says Foucault:

> He who is subjected to a field of visibility and who knows it, assumes responsibility for the constraints of power; he makes them play spontaneously upon himself; it inscribes in himself the power relation in which he simultaneously plays both roles; he becomes the principle of his own subjection. (pp. 202–203)

Foucault encourages us to resist, and so do the MBPs—if we listen. The classroom is a site of resistance, and the confluence is a counter-culture in which it is possible to identify and experience other ways of being.

Non-hierarchical

This virtue, too, can be seen as contested. Coming from a culture of expertise, participants assume that the teacher is the expert with a repository of knowledge to share with those who lack. There is much work to be done in the pedagogy to shift this view. Seating the group in a circle is a useful move that sends a non-hierarchical signal—no one is lifted up, put forward, or preferred, not even the teacher. In fact, the pedagogy directs participants toward each other in the dialogue of the gathering. From the start, teachers ask that participants speak to the whole group, not just to the teacher, and reinforce this with nonverbal cues. Another useful strategy is to have participants regularly explore dialogue in dyads and small groups. There is a non-hierarchical message in the fact that the teacher is not privy to these conversations. Such actions work toward dissolving not only the hierarchy of teacher and participant, but also of the more extroverted and less extroverted participants.

The non-hierarchical disposition can also be revealed in the language choices of the teacher—which shape the dialogue of the confluence. Kabat-Zinn (2004) identified a list of difficulties that can be introduced through verbal and non-verbal communication. The one he calls "idealizing" is important to reflect on here. It describes an approach and tone of "I know how to do this and I'm going to teach you," when the language should propose shared exploration, as in, "Let's try this together and see what happens."

The key move of the pedagogy is the great leveler: the group practices mindfulness by turning toward the experience of the moment to be with and in it—and no one knows how it will be, for anyone.

Not knowing is the key to the non-hierarchical disposition. There are not "right" answers, there are only meanings negotiated by each participant—perhaps in dialogue out loud, or maybe in the "unfinished dialogue" of thinking shaped within the confluence. In guidance of practices, the language opens and invites, neither imposing nor assuming any particular quality of experience. In inquiry dialogue, participants have the opportunity to speak and reflect on the experience, to have it witnessed by all, and to have it corrected by none. In a curriculum, whether presented as secular or grounded in Buddhist thought, no particular meaning for a participant's experience is set—in course materials, in the recommended activities in the class, or even in the use of poems or stories. The course is ultimately an object of reflection, and participants are free to ascribe meaning to their experiences, or not, within or outside any spiritual or philosophical tradition. We are in the realm of poetics, together.

Non-instrumental

This is a revelation of the radical nature of the MBPs. It is the basic orientation toward participants in the MBPs: it's not about fixing something that is broken, but about turning toward and being with/in the experience of the moment. It's not about trying to have a particular experience, but about being friendly toward the one you are having. Kabat-Zinn describes it as

> This challenge we pose to our patients in the Stress Reduction Clinic at the very beginning, and with the introduction to the body scan meditation, or even the process of eating one raisin mindfully: namely, to let go of their expectations, goals, and aspirations for coming, even though they are real and valid, to let go—momentarily, at least—even of their goal to feel better or to be relaxed in the body scan, or of their ideas about what raisins taste like, and to simply "drop in" on the actuality of their lived experience and then to sustain it as best they can moment by moment with intentional openhearted presence and suspension of judgment and distraction, to whatever degree possible. (2003, p. 148)

In pedagogical practice, the encounter with the raisin, the body scan, and the other formal meditations are offered in the spirit of "Let's try this together and see what happens." This disposition shapes the language of the classroom, helping participants to explore their experience as it unfolds in the moment—however it might be. The sometimes profound inquiry dialogues between teacher and participant work in this way, taking a fluid path to stay with what is arising, not leaping toward what would be preferred. As this language saturates the confluence, participants begin to apply the approach in their own "unfinished" dialogues, as well—attending to their thinking in a different way. They also attend differently within their dialogues in dyads and small groups, being non-instrumental with themselves and each other.

Relations between participants are regulated by suppression of the impulse to "fix" others—to give advice rather than to be curious about one's own experience of the moment. When moments of suffering arise out loud, as Rebecca Crane and David Elias (2006) have suggested, teacher and participants can

> work to subvert a strong internal and external tendency to look for certain (sometimes quite fixed) kinds of improvement or resolution of difficulties. This is a tendency that can play out in therapeutic and mental health contexts in familiar and unhealthy ways for both practitioners and clients at times. In comparison, the possibility to experience a sense of "OKness" in the midst of "not-OKness," is a broader influence offered by the meditative traditions, which can inform not merely process but also potentially a different approach to content. (p. 32)

Implicit within this choice to be with and in is its obverse—the choice to change what can be changed. This also reflects the non-instrumental disposition. That is, the teacher makes the concept of choice available, but leaves alone what the participant changes or how. On both sides of the coin, curiosity and courage are required, and are essential to this virtue.

And They Make One Whole

These dispositions are interdependent (McCown, 2013). If any one of them is compromised, all of them are compromised. For example, to label a participant with pathology is also to assume a superior place in a hierarchy, and to imply an instrumental intention behind the curriculum. Understanding the costs of compromise, then, is extremely important. The balancing of the three dispositions is precarious and requires significant care, in both curriculum design and teaching. This is another way of considering the poetics of the MBPs.

As the result of such a poetics, an MBP confluence in its practice would have the know how to bring forth a virtuous community. The bonds among participants would be strong enough that all may feel safe and cared for, yet weak enough that any in dissent from the others (even if only in the unfinished dialogue of thought) may also feel safety and caring extended to them. If this is the telos, the end that we have been moving toward, what shall we call it? How shall we characterize it? The deep resources of thought that lie beyond the dominant disciplines of the MBPs are being brought into greater play by the ethical critique, and may be valuable in this process.

Love Will Keep Us Together

I have suggested (McCown, 2013) that what ultimately results from the practice of the pedagogy of mindfulness, within a virtuous community as described above, is *friendship*. Friendship is not a characteristic of one person, not a virtue inside, but rather a quality saturating a confluence. It does not refer to knowledge of how to "get along" with others, but rather refers to the know-how of "going on" together.

It is understood in such a spacious way in two descriptions from the axial age (800 to 200 BCE), when wisdom arose simultaneously in different cultures with little evidence of common influence (Jaspers, 1953; for verifiable East–West influences, see McEvilley, 2002). Greek philosophical thought and the streams of philosophical thought in India leading to Buddhism both seem to offer friendship as an exalted virtue or ultimate good.

Aristotle describes three types of friendship in the *Nicomachean Ethics*. First are the friends you cultivate for pleasure, because they are fun; next are friends who can bring you advantages in business or politics, because of their positions; third are the ones you wish to be with, because of their own goodness—their virtues, their very being. In all three cases, friendship is based on mutual well-wishing; however, in the third case, you wish the other well without expectation of advantage for yourself, and such a wish is returned in the same way. For Aristotle, the third is the perfect form of friendship.

This perfect friendship of mutual well-wishing, for Aristotle and contemporary Aristotelian thinkers (e.g., MacIntyre, 2007; Nussbaum, 1986), is a model for how members of a community (*polis*) should relate to each other. MacIntyre (2007), pointing toward the kind of strong relational view of a confluence, suggests that smaller groups of friends of this type are the very stuff of which the polis is made.

In Buddhist sources, friendship is the paradigm for interpersonal relationships in community (Keown, 1995). In the Upaddha Sutta (Thanissaro, 1997), the Buddha himself states that the whole of the holy life is the life shared with friends. The earlier tradition actually spells out particular virtues that help to bond the community, and in the four divine abodes (*Brahmavihara*) provides separate practices to encourage them—friendliness (metta), compassion (karuna), sympathetic joy (mudita), and equanimity (upekkha). Keown (1995) reminds us that these practices are prescribed to overcome *unfriendly* attitudes. Preferring friendship as the paradigm for relating, he is essentially an Aristotelian thinker, one of a number (e.g., Flanagan, 2011; Harvey, 2000; Whitehill, 1994) who suggest a virtue ethics for Buddhism.

Compassion, while central to the later Mahayana tradition, is a more specific construct, and is neither a day-to-day nor a mutually shared mode of relating. It can be defined as recognizing and wishing to end the suffering of others, which is certainly both useful and admirable (for a thoroughgoing discussion, see Chap. 10). However, it may not be required continually within a small community. Rather, a confluence is more likely to reflect a disposition such as friendship in its day-to-day, moment-to-moment "going on together." Perhaps the prevalence and increasing frequency of *metta* practice within the MBPs (e.g. Feldman & Kuyken, 2011; Horrigan, 2007) is indicative of the ubiquity of friendship as a disposition—or, at least, an aspiration.

A Community that Matters

Friendship binds together the gathered folks in an MBP class. It is not an imposed way of being, not an ethic in itself. Rather, as the embodiment of the non-pathologizing, non-hierarchical, and non-instrumental dispositions that make the pedagogy possible, friendship is what makes ethics—and even a dialogue about ethics—possible. Friendship itself creates community in which all can thrive. Its bonding is strong enough to hold with care all of the questioning, yearning, and suffering that participants bring, while it is weak in ways that allow it to hold difference without penalty or exclusion.

In Gergen's (2009) terms, the first-order morality that binds the MBP confluence together is actually a second-order morality, as well. First-order moralities naturally create conflicts between them; they generate in- and out-groups that are set in their own "right" ways of being, and thus oppose other first-order moralities. Second-order moralities then provide the possibility of overcoming the conflicts of the first order, by tending to relationships. That is, the focus in a second-order morality is not on imposing the discipline and boundaries of the group, but rather is on finding ways of including the otherwise alienated. It seems to me that the friendship of the MBP confluence is a model for this.

In this time of great growth, opportunity, and tension in the MBPs, a question arises for me—and I suspect for many others. Can we, its diverse community of scholars, researchers, and teachers, apply the second-order morality that arises from our work? Can we embody the non-pathologizing, non-hierarchical, and non-instrumental dispositions that comprise friendship? I would very much like to think so. The way that the community receives critique from those who dissent within it is of great consequence. This volume, which brings powerful, valuable, and diverse new resources to the practice and poetics of the pedagogy of the MBPs, is an offering made in friendship—how it is received will tell us much. As we tend our relationships together, may we find a new hope.

References

Amaro, A. (2015). A holistic mindfulness. *Mindfulness, 6*, 63–73.

Baer, R. (2015). Ethics, values, virtues, and character strengths in mindfulness-based interventions: A psychological science perspective. *Mindfulness, 6(4)*, 956–969.

Baracchi, C. (2008). *Aristotle's ethics as first philosophy*. Cambridge: Cambridge University Press.

Bell, S. (2002). Scandals in emerging Western Buddhism. In C. S. Prebish & M. Baumann (Eds.), *Westward dharma: Buddhism beyond Asia*. Berkeley, CA: University of California Press.

Brown, K. W., Ryan, R. M., Loverich, T. M., Biegel, G. M., & West, A. M. (2011). Out of the armchair and into the streets: Measuring mindfulness advances knowledge and improves interventions: Reply to Grossman. *Psychological Assessment, 23*, 1041–1046.

Caputo, J. D. (2003). *Against principles: A sketch of an ethics without ethics*. In E. Wyschogrod & G. McKenny (Eds.), *The Ethical*. Malden, MA: Blackwell.

Crane, R., Kuyken, W., Hastings, R., Rothwell, N., & Williams, J. M. (2010). Training Teachers to Deliver Mindfulness-Based Interventions: Learning from the UK Experience. *Mindfulness, 1(2)*, 74–86. https://doi.org/10.1007/s12671-010-0010-9.

Crane, R. S., Brewer, J., Feldman, C., Kabat-Zinn, J., Santorelli, S., Williams, J. M. G., & Kuyken, W. (2016). What defines mindfulness-based programs? The warp and the weft. *Psychological Medicine*. https://doi.org/10.1017/S0033291716003317. Retrieved from http://www.cambridge.org/core

Crane, R., & Elias, D. (2006). Being with what is. *Therapy Today, 17(10)*, 31–33.

Crane, R. S., Soulsby, J. G., Kuyken, W., Williams, J. M. G., & Eames, C. (2016). *2016-last update, The Bangor, Exeter & Oxford Mindfulness-Based Interventions Teaching Assessment Criteria (MBI-TAC) for assessing the competence and adherence of mindfulness-based class-based teaching.* Retrieved from https://www.bangor.ac.uk/mindfulness/documents/MBITACmanualsummaryaddendums05-16.pdf

Cullen, M. (2011). Mindfulness-based interventions: An emerging phenomenon. *Mindfulness, 2,* 186–193.

Downing, M. (2001). *Shoes outside the door: Desire, devotion, and excess at San Francisco Zen Center.* Washington, DC: Counterpoint.

Feldman, C., & Kuyken, W. (2011). Compassion in the landscape of suffering. *Contemporary Buddhism, 12*(1), 143–155.

Flanagan, O. (2011). *The Bodhisattva's brain: Buddhism naturalized.* Cambridge, MA: MIT Press.

Foucault, M. (1995). *Discipline and punish.* New York: Vintage.

Gergen, K. (2009). *Relational being: Beyond self and community.* Oxford, England: Oxford University Press.

Gergen, K. (2011). From moral autonomy to relational responsibility. *Zygon, 46*(1), 204–223.

Gergen, K. (2015). *An invitation to social construction* (3rd ed.). London, England: Sage.

Gombrich, R. (2009). *What the Buddha thought.* London: Equinox.

Grossman, P. (2010). Mindfulness for psychologists: Paying kind attention to the perceptible. *Mindfulness, 1,* 87–97.

Grossman, P. (2011). Defining mindfulness by how poorly I pay attention during everyday awareness and other intractable problems for psychology's (re)invention of mindfulness: Comment on Brown, et al., (2011). *Psychological Assessment, 23,* 1034–1040.

Grossman, P. (2015). Mindfulness: Awareness informed by an embodied ethic. *Mindfulness, 6*(1), 17–22.

Harrington, A. & Dunne, J. (2015). *American Psychologist, 70*(7), 621–631.

Harvey, P. (2000). *An introduction to Buddhist ethics.* Cambridge: Cambridge University Press.

Hölzel, B. K., Lazar, S. W., Gard, T., Schuman-Olivier, Z., Vago, D. R., & Ott, U. (2011). How does mindfulness meditation work? Proposing mechanisms of action from a conceptual and neural perspective. *Perspectives on Psychological Science, 6*(6), 537–559.

Horrigan, B. J. (2007). Saki Santorelli, EdD, MA: Mindfulness and medicine. *Explore, 3*(2), 137–144.

Jaspers, K. (1953). *The origin and goal of history.* New Haven: Yale University Press.

Kabat-Zinn, J. (2003). Mindfulness-based interventions in context: Past, present and future. *Clinical Psychology: Science and Practice, 10,* 144–156.

Kabat-Zinn, J. (2004). *[audio recording] The uses of language and images in guiding meditation practices in MBSR.* Second annual conference sponsored by the center for mindfulness in medicine, health care, and society at the University of Massachusetts Medical School, March 26.

Kabat-Zinn, J. (2011). Some reflections on the origins of MBSR, skillful means, and the trouble with maps. *Contemporary Buddhism, 12*(1), 281–306.

Keown, D. (1992). *The nature of Buddhist ethics.* New York: Palgrave.

Keown, D. (1995). *Buddhism and bioethics.* New York: Palgrave.

Keown, D. (2006). Buddhism: Morality without ethics? In D. Keown (Ed.), *Buddhist studies from India to America* (pp. 40–48). New York: Routledge.

Krznaric, R. (2017, May 26). How we ruined mindfulness. *Time.* Retrieved from http://time.com/4792596/mindfulness-exercises-morality-carpe-diem/

Lindahl, J. (2015). Why right mindfulness may not be right for mindfulness. *Mindfulness, 6,* 57–62.

MacIntyre, A. (2007). *After virtue* (3rd ed.). Notre Dame, IN: University of Notre Dame Press.

McCown, D. (2013). *The ethical space of mindfulness in clinical practice.* London: Jessica Kingsley.

McCown, D. (2016). Being is relational: Considerations for using mindfulness in clinician-patient settings. In E. Shonin, W. VanGordon, & M. Griffiths (Eds.), *Mindfulness and Buddhist-derived approaches in mental health and addiction.* New York: Springer.

McCown, D. & Billington, J. (under review). *Correspondence: Sitting and reading as two routes to community.*

McCown, D., Reibel, D., & Micozzi, M. (2010). *Teaching mindfulness: A practical guide for clinicians and educators.* New York: Springer.

McCown, D. & Wiley, S. (2008). *Emergent issues in MBSR research and pedagogy: Integrity, fidelity, and how do we decide?* 6th annual conference: integrating mindfulness-based interventions into medicine, health care, and society, Worcester, MA, April 10–12.

McCown, D. & Wiley, S. (2009). *Thinking the world together: Seeking accord and interdependence in the discourses of mindfulness teaching and research.* 7th annual conference: Integrating mindfulness based interventions into medicine, health care, and society, Worcester, MA, March 18–22.

McEvilley, T. (2002). *The shape of ancient thought: Comparative studies in Greek and Indian philosophies.* New York: Allworth Press.

Monteiro, L. (2017). The moral arc of mindfulness: Cultivating concentration, wisdom, and compassion. In L. Monteiro, R. F. Musten, & J. Compson (Eds.), *A practitioner's guide to ethics in mindfulness-based programs.* New York: Springer.

Monteiro, L., Musten, R. F., & Compson, J. (2015). Traditional and contemporary mindfulness: Finding the middle path in the tangle of concerns. *Mindfulness, 6*(1), 1–13.

Nussbaum, M. (1986). *The fragility of goodness.* Cambridge: Cambridge University Press.

Porges, S. W. (2011). *The polyvagal theory: Neurophysiological foundations of emotions, attachment, communication, and self-regulation.* New York: Norton.

Purser, R. E. (2015). Clearing the muddled path of traditional and contemporary mindfulness: A response to Monteiro, Musten, and Compson. *Mindfulness, 6,* 23–45.

Purser, R., & Loy, D. (2013). Beyond McMindfulness. *Huffington Post.* Retrieved from http://www.huffingtonpost.com/ron-purser/beyond-mcmindfulness_b_3519289.html website: http://www.huffingtonpost.com. Retrieved from http://www.huffingtonpost.com

Santorelli, S., Goddard, T., Kabat-Zinn, J., Kesper-Grossman, U., Reibel, D. (2011). *Standards for the formation of MBSR teacher trainers: Experience, qualifications, competency and ongoing development.* Ninth annual conference: Integrating mindfulness-based interventions into medicine, health care, and society, Norwood, MA, March 30–April 3.

Sauer, S., Lynch, S., Walach, H., & Kohls, N. (2011). Dialectics of mindfulness: Implications for Western medicine. *Philosophy, Ethics, and Humanities in Medicine, 6,* 10.

Schwartz, T. (1995). *What really Matters: Searching for wisdom in America.* New York: Bantam.

Shonin, E. (2016, February 29). This is not McMindfulness by any stretch of the imagination. *The Psychologist.* Retrieved from https://thepsychologist.bps.org.uk/not-mcmindfulness-any-stretch-imagination

Shotter, J. (2011). *Getting it: Withness-thinking and the dialogical…in practice.* New York: Hampton Press.

Thanissaro, B. (trans.). (1997). *Upaddha Sutta (Samyutta Nikaya 45.2).* Retrieved from www.accesstoinsight.org/tipitaka/sn/sn45/sn45.002.than.html

Van Gordon, W., Shonin, E., & Griffiths, M. D. (2015). Towards a second generation of mindfulness-based interventions. *Australian and New Zealand Journal of Psychiatry, 49,* 591–592.

Whitehill, J. (1994). Buddhism and the virtues. *Journal of Buddhist Ethics, 1,* 1–22.

Williams, M., & Kabat-Zinn, J. (2011). Mindfulness: Diverse perspectives on its meaning, origins, and multiple applications at the intersection of science and dharma. *Contemporary Buddhism, 12*(1), 1–18.

Part I
Issues in the Ethics of Mindfulness

Chapter 2
Is Mindfulness Secular or Religious, and Does It Matter?

Jane F. Compson

There are a number of intersecting questions that arise when considering the role of ethics in mindfulness-based interventions (MBIs) and the ethics of their implementation in secular contexts. Each of them brings a layer of depth and complexity to the issue. For example, the chapters in this section are about the role of ethics in mindfulness-based programs. However, they each explore a different dimension. Some of the questions they bring to the fore include: Are there implicit or explicit ethics in MBIs? If they are there explicitly, which values are they rooted in, and is it ethical to impose ethical values on clients or patients? If they are implicit, where do they come from, and do providers of MBIs have a moral obligation to make the implicit visible? Is it ethical to teach ethics? Whose ethics? Who is an appropriate teacher of ethics? Do you have to attain a certain level of ethical embodiment before you are qualified to teach?

One of the insights from the social sciences and philosophy is that the way that we conceptualize the world is to some degree at least (and the extent is the subject of much discussion and disagreement) socially constructed. In other words, the concepts that we use to describe and understand the world have a history and their meaning and significance usually evolve over time. We use concepts to help navigate and function in the world; changing concepts can determine the way we interact with phenomena, and by the same token when our needs and actions vary, then this might change the way we conceptualize things. In the context of this discussion, concepts such as "religion" and "secular" are telling examples of constantly evolving concepts. Often a concept is defined in terms of its supposed opposite.

J.F. Compson, PhD (✉)
University of Washington, Tacoma, 1900 Commerce Street, Tacoma, WA 98402, USA
e-mail: jcompson@uw.edu

© Springer International Publishing AG 2017   23
L.M. Monteiro et al. (eds.), *Practitioner's Guide to Ethics and Mindfulness-Based Interventions*, Mindfulness in Behavioral Health,
DOI 10.1007/978-3-319-64924-5_2

Examples of these kinds of binaries include religious/secular, scientific/religious, facts/values, private/public, and so on. Nested within these concepts are value judgments, such as about the appropriate domains for "religious" and "secular" activities. As we will see, how one understands a term can have behavioral and ethical ramifications. Contemporary mindfulness inhabits this zone of contested meanings, values, and contexts. As contexts evolve, so meanings and values adapt to the new situation, giving rise to the kind of challenging questions mentioned above. The three chapters in this section each bring to the fore different ways of contextualizing and framing mindfulness. In so doing they present varying ideas about what is ethically appropriate in the way MBIs are taught and framed.

In this chapter I will lay out some of the contexts for the positions argued in the rest of this section, locating them within a historical or philosophical framework. We will see how many of the ethical judgments about the appropriate application of mindfulness rest on various assumptions and value judgments about what it means for something to be "religious" or "secular," and so on. I will discuss how the framing of concepts such as the religious and the secular have evolved through the modern period to the postmodern period, and how this has a bearing on the contemporary mindfulness debates. I will argue that the contemporary mindfulness debates are most fruitfully understood in postmodern, postsecular terms, and that doing so opens the door to mutually beneficial dialogue between narratives and disciplines.

Mindfulness and Religion: A Complicated Relationship

The study and application of mindfulness is a truly multidisciplinary realm, drawing contributions from religious studies, cognitive and psychological sciences, social sciences, medicine, and education. In addition to being practiced within religious and contemplative contexts, it is now found in various professional and vocational domains, including business, healthcare, education, law enforcement, and the military. Contributors to this volume offer perspectives from a wide range of these contexts. The authors of the chapters in this section are a professor of religious studies (Gunther Brown), a professor of psychology (Baer), and two physicians, one a professor of clinical internal medicine (Krasner), and the other a palliative care specialist (Lück).

Krasner and Lück are also trained and active teachers of mindfulness-based stress reduction (MBSR), and advocate for and practice the integration of mindfulness training or interventions in the medical profession and among their patients. In their chapter, they make the case for the continued and increasing integration of mindfulness-based training into medical education as a way of addressing provider burnout and ensuring a better quality of care for patients. From her perspective as a psychologist, Baer acknowledges the therapeutic value and efficacy of many mindfulness-based practices (MBPs). However, she argues that MBIs should be, as much as possible, distanced from explicitly Buddhist frameworks and made more consistent with secular ethical norms and assumptions. This will prevent the imposition of values on the client, and respect their autonomy in choosing their own values. MBPs will be more widely accessible if they are "genuinely secular."

Gunther Brown is more skeptical of the appropriateness of introducing mindfulness in secular contexts such as healthcare. She argues that even so-called secularized versions of mindfulness are still essentially rooted in Buddhist philosophy (i.e. in religious ideals). She calls into question whether mindfulness can ever be "genuinely secular," as Baer proposes. In certain secular contexts, the introduction of mindfulness may be inappropriate or unethical, since it is a religious practice. She argues that in the interests of transparency and to preserve informed consent, mindfulness teachers should "own" and be explicit about the religious nature of the intervention.

In their chapter on mindfulness in health care, Lück and Krasner mention the Buddhist foundations of mindfulness once, and do so in a way that is intended to *legitimize* its use in medicine: "The original purpose of mindfulness in Buddhism is to alleviate suffering and cultivate compassion. This suggests a role for mindfulness in medicine." In contrast, it is precisely the Buddhist framing and context of mindfulness that makes Gunther Brown, and, to a lesser extent, Baer, wary of the role of mindfulness in medicine because of its introduction of non-secular values. This approach highlights one of the key "sticking points" in this discussion—to what extent is mindfulness "secular" or "religious," and how do or should the secular and religious relate to each other? How one answers these questions has important ethical implications. If mindfulness is a religious practice, and introducing a religious practice into a secular sphere is ethically unacceptable, then this clearly has implications in terms of a professional's ethical obligations.

Defining Our Terms: Religious and Secular

To understand and negotiate these diverse perspectives, it is helpful to unpack some of the concepts, particularly "secular" and "religion," and explore some assumptions about them.

Earlier we talked about binaries—how words are often defined by their opposites. One such binary is "religious" versus "secular" and the development of this binary has a history. The concepts of religion and secularism as they are commonly used today arose during the modern period in Western Europe. Broadly, this refers to a time in history between the premodern period and the current, postmodern period. The early modern period began in the early sixteenth century and included the Renaissance in Europe and the "Age of Discovery" where European countries engaged in extensive overseas exploration and colonized many other cultures. The late modern period began in the eighteenth century and included the French and American revolutions and the industrial revolution.

In the premodern period, what we now describe as "religion" was deeply imbued into everyday life and culture, and was the primary lens for understanding the world and for ordering social and cultural affairs (Esposito, Fasching, & Lewis, 2002). The idea of "religion" as a noun indicating a set of beliefs and practices distinct from other aspects of life would have been entirely unfamiliar to premoderns. "Religious" as an adjective, though, is more applicable to the premodern world if it is understood as a loyal orientation and obligation to the powers that were thought to govern existence and destiny. Etymologically the Latin word *religare*, from which "religion" is derived, means "to tie and bind," suggesting a sense of commitment and affiliation (Esposito et al., 2002). Religious historian Karen Armstrong explains that the Greek word *pistis*, translated from the New Testament as "faith," means "trust, loyalty, engagement, commitment." In Latin, it was translated to *fides*, meaning "loyalty," and the verbal form used was "*credo*" meaning "I give my heart." When the Bible was translated into English in the middle ages, this was translated as "I believe," but at that time the word "belief" meant "loyalty to a person to whom one is bound in promise and duty" (Armstrong, 2009, p. 87). In other words, terms such as "faith", "belief," or "religious" were associated with a sense of personal orientation and value rather than propositional assent to a set of creeds and doctrines. Cantwell Smith (1963) describes how the meaning of the word "religion" has radically changed since the fourteenth century. It began as signifying a human quality of inner life, such a sense of commitment or an effort to be guided by the example of a model group or teachers (such as Christ). For example, to be "Christian" meant to be "Christ-like." Over time this evolved to take on the connotation of an ideal or aspiration— "Christian," for example, would signify the ideal way that people should learn to live. "Christianity" meant "Christendom," and "Christian" meant "Christlikeness." During the Enlightenment, the meaning "religion" shifted again to signify a system of beliefs. At the same time, the meaning of "belief" had shifted from signifying a sense of loyalty to instead meaning "opinion" or intellectual assent to a set of propositions. "Religion" also came to signify a historical phenomenon and a set of institutions, and it was around this time that the idea of different and competing world religions appeared and disparate phenomena were reified into "isms" such as "Buddhism" or "Hinduism." No equivalent for these terms exists in Hindu or Buddhist texts. The introduction of these terms was one of the many consequences of European colonialism; categories born out of Western European concepts were applied to the cultural phenomena in "discovered" lands. This included an increasing reification of practices into discrete and competing "isms," and identification of creeds and doctrines (as opposed to inner faith or piety) with "religion":

> Crucially, just as the multiple forms of Christianity were presumed to be mutually exclusive, so too were these other "religions." The world religions, in short, were created through a projection of Christian disunity onto the world. Their fabrication in the Western imagination is registered in the terms that indicate their birth: "Boudhism" makes its first appearance in 1821, "Hindooism" in 1829, "Taouism" in 1829, and "Confucianism" in 1862. (Harrison, 2006, p. 42)

Evolving Relationships: The Modern Period The concept of "religion," then, is the product of particular cultural and historical forces that are not universal.

Specifically, the sense of "world religions" as discrete institutions of systematic beliefs and practices is a product of the European Enlightenment. Another characteristic of this time was the birth of the modern discipline of "science" as we know it, and the separation of science and religion. The Enlightenment brought increasing interest in the natural sciences, but even so, natural history and philosophy were pursued from religious motives (Harrison, 2006). Since it was generally assumed that God created the world, learning about nature was a way of learning about God; many key natural historians were clergymen. In the nineteenth-century Europe, this began to change and science became more autonomous from religion. Armstrong describes this process in terms of changing relationship between *mythos* and *logos*. These describe two different ways of being in and relation to the world that existed in most premodern cultures. *Mythos* refers to ways of making meaning and coping with the world. This might present as epic stories, poetry, art work, myths, "designed to help people navigate the obscure regions of the psyche, which are difficult to access but which profoundly influence our thought and behavior." (Armstrong, 2009, p. xi). Myths, argues Armstrong, are essentially programs of action, enacted through rites and rituals, which *when put into practice* "could tell us something profoundly true about our humanity ... how to live more richly and intensely, how to cope with our mortality, and how to creatively endure the suffering that flesh is heir to." (p. xii). *Logos*, on the other hand, refers to a "pragmatic mode of thought" that enables us to be in the world, manipulate reality and meet our needs for physical and social survival. During premodern times, both forms of knowledge coexisted and were equally valued. However, during the early modern period in the West, logos became increasingly valued, and mythos increasingly discredited. The modern scientific method became prized as "the only reliable means of attaining truth." Mythos became discredited because the criteria for "truth" became rational, empirical, and scientific; viewed through these lenses, myths became "false" and "meaningless." Through the lens of logos, scientists could not see the point of rituals, and rather than being understood as programs of action, religious myths became understood as theoretical knowledge claims which often failed the test of empirical truth. Confronted with this rise of logos, religious advocates were faced either with seeing their traditions as "not true," or trying to present their traditions as rival "scientific" descriptions of reality. This, in turn, led to fundamentalism and atheism. In Christianity, for example, fundamentalists interpreted the mythos in the Bible (such as the creation story, or the virgin birth) as though they were empirical claims. The backlash against this literalism gave rise to a new kind of atheism, a rejection of religion when being "religious" meant interpreting sacred texts as though they were literal and empirically verifiable accounts of reality (Armstrong, 2009).

In this respect, modern concepts of science and religion co-created each other:

> For if this is the period during which "science" was eventually to emerge as a discipline evacuated of religious and theological concerns, logically "religion" was itself now understood as an enterprise that excluded the scientific. The birth of "science" was part of the ongoing story of the ideation of "religion." (Harrison, 2006, p. 93)

Whereas in premodern times, religion undergirded every aspect of public life, during the modern period, science became understood as the most reliable form of knowledge. Theology was deposed from its centuries-long reign as "queen of the sciences" and the powers of church and state were separated. Religion became seen as more of a matter of personal faith than objective knowledge as the shared and pervasive religious worldviews of premodern times retreated. At the same time, the concept of "secular" took on a new meaning. In medieval Europe, secular referred to the "temporal-profane" world, in contrast to the "religious-spiritual-sacred world of salvation," the existence of which was taken for granted (Casanova, 2013, p. 29). However, during the modern period "secular" took on the meaning of "devoid of religion." Cosmic, social, and moral orders were no longer understood as transcendent and religious, but this-worldly and immanent. On this understanding, which persists today, "secular" and "religious" are oppositional—the more secular a society, the less religious it is, and vice versa. Casanova identifies another connotation of secularism, one which reflects Armstrong's discussion about the rise of logos over mythos. This is the idea that secularism is a coming of age, a progressive emancipation from religion:

> The historical self-understanding of secularism has the function of confirming the superiority of our present secular modern outlook over other supposedly earlier and therefore more primitive religious forms of understanding. To be secular means to be modern, and therefore by implication to be religious means to be somehow not yet fully modern.
> (Casanova, 2013, p. 32)

This is another key characteristic of the modernist period—a sense of confidence and optimism in science and technology which are framed in a narrative of progress. There is a sense that religion has been "outgrown" and is seen as regressive and even oppressive. This kind of perspective on religion is exemplified by Christopher Hitchens:

> Religion comes from the period of human prehistory where nobody—not even the mighty Democritus who concluded that all matter was made from atoms—had the smallest idea what was going on. It comes from the bawling and fearful infancy of our species, and is a babyish attempt to meet our inescapable demand for knowledge (as well as for comfort, reassurance, and other infantile needs). Today the least educated of my children knows much more about the natural order than any of the founders of religion.
> (Hitchens, 2008, p. 64)

This quote contains many typical attitudes of modernism toward religion. It is assumed that religion's role is to explain the natural order, and that it does so very poorly. It is associated with an early developmental stage of our species that has been outgrown; it is portrayed as inferior to science, and obsolete.

> Religion has run out of justifications. Thanks to the telescope and the microscope, it no longer offers an explanation of anything important. Where once it used to be able, by its total command of a worldview, to prevent the emergence of rivals, it can now only impede and retard—or try to turn back—the measurable advances that we have made.
> (Hitchens, p. 282)

The diminishing power of religion in the modern period had major implications for ethics. Before the rise of Christianity in the West, Platonic, and Aristotelian systems of natural law provided the foundation for ethics. As Christianity became increasingly dominant in the West in the premodern period, ethics became grounded in religious doctrines and metaphysics. With the falling status of religion during the Enlightenment period and beyond, ethical systems began to emerge that did not depend on religious beliefs, but were grounded in naturalistic understandings of reality. These included the social contract theory, Kantian ethics grounded in principles of reason, and utilitarianism. These superseded ethics grounded in religion, as they were more compatible with contemporary naturalistic understandings of the cosmos.

So far, then, we have seen how contemporary understandings of concepts such as "religion/religious," "secular," and "belief" were shaped by the cultural forces of the modernist period. Shortly, we will explore some of the ways these modernist assumptions play out in the contemporary mindfulness debate. First, though, it is important to briefly consider the challenges to modernism that have characterized the postmodern era. This will help to provide further context for the mindfulness debates in this volume.

Postmodernism Modernism's confidence in perpetual progress delivered by science and technology was shaken to the core by the two World Wars. The very forces thought to bring emancipation from premodern ignorance were shown to be capable of cataclysmic destruction. Colonial powers withdrew from their empires, leaving instability and poverty in the wake of their exploitative practices. The US and Europe entered a Cold War with the USSR, with the constant threat of nuclear holocaust. At the same time, increasing globalization meant that, to an unprecedented degree, people were now aware of multiple alternative ways of living and seeing the world. All this had the effect of undermining confidence in the scientific rationalism and the narrative of progress that characterized modernism (Esposito et al., 2002). The scientific worldview in modernism had replaced premodern metaphysics as the authoritative "truth" about reality. One of the most fundamental characteristics of postmodernism is the erosion of the idea that there is a discoverable objective truth about the way the world really is. Increased globalization gave access to many different cultural and individual ways of understanding the world, raising questions about the extent to which our reality is socially constructed.

> The postmodern individual is continually reminded that different peoples have entirely different concepts of what the world is like. The person who understands this and accepts it recognizes social institutions as human creations and knows that even the sense of personal identity is different in different societies. Such a person views religious truth as a special kind of truth and not an eternal and perfect representation of cosmic reality. And—going beyond secular humanism—he or she sees the work of science as yet another form of social reality construction and not a secret technique for taking objective photographs of the universe. (Anderson, 1990, p. 8)

A postmodern view of science rejects the idea of it being "the Truth" and sees it as one of many possible narratives for making sense of the world. "Religious" worldviews are also meaning-making narratives which may or may not be compatible with scientific ones. Neither, though, has a privileged position as corresponding the best to "objective" reality, although some may be more useful or effective than others in promoting certain individual or cultural purposes. In fact, postmodernism challenges the very concept of "objective reality" as it implies that it is possible to have a standpoint free from bias and interpretation from which we can see how things really are. In other words, postmodernism does more than challenge certain beliefs about the world—it raises questions about the nature of knowledge itself. For example, a postmodern account of science rejects the idea that it provides uniquely objective access to the truth about the world:

> The history of the term shows that "science" is a human construction or reification. This is not necessarily to say that scientific knowledge is socially constructed: rather, it is the category "science"—a way of identifying certain forms of knowledge and excluding others—that is constructed. (Harrison, 2006, p. 90)

Earlier in this chapter, we saw how the concepts such as "religious" and "secular" have evolved over time. A postmodernist would point to this as evidence that the way the world appears to us is not a *given*—rather, in the way that we construct categories for understanding it we shape it. As Harrison explains, social construction not only shapes the shifting relationship between science and religion but is responsible for the creation of the very categories that make such debates possible:

> In much the same way that the objectifying and logocentric tendencies of the Enlightenment produced the "other religions," creating at the same time the vexed question of their relation to each other, so too "science and religion" is a relationship that has come about only because of a distorting fragmentation of sets of human activities. (Harrison, 2006, p. 99)

If these categories of science and religion are social constructions, rather than "givens," then the boundaries between them can be negotiated or even dissolved altogether. An example where this kind of renegotiation is happening is described as postsecularism (Casanova, 2013). The term "postsecularism" can be applied both descriptively and normatively. Descriptively, it can refer to the fact that the rise of scientific humanism did not, in fact, lead cultures to "outgrow" religion. Instead, religious forms and practices are still thriving even in the most "secularized" societies of Western Europe and religion is gaining influence both worldwide in national public spheres. Normatively, postsecularism can refer to the position that the domains of faith and reason should not be separated and stratified from each other, but should dialogue and learn from each other (Habermas, 2008). Postsecularism is not arguing that secularism is dead, but that the sharp separation between the religious and the secular has—and/or should be—deconstructed. This could take various forms. For example, to use Armstrong's terms, it could mean turning to religion to help redress the imbalance between logos and mythos.

The interplay between the different forces and perspectives of the premodern, the modern and the postmodern can be clearly seen in debates about contemporary mindfulness practice, including those in the section of this volume. In particular, the tension between the modern and the postmodern is helpful lens through which to frame some of the discussions.

Mindfulness and Modernism

There is a case to be made that the growing popularity of mindfulness in the West has its roots in the modernist project. We have seen how the idea of "Buddhism" as a "world religion" arose in the nineteenth-century Europe. As David McMahan explains, many of the Western "early adopters" of Buddhism saw it as being compatible with modern science at a time when the relationship between science and Christianity was increasingly troubled. At the same time, pressures of colonization meant that Asian Buddhists themselves highlighted those elements of Buddhist teachings most compatible with scientific humanism to increase its appeal. Cosmological claims were downplayed as cultural artifacts, and the "universal essence" of Buddhism extracted from it: "Buddhism itself had to be transformed, reformed, and modernized-purged of mythological elements and "superstitious" cultural accretions." (McMahan, 2008). This is a typical modernist move.

> Detraditionalization embodies the modernist tendency to elevate reason, experience, and intuition over tradition and to assert the freedom to reject, adopt, or reinterpret traditional beliefs and practices on the basis of individual evaluation. Religion becomes more individualized, privatized, and a matter of choice-one has the right to choose and even construct one's own religion. (McMahan, 2008, p. 43)

Mindfulness was one of these elements that was "extracted" from tradition and seen as having universal appeal. Prior to the nineteenth century, mindfulness practice was generally reserved for monastics in Asian Buddhism, and in fact the practice of meditation had almost died out in Theravada Buddhism by the tenth century (Gleig, 2018; Wilson, 2014). It was revived and made popular among lay people as a result of the modernist reforms that accompanied colonization. Burmese monk Ledi Sayadaw and his students popularized lay meditation and his trainings were taken by Westerners who transmitted this interest in meditation back to Europe and the USA (Braun, 2013). Among these Western students of Asian Buddhist teachers were Joseph Goldstein, Jack Kornfield, Sharon Salzberg, and Jacqueline Schwartz, who went on to set up the Insight Meditation Society and Spirit Rock Meditation Center in the US. In true modernist fashion, these founders intentionally taught meditation in a way assumed more accessible to Western audiences, "as simply as possible without the complications of rituals, robes, chanting and the whole religious tradition" (Fronsdal, 1998, p. 167). Among the students at IMS was Jon Kabat-Zinn. During a vipassana retreat he had a vision of bringing mindfulness into the medical system, a vision he realized in the creation of Mindfulness-Based Stress Reduction, which is the first and best-known mainstream "secular" MBI (Gleig, 2018). As Gunther Brown notes in her chapter in this volume, Kabat Zinn shared the vision of making "essential" teachings found in Buddhism palatable to Western audiences by decontextualizing them from "cultural" or "traditional" Buddhism. He saw MBSR as a method to:

> Take the heart of something as meaningful, as sacred if you will, as Buddha-dharma and bring it into the world in a way that doesn't dilute, profane, or distort it, but at the same time is not locked into a culturally and tradition-bound framework that would make it absolutely impenetrable to the vast majority of people. (Kabat-Zinn, 2000, p. 227)

In a way, this continues a trajectory of how Western scholarship constructed Buddhism. Masuzawa explains how the emphasis has typically been placed on the teachings of the historical Buddha, and particularly on his rejection of prevailing traditions and dogmas, presenting it as a "world" religion in the sense of having universalistic appeal that transcends national boundaries (Masuzawa, 2005). Thus, the way Buddhism has been framed in the west, and the way that "secular" mindfulness has evolved out of this lineage can be understood as part of a modernist tradition.

Criticisms of Popular Mindfulness

The framing of mindfulness as an universal "essence" of Buddhism stripped of its tradition and applied to secular realms has received criticism from both within and outside Buddhist communities. Gleig identifies two types of critique of secular mindfulness; from within Western Buddhism that it is canonically unsound, and from both within and outside Buddhist communities, arguments that it is socioculturally unsound.

The canonically unsound critique of popular mindfulness argues that neither the understanding of mindfulness as neutral "bare attention," nor the idea that mindfulness alone is sufficient for awakening are supported by the canonical Buddhist texts. In traditional Buddhism, "right mindfulness" (*samma sati*) is distinguished from "wrong mindfulness" (*miccha sati*); it is right to the extent that it supports the development of all aspects of the eightfold path toward liberation, and wrong if it does not (Compson & Monteiro, 2015). The eight elements of the path can be divided into the categories of mental development, wisdom, and ethics. Mindfulness belongs in the first category, but if it is not fundamentally supportive of right wisdom and right ethics, it is not "right" mindfulness. In other words, mindfulness in the Buddhist canonical sense is not ethically neutral—it is more than just "bare attention," but an attention framed within the intention and conduct that leads to the liberation from suffering (Monteiro, Musten, & Compson, 2015).

For the critics of popular mindfulness, this distinction between right and wrong mindfulness has important ethical implications; when mindfulness is no longer nested in the context of the eightfold path, then it is vulnerable to misuse. This leads to the critiques of popular mindfulness as unsound for sociocultural reasons. Buddhist psychotherapist Miles Neale coined the term "McMindfulness" to describe "a kind of compartmentalized, secularized, watered-down version of mindfulness … Meditation for the masses, drive-through style, stripped of its essential ingredients, prepackaged and neatly stocked on the shelves of the commercial self-help supermarkets" (Neale, 2015).

Critiques from outside Buddhist communities also have ethical misgivings about the popularization of secular mindfulness, but in a kind of negative image of the McMindfulness critique. These objections cluster around the fact that it is precisely the Buddhist roots of mindfulness that make it inappropriate for application in secular contexts unless these ethical and ideological roots are expressly "owned" and made visible. Sometimes called the "stealth Buddhism" critique, this kind of objection is offered by Candy Gunther Brown later in this volume.

Gleig identifies three themes in the sociocultural critiques of popular mindfulness: capitalism, scientism, and colonialism. An example of the capitalism critique is offered by Purser and Loy (2013), who warn that instead of challenging the roots of suffering, a decontextualized mindfulness could reinforce exploitative and antisocial practices:

> Mindfulness training has wide appeal because it has become a trendy method for subduing employee unrest, promoting a tacit acceptance of the status quo, and as an instrumental tool for keeping attention focused on institutional goals. (Purser & Loy, 2013)

A similar critique is offered by Stone (2014) who argues that the use of mindfulness in the military is at odds with its Buddhist ethical roots rooted in the principle of non-harm (*ahimsa*).

Another type of critique of popular mindfulness laments how science has been marshaled to legitimize and validate mindfulness, as this smacks of scientism. Scientism has its roots in modernism and describes the view that the most authoritative and valid forms of knowledge are scientific and other ways of knowing (religious, for example) are inferior and incomplete. On this view, "religious practices and beliefs remain conditional until granted the imprimatur of empirical verification" (Harrison, p. 65). This exclusive confidence in science dismisses other narratives about what it means to be human. Framing mindfulness in this scientific narrative limits it in this way, and can subsume it under foundational assumptions of science—such as materialism—assumptions that are not shared by, and in some cases, may be anathema to, Buddhist narratives (Heuman, 2014).

From outside Buddhist communities, critiques about science come from a different angle. Gunther Brown, for example, notes that the cultural cache of science is used to prove that mindfulness is legitimately secular, with the implication that if it is "scientific," it is "not religious". She argues that scientific claims made about mindfulness actually exceed the evidence about them, which is ethically problematic in itself, and especially because these scientific validation claims serve to cloak the Buddhist nature of mindfulness. Appealing to science is one of the stealth methods for introducing Buddhist ideas into secular spaces.

Just as critics of scientism see science as colonizing and effacing other disciplines and ways of knowing, so issues of colonialism provide the basis for a critique on secular mindfulness. In her chapter, Gunther Brown argues that: "In the case of MBIs, the interests and worldviews of socially privileged European American Buddhists hegemonically pass for universal truths and values needed by all of society." She is referring to the Buddhist modernist project of stripping mindfulness of its "cultural accretions" and identifying it as the "universal truth" that will benefit everyone. This framing as "universalism" is hegemonic—a way of imposing the "interests and worldviews of socially privileged European American Buddhists" onto other less privileged groups. It also "condescends to racial and ethnic others as having unenlightened cultural practices" that can be replaced or improved upon by mindfulness.

Defenses of popular mindfulness against these critiques arise from within and outside Buddhist communities. In the remainder of this chapter, I will make the argument that some of the critiques arise from the modernist framing of distinctions such as religious/secular and so on, and that framing the discussion in these terms is not helpful. Instead, I will argue that we are in a postsecular, postmodern condition where these binaries are—and should be—deconstructed.

Religion, Science, and the Secular Harrison (2006) makes this point in the context of both science and religion. He notes that just like the concept of "religion," the definition of "science" has a dynamic history and that the sciences are "plural and diverse." How one views the relationship between science and religion depends upon how they are conceptualized:

> …once the constructed nature of the categories is taken into consideration, putative relationships between science and religion may turn out to be artifacts of the categories themselves. Whether science and religion are in conflict, or are independent entities, or are in dialogue, or are essentially integrated enterprises will be determined by exactly how one draws the boundaries within the broad limits given by the constructs (Harrison, 2006, p. 102).

Harrison finds it informative that these categories are historically and culturally contingent, and suggests moving beyond these categories:

> There is something to be learned from the relative indifference of those in other faith traditions to the issue of science and religion—and I refer here to those who have remained immune to the Western concept "religion" and the cultural authority of science. It might be better simply to emulate this indifference than to export a set of problems that are to a large degree creatures of the categories of Western knowledge. (Harrison, 2006, p. 104)

In fact, the porosity of boundaries between science and religion is already evident in fields such as medicine and psychology. In psychology, approaches such as transpersonal psychology have introduced spirituality back into mainstream therapeutic contexts. In medicine, there is increasing interest in complementary and alternative medicine. Medical humanities and narrative medicine resist the tide of scientism. They re-animate the realm of mythos in medicine:

> From a narrative medicine perspective, truth and construction are always co-constitutive. Even the most rigorous medical science still contains human perspectives, interests, and goals imbedded in the way the knowledge is selected, organized, and prioritized. (Lewis, 2016, p. 8)

This contention from narrative medicine challenges the notion that science is somehow "value free"; in fact, it makes all kinds of foundational assumptions. In their chapter in this volume, Luck and Krasner write about their experiences as practicing physicians. Both describe grappling with a medical model, where patients are depersonalized and a "hidden curriculum" of medical training where physicians lose idealism, can experience erosion of their ethical integrity, and become emotionally numbed or neutral. They refer to the seminal article by Eric Cassell about the legacy of Cartesian mind/body dualism on this hidden curriculum (1998). Earlier we saw how logos triumphed over mythos during the modern period. Cassell illuminates the extent to which this happened in modern medicine. He identifies the Cartesian heritage of a mind/body dualism in modern Western medicine. Western scientific materialism has difficulty in accounting for emergent, nonphysical properties that cannot be explained in reductionist terms. One of these properties is mind. Cassell argues that because mind is "problematic" (he defines this as being "not identifiable in objective terms"), "its very reality diminishes for science, and so, too, does the person." This partly accounts for the depersonalizing tendency to view only a patient's physical pain as the province of the modern physician: "So long as the mindbody dichotomy is accepted, suffering is either subjective and thus not truly "real"—not within medicine's domain—or identified exclusively with bodily pain."

One effect of the mind/body dualism was to contribute to the stratification between science and religion:

> Cartesian dualism made it possible for science to escape the control of the church by assigning the noncorporeal, spiritual realm to the church, leaving the physical world as the domain of science. In that religious age, "person", synonymous with "mind" was necessarily off-limits to science. (Cassell, 1998, p. 132)

Cassell argues that a consequence of this stratification is that in Western medical education, research and practice, very little attention is paid to the issue of suffering, or, that it is too narrowly defined. One of the reasons for this is that in the medical literature, suffering is equated with physical pain or disease, so that treating these pathologies is seen as the only remit of the physician. However, Cassell points out that suffering is not limited to the experience of physical symptoms. Indeed, sometimes the treatment for an illness can cause extreme suffering, as can the loss of personhood in the form of changing social roles, increased dependence on others, changing functionality of the body, and so on. In his research, Cassell was surprised by the following phenomenon:

> The relief of suffering, it would appear, is considered one of the primary ends of medicine by patients and lay persons, but not by the medical profession. As in the care of the dying, patients and their friends and families do not make a distinction between physical and non-physical sources of suffering in the same way that doctors do. (Cassell, 1998, p. 130)

Cassell argues that this equating of "suffering" with pain is an impoverished and inadequate understanding. He maintains that three factors, currently neglected in medical understandings of suffering, need to be taken into account when considering suffering—it happens to persons, who consist of more than just bodies that experience pain and disease; it occurs when this personhood is perceived as being under threat; and it can occur in relation to any aspect of the person (i.e. not just its physical aspect).

Related points are made by Loewy (1986) in his discussion of medical ethics education. He notes that the practice of ethics has always been an integral part of medicine since antiquity, and considered just as important as the disease-curing aspects. Loewy mentions Plato's distinction between an art and a craft. In a craft, the technical activity is an end itself—an art, on the other hand, has a moral end (Loewy 661). An example of this moral end in medicine might be the alleviation of suffering, as it is understood in its broad sense by Cassell. Loewy argues that until modern times, the "art" and "craft" aspects of medicine were always understood to be inextricably entwined. However, things changed in the modern era, with the advent of increasing technology:

the art of medicine, with its emphasis on the moral end, tended to be swamped by technology…. Medicine, as an art, uses technology as a means to serve its moral end. Advances in the technology of medicine changed what had been a paternalistic basis of medical practice to a scientific one. That is, physicians saw themselves less as benevolent and wise counselors overseeing the patient's welfare … and more as objective scientists applying the latest technical methods to bring about desired ends. (Loewy, p. 661)

This depersonalization—and its corrosive effects on morale in the medical profession—are described by Lück and Krasner later in this volume. Both call for a shift toward a more holistic understanding of suffering, and more relationship-centered care. They make a favorable reference to various approaches to medical training and care that are indicative of a move away from the depersonalized, technical approach toward a more emotionally and spiritually integrated one. One of these movements is narrative medicine, which recognizes that patients and their caregivers enter into the experience of sickness and healing not just as physical bodies, but as individuals with a complex of values, histories, relationships, and beliefs. These are all intricately woven into unique narratives about what health and illness means to them. Offering compassionate care and understanding the patient requires more than just technical proficiency, but a sensitivity to their narratives: without understanding this, "the caregiver might not see the patient's illness in its full, textured, emotionally powerful, consequential narrative form" (Charon, 2006, p. 13).

Another recent shift within medicine is an increasing focus on the importance of spirituality. Many illustrative examples of this are provided by the George Washington Institute for Spirituality and Health. Their founder, Christina Puchalski, advocates for spirituality in medicine as an antidote to the kind of depersonalization and technologizing that Cassell laments:

Spirituality is the basis for the deep, caring connections physicians and healthcare professionals form with their patients. While cure may result from technical and disease oriented care, healing occurs within the context of the caring connection patients form with their physicians and healthcare professionals. This is why spirituality is essential to all of medicine and healthcare. (Puchalski, 2016)

Lück and Krasner (Chap. 5) found that mindfulness training was very effective in helping physicians attune themselves to their patients' narratives, and to their own experience. In the Mindful Practice course that is part of the medical school curriculum at the University of Rochester, mindfulness, narrative medicine, and appreciative inquiry are combined to help improve well-being, decrease the chances of professional burnout, and to enhance personal characteristics better oriented to patient-centered care.

The Postmodern, Postsecular Turn

Earlier we discussed the deconstruction of conceptual boundaries associated with the modern period and a renewed interest in spiritual and religious values and ways of knowing are symptomatic of postmodernism and postsecularism. Narrative medicine is one example of a move toward the postsecular, but there are various other examples within medicine, psychology and the mindfulness movement itself. One such example is in the domain in ethics. For example, medical ethics have typically been dominated by principlism; the idea that ethical actions should be guided by adherence to principles—most commonly, the principles of autonomy, beneficence, non-maleficence, and justice (Beauchamp & Childress, 2001). Increasingly, though, this reliance on principlism is critiqued as being too rigid and lacking sensitivity to context and there has been a surge of interest in other ethical approaches such as care ethics and virtue ethics. Both of these are relationship-centered and context-dependent—rather than advocating solely the use of reason to apply principles to cases, they emphasize the importance of character, relationship, and particularly *emotion* in making ethical judgments. In reason-based ethics, emotion is often seen as clouding judgment, or getting in the way of making "rational decisions." Care and virtue ethics challenge this perspective, maintaining that in fact ethical perception is both a cognitive and emotional affair. Furthermore, principlism does not give adequate account to the role of emotion in human experience (Gardiner, 2003). Interestingly, there is a tendency to see different ethical theories as complementing, rather than conflicting with each other—in other words, a kind of ethical pluralism is emerging. This too is suggestive of a postmodern turn—moving from focus on a particular perspective as true, a "grand narrative," to a cosmopolitan openness to a variety of narratives. A variety of historical lineages of ideas bring a richness rather than a sense of competition. For example, Benner (1997) argues that virtue ethics is grounded in ancient Greek philosophy, where the focus is on the character of the agent. Care ethics draws more on Judeo-Christian traditions where the focus is *relational* on how the virtues are expressed in specific relationships. Both these streams come together and make for a richer, more comprehensive moral philosophy. On this cosmopolitan, pluralistic model, drawing and synthesizing from different philosophical backgrounds is perceived as a strength, rather than a threat to the integrity of a particular tradition.

We see this phenomenon, too, in the "second generation" of MBIs. Second-generation mindfulness practices are those which have responded and evolved in response to the critiques of popular mindfulness. Gleig identifies four "turns" represented in these second-generation movements—the social justice turn, the explicit Buddhist turn, the implicit Buddhist turn, and the human turn. Characteristic of all of these is a revalorization of ethics, and to varying degrees, open engagement with Buddhist narratives and values. In the social justice turn, the ethical dimensions and implications of mindfulness are emphasized and attempts made to engage social justice and create more diversity and inclusion in mindfulness. In Buddhist communities, this is exemplified by movements such as Engaged Buddhism, or organizations such as the Buddhist Peace Fellowship; in terms of MBIs that are not explicitly Buddhist, examples are the Inward Bound Mindfulness Education and Peace in Schools. The explicit Buddhist turn describes a move toward openly embracing or engaging with Buddhist teachings as increasing the transformative power of mindfulness. This may include explicit reference to Buddhist teachings, such as the four noble truths and the eightfold path, or in a "softer" form, may be influenced in structure and content by engagement with Buddhist traditions (see Chap. 7). For example, Gleig cites the Compassion Cultivation Training at Stanford and the Cognitively Based Compassion Training at Emory as programs which, as a direct result of their dialogue with Tibetan Buddhism, have incorporated compassion into their mindfulness training (see Chap. 6).

The implicit Buddhist turn refers to an approach that draws on a wide range of Buddhist teachings to deepen mindfulness teachings with more ethical and relational content, found within Buddhist traditions. However, the language and terms of traditional Buddhism are often translated into contemporary, secular language. The intent is not to "hide" the Buddhist associations, but to use language that is more accessible to their audiences (Monteiro, Musten, & Compson, 2015). There is an emphasis, too, on seeing these teachings as referring to the broad human condition, and having wisdom that is present in other traditions too. Gleig cites The Mindfulness Institute, and Sati: Mindfulness Coaching and Workshops as organizations that take this kind of approach.

The human turn approach emphasizes shared human values and needs such as love, interconnection, and compassion, and sees mindfulness as effective in realizing these. In this approach, teachings are disassociated from Buddhism on the grounds that the teachings move beyond specific religious forms and transcend religious and secular differences. An example of this approach is found in the Peace in Schools group.

What is interesting about these approaches is that they represent neither a modernist approach of detraditionalization, nor a "fundamentalist" reclaiming of traditional Buddhism. Instead they represent a hybridization. They have responded from critiques rooted variously in modernism, post-colonialism, and canonical Buddhism.

One of the defenses against both the "McMindfulness" and "Stealth Buddhism" critiques is what Gleig describes at the experiential/functional argument. To put it simply, this defense focuses on the fact that mindfulness *works*. This defense tends to be forwarded by people who are actively teaching mindfulness to different populations, and seeing its transformative effects in reducing suffering. This rests on an understanding of mindfulness having an intrinsic power, whether or not it is associated with Buddhism. As we have seen in the "explicitly Buddhist" turn, some maintain that overtly integrating other Buddhist teachings into MBIs make them more potent transformative programs. Others, though, see "secular" versions of mindfulness, such as MBSR, as different (but complementary) ways of training toward the liberation of suffering, with some framing them as evolutionary advances over Buddhist approaches. Connected to these defenses is often the idea that mindfulness, and the capacity to develop wisdom and compassion, are universal human qualities, accessible from within both secular and religious traditions—it is not the "property" of Buddhism. However one frames this "mindfulness works" perspective, its pragmatic approach is instructive and, as I will now argue in this concluding section, a good model for navigating the fraught territory of contemporary mindfulness debates.

The Case for a Pragmatic, Postsecular Approach

We have seen how one of the characteristics of postmodernism is the recognition that our concepts are socially constructed and change over time. Asking questions about whether mindfulness is "too religious" or "not secular enough" rests on a binary of "religious" and "secular" that is culturally specific to the West. The meaning of these terms is contested and evolving. Often claims that mindfulness is "too religious" rest on the reification of "Buddhism" as an institutionalized "religion" and assume that its association with religions makes it inappropriate for inclusion into secular realms.

One of the "stealth Buddhism" critiques of popular mindfulness is that in presenting itself as secular, it is implying that it is ethically neutral or value-neutral, when in fact it is either implicitly or explicitly promoting Buddhist values. Many assumptions in this critique are problematic. For example, it assumes that "secular" somehow means "value-free," but it is not at all clear that this is the case. Bioethicist Robert Veatch explains, for example, that "mainstream American physicians, nurses, pharmacists, and social workers are likely to acknowledge that they hold certain truths to be self-evident and that, among these, they accept that all people are created equal and endowed with certain inalienable rights." These are not value-free beliefs, but ones grounded in US liberal political philosophy—a particular worldview and tradition. His point is that even professional medical codes rely on normative values external to their fields: "The problem for these secular physicians, like their religious brothers and sisters, is that these moral theories have metaethical and normative commitments that have nothing to do with Hippocratic and other professionally generated ethics." (Veatch, 1981, p. 138).

If secular means "not religious," then it is presumably *religious* values that it is meant to be free from. But what exactly is a *religious* value as opposed to any other kind of value? Is it the historical provenance of a value, or the nature of a value itself that makes it "religious"? For example, is mindfulness necessarily religious because it has historical roots in Buddhist traditions, or because it somehow embodies "Buddhist values"? What is it that makes a value a *Buddhist* value, and who decides? There are countless expressions of Buddhist teachings and they continue to morph and adapt over time, such that a quest for an authoritative version is problematic (Sharf, 2015). For that matter, what makes a value a *secular* one, and who decides? How one answers these questions is contingent on many other culturally conditioned assumptions.

Rather than debating whether mindfulness is or is not Buddhist or religious, my suggestion is that a better question to focus on is "is mindfulness helpful in reducing suffering?", be that on an individual or corporate level. Psychologist and Zen priest Seth Segall makes this point:

> The more important question isn't semantic, but empirical: Is mindfulness, as currently construed, useful or not? Does it reliably and meaningfully impact matters that human beings care deeply about, things like the perennial Buddhist concerns of sickness, old age, and death? (Segall, 2013)

He goes on to list empirical answers to some of these questions, citing studies that show mindfulness being effective in lowering sensitivity to pain, reducing age-related decline in the brain, and improving subjective well-being (Segall, 2013). This kind of response is more helpful, I argue, than one that rules out the use of mindfulness, for example, insofar as it is "Buddhist."

This is not to dismiss the concerns of the "Stealth Buddhism" or the "McMindfulness" critics, but to advocate addressing each one pragmatically on a case-by-case basis. For example, one of the McMindfulness critiques is that mindfulness can be a tool for corporate interests, pacifying workers. Baer (2015) describes a series of studies pointing to the fact that engagement in MBIs is associated with increasing prosocial and values-consistent behavior and concludes that it "seems unlikely that worksite mindfulness training will encourage passive acquiescence with corporate wrongdoing." (p. 964). When the question moves from a principled one to a practical or empirical one, the predictions of the McMindfulness critics are not, in this case at least, supported. Rather than getting tangled in the theoretical objections, it is better to explore if and how these concerns play out in practice. For example, later in this volume, Gunther Brown expresses concern about mindfulness being implemented in secular contexts. Her in-principle objection rests mainly on the idea that mindfulness is inescapably Buddhist, or at the very least, religious. The reasons she gives for why this matters are more praxis-based. For example, she is concerned that not fully disclosing the Buddhist roots of mindfulness violates contemporary ethical norms such as informed consent. She argues that potential participants should be told warned that engaging in MBIs may have "religious effects" that may be at odds with their current values. This concerns patient or client autonomy—people should be free to choose their own religious or spiritual resources, and encouraging them to undertake a "spiritual" practice like mindfulness without explaining that it is spiritual violates their ability to make autonomous decisions. Another objection is that mindfulness meditation can have adverse emotional, psychological, or spiritual effects, and participants are given insufficient warning about these risks.

Many of these claims are loaded with assumptions and make for *a priori* rather than *a posteriori* objections. For instance, Gunther Brown cites the following quote from Farias and Wikholm in support of her argument that mindfulness transgresses secular boundaries:

> Meditation leads us to become more spiritual, and that this increase in spirituality is partly responsible for the practice's positive effects. So, even if we set out to ignore meditation's spiritual roots, those roots may nonetheless envelop us, to a greater or lesser degree. Overall, it is unclear whether secular models of mindfulness meditation are fully secular. (2015, loc. 3293)

It seems unclear, though, why this should be problematic, particularly as this "increase in spirituality" has a positive effect. For Gunther Brown, the problem again comes down to informed consent: "Marketing mindfulness as secular, implicitly defined as resulting in empirically validated effects, may both veil and heighten religious effects by *inducing participation by those who might otherwise object to joining in a Buddhist practice.*" (Gunther Brown, p. x, emphasis added). This objection rests on strong (and as we have seen, contested) binaries between "religious" and "secular," the equating of spirituality and religion and the equating of mindfulness and Buddhism. Even if these conceptualizations are correct, the underlying assumption that different spirituality or religious forms are incommensurable or mutually exclusive. Gunther Brown elaborates on this latter theme in her chapter, rejecting the claims that values such as compassion are universal ideas. For example, she argues that while Buddhists and Christians both see compassion as a core value, they frame it so differently that to equate them is to distort both conceptions, and to efface important distinctions. Certainly, it is true that different traditions and narratives bring varying nuances and meanings that should be respected, not merged into a bland universalism. My argument, however, is that awareness of these differences should be the *start* of a conversation, not the end of it. If different traditions have contrasting accounts of virtues, this does not necessarily mean they are incommensurable—on the contrary, mutual exploration and dialogue may lead to great enrichment. I contend the same is the case for discussions about spiritual/secular boundaries—where disagreements arise about where to draw them, this is an invitation for looking more deeply rather than walking away. All this is with the proviso that efforts are made to minimize harm and distress. One of Gunther Brown's most compelling arguments for caution around MBIs is the risk of adverse psychological experiences. This has, indeed, been a neglected area and the research on this is in its early stages and rightly should continue to develop. Just as with any intervention, prescribers have an ethical obligation to identify contraindications and protect the vulnerable. The point, though, is that these decisions should be based on empirical evidence, not *a priori* conceptualizations.

In our postsecular age, the case for separation of "religion and "secular" is not as strong as the case for porosity and mutual dialogue. These narratives are constantly interacting and modifying each other. The renewed valorization of spirituality and religion within the contexts of psychology and medicine are symptomatic of a movement toward engagement between these spheres. The contemporary debates about mindfulness show different points along the spectrum of convergence and divergence. Gunther Brown's position takes a more "segregationist" approach, suggesting that mindfulness can never be secular. Baer's position is further on the spectrum toward convergence. She acknowledges that explicitly Buddhist MBIs have their place, but argues that presenting mindfulness in a more secular format makes it more accessible and user-friendly, maximizing the opportunities for it to benefit people.

> As the demand for MBPs expands, the diversity of people seeking professional training in how to provide them will also increase. Training that requires participation in overtly Buddhist practices or relies heavily on Buddhist frameworks or belief systems may create barriers to teachers from other traditions. For these reasons, while acknowledging that explicitly Buddhist-based programs may be beneficial in some settings, we have argued that mindfulness-based training will be more widely accessible if genuinely secular MBPs, with secular foundational ethics, are available. (Baer, Chap. 4)

Divergence does not have to mean incommensurability; it can imply complementarity.

It is important for religious and scientific discourse to maintain a critical distance from each other. This does not mean that their spheres should be entirely discrete, but that neither becomes subsumed by the foundational values of the other. Harrison gives the example of how sometimes bioethics has been a source of legitimation for medicine, contributing to questionable trends such as the medicalization of society. He also gives the example of how scientific studies of Buddhist meditation have prioritized agendas of physical health while neglecting to explore the wider spiritual or religious teachings. Rather than trying to subsume the religious or the secular into one or the other grand narrative, critical distance between them should be maintained and celebrated:

> The suggestion is rather that it will be impossible for theology to exercise a critical or, in religious terms, "prophetic" role in a society unless it maintains an appropriate distance from dominant cultural forces. This is an independence of theology from science that leaves room for legitimate conflict. (Harrison, 2006, p. 104)

Veatch makes a compelling point in this regard about professional or secular ethics, which is worth quoting in some length because it highlights some of the difficulties with relying on professional ethics:

> Even if we assume that the physician is the presumed expert in describing the medical facts, the presumption that the individual physician or a group of physicians has expertise in developing a moral code for their profession is baseless. To the contrary, we have every reason to believe that physicians (or any other specialized group) would be expected to make distorted choices when they put forward a moral code. In the case of classical professional medical ethics, their theory is unacceptably overcommitted to consequences at the expense of nonconsequentialistic moral principles such as autonomy and justice. Their theory is unacceptably overcommitted to the consequences for the patient to the exclusion of those for all others in society. Their theory is unacceptably overcommitted to the place of the physician in deciding what counts as a good consequence for the patient. (Veatch, 2012, p. 149)

Lück and Krasner's account of mindfulness in medical practice provides an example of how norms and practices from outside the realm of scientific medicine reinvigorated their experience of their profession and offer immense benefits to caregivers and patients.

One of the strengths of mindfulness is that it has the capacity to be interpreted and applied at different stages along the spectrum of "spiritual" to "secular." In this respect, it has versatility and broad appeal. On a postsecular view, its connection with spirituality is to be celebrated, not mistrusted:

> Mindfulness has the potential to be more than a medical and psychological tool for reducing stress. It can also connect us to a form of mystical wisdom that has been lost to modern health care. Indeed, mindfulness signals an opening between secular and spiritual approaches to suffering, and, more important, mindfulness provides a discursive bridge between these two worlds. (Lewis, 2016, p. 15)

To conclude, debates about the role of ethics in MBIs and the ethics of their implementation in various spheres are very complicated and multidimensional. I have argued that modernist assumptions about the nature of religion or spirituality in relation to science and secularity are outdated and shut down dialogue between these spheres. In contrast, a postmodern, postsecular openness to interplay and dialogue between narratives is more generative and inclusive.

References

Anderson, W. T. (1990). *Reality is not what it used to be: Theatrical politics, ready-to-wear religion, global myths, primitive chic, and other wonders of the postmodern world.* San Francisco: Harper & Collins.

Armstrong, K. (2009). *The case for God.* New York: Knopf.

Baer, R. (2015). Ethics, values, virtues, and character strengths in mindfulness-based interventions: A psychological science perspective. *Mindfulness, 6*(4), 956–969.

Beauchamp, T. L., & Childress, J. F. (2001). *Principles of biomedical ethics.* New York: Oxford University Press.

Benner, P. (1997). A dialogue between virtue ethics and care ethics. *Theoretical Medicine, 18*(1), 47–61.

Braun, E. (2013). *The birth of insight: Meditation, modern Buddhism, and the Burmese monk Ledi Sayadaw.* Chicago: University of Chicago Press.

Casanova, J. (2013). Exploring the postsecular: Three meanings of the "Secular" and their possible transcendence. In C. Calhoun, E. Mendieta, & J. VanAntwerpen (Eds.), *Habermas and religion.* Cambridge: Polity Press.

Cassell, E. J. (1998). The nature of suffering and the goals of medicine. *Loss, Grief and Care, 8*(1–2), 129–142.

Charon, R. (2006). *Narrative medicine: Honoring the stories of illness.* New York: Oxford University Press.

Compson, J., & Monteiro, L. (2015). Still exploring the middle path: A response to commentaries. *Mindfulness, 7*(2), 548–564.

Esposito, J. L., Fasching, D. J., & Lewis, T. T. (2002). *World religions today.* New York: Oxford University Press.

Farias, M., & Wikholm, C. (2015). *The Buddha pill: Can meditation change you?* London: Watkins.

Fronsdal, G. (1998). Life, liberty and the pursuit of happiness in the American insight community. In C. S. Prebish (Ed.), *The faces of Buddhism in America.* Berkeley: University of California Press.

Gardiner, P. (2003). A virtue ethics approach to moral dilemmas in medicine. *Journal of Medical Ethics, 29*(5), 297–302.

Gleig, A. (2018, forthcoming). WORKING TITLE: *Enlightenment after the enlightenment: American Buddhism after modernity.*

Habermas, J. (2008). Notes on post-secular society. *New Perspectives Quarterly, 25*(4), 17–29.

Harrison, P. (2006). "Science" and "religion": Constructing the boundaries. *The Journal of Religion, 86*(1), 81–106.

Heuman, L. (2014). The science delusion: An interview with cultural critic Curtis White. *Tricycle Magazine,* Spring 2014. Retrieved on March 7, 2017 from https://tricycle.org/magazine/science-delusion/

Hitchens, C. (2008). *God is not great: How religion poisons everything.* Toronto: McClelland & Stewart.

Kabat-Zinn, J. (2000). Indra's net at work: The mainstreaming of Dharma practice in society. In G. Watson, S. Batchelor, & G. Claxton (Eds.), *The psychology of awakening: Buddhism, science, and our day-to-day lives* (pp. 225–249). York Beach, ME: Weiser.

Lewis, B. (2016). Mindfulness, mysticism, and narrative medicine. *Journal of Medical Humanities, 37*(4), 401–417.

Loewy, E. H. (1986). Teaching medical ethics to medical students. *Academic Medicine*, *61*(8), 661–665.

Masuzawa, T. (2005). *The invention of world religions: Or, how European universalism was preserved in the language of pluralism*. Chicago: University of Chicago Press.

McMahan, D. L. (2008). *The making of Buddhist modernism*. New York: Oxford University Press.

Monteiro, L. M., Musten, R. F., & Compson, J. (2015). Traditional and contemporary mindfulness: Finding the middle path in the tangle of concerns. *Mindfulness*, *6*(1), 1–13.

Neale, M. (2015). *Frozen Yoga and McMindfulness: Miles Neale on the mainstreaming of contemplative religious practices*. Retrieved March 3, 2017 from https://www.lionsroar.com/frozen-yoga-and-mcmindfulness-miles-neale-on-the-mainstreaming-of-contemplative-religious-practices/

Puchalski, C. (2016). *A message from Dr. Puchalski. George Washington Institute for Spirituality and Health*. Retrieved from https://smhs.gwu.edu/gwish/about/message

Purser, R. & Loy, D. (2013, July 1). Beyond McMindfulness. *Huffington Post*. Retrieved March 3, 2017, from http://www.huffingtonpost.com/ron-purser/beyond-mcmindfulness_b_3519289.html

Segall, S. (2013). In defense of mindfulness. The Existential Buddhist, December 19, 2013. Retrieved on February 28, 2017 from http://www.existentialbuddhist.com/2013/12/in-defense-of-mindfulness/

Sharf, R. H. (2015). Is mindfulness Buddhist? (and why it matters). *Transcultural Psychiatry*, *52*(4), 470–484.

Smith, W. C. (1963). *The meaning and end of religion*. New York: Macmillan.

Stone, M. (2014). Abusing the Buddha: How the U.S. Army and Google co-opt mindfulness. *Salon*, March 17, 2014. Retrieved on March 6, 2017 from http://www.salon.com/2014/03/17/abusing_the_buddha_how_the_u_s_army_and_google_co_opt_mindfulness/. Accessed X.

Veatch, R. M. (1981). *A theory of medical ethics*. New York: Basic Books.

Veatch, R. (2012). Hippocratic, religious, and secular medical ethics : The points of conflict. Washington, DC: Georgetown University Press.

Wilson, J. (2014). *Mindful America: Meditation and the mutual transformation of Buddhism and American culture*. Oxford: Oxford University Press.

Chapter 3
Ethics, Transparency, and Diversity in Mindfulness Programs

Candy Gunther Brown

Introduction

Mindfulness-Based interventions (MBIs) are everywhere: hospitals, psychology clinics, corporations, prisons, and public schools. Mindfulness entered the American cultural mainstream as promoters downplayed its Buddhist origins and ethical contexts, and linguistically reframed it as a secular, scientific technique to reduce stress, support health, and cultivate universal ethical norms. Despite their secular framing, many MBIs continue to reflect their Buddhist ethical foundations. The effects are far-reaching, though largely uninterrogated. This chapter argues that if MBIs are not fully secular, but based on Buddhist ethics (whether explicitly or implicitly), then there should be transparency about this fact—even if transparency comes at the expense of no longer reaping benefits of being perceived as secular. The ethical grounds for transparency may be articulated using principles internal or external to a Buddhist framework: (1) fidelity to the Noble Eightfold Path, including right mindfulness, right intention, and right speech; (2) intellectual integrity, cultural diversity, and informed consent.

Transparency Defined

The scope of this chapter extends to all mindfulness-Based interventions (MBIs), because the term "mindfulness" is remarkably opaque. By design of its popularizers, mindfulness has cultural cachet as a scientifically validated, religiously neutral

C.G. Brown, PhD (✉)
Department of Religious Studies, Indiana University,
Sycamore Hall 230, 1033 E. Third St., Bloomington, IN 47405-7005, USA
e-mail: browncg@indiana.edu

© Springer International Publishing AG 2017   45
L.M. Monteiro et al. (eds.), *Practitioner's Guide to Ethics and Mindfulness-Based Interventions*, Mindfulness in Behavioral Health,
DOI 10.1007/978-3-319-64924-5_3

technique of "bare attention," yet gestures toward a comprehensive worldview and ethical system. Even in its most secular guises, part of the appeal of mindfulness is that it vaguely connotes ancient, quasi-religious wisdom; it seems the cutting edge of low technology to heal what ails modern, hyper-technical society. This chapter advocates full disclosure of all that mindfulness entails—including its Buddhist ethical foundations and range of potential physical, mental, and religious effects—to MBI administrators (e.g., CEOs of hospitals and corporations, prison wardens, public-school superintendents), providers (e.g., nurses, public-school teachers), and clients (e.g., patients, employees, prisoners, school children and their parents). Transparency encompasses the volunteering of material information, negative as well as positive, in a manner that promotes clear understanding. The goal of transparency is not achieved merely by acknowledging that mindfulness has Buddhist roots. This is because historical framing may imply a secularization narrative, suggesting that once-religious practices have since outgrown their religious roots and are now completely secular, much like modern medicine. The position of this chapter is that if MBIs are to benefit from positive cultural associations with the term mindfulness, then program directors and instructors have an ethical obligation to fully own the term.

Buddhist Associations of Mindfulness

Mindfulness-Based interventions are relatively recent inventions, developed by Buddhists and individuals influenced by Buddhism who wanted to bring Buddhist assumptions, values, and practices into the American cultural mainstream. One of the most important figures in this regard is Jon Kabat-Zinn, a Jewish-American molecular biology PhD, "first exposed to the dharma" in 1966 while a student at MIT (2011, p. 286). Kabat-Zinn trained as a Dharma teacher with Korean Zen Master Seung Sahn, and draws eclectically on Soto Zen, Rinzai Zen, Tibetan Mahamudra, and Dzogchen; a modernist version of Vipassana, or insight meditation, modeled after Burmese Theravada teacher Mahasi Sayadaw; as well as hatha yoga, Hindu Vedanta, and other non-Buddhist spiritual resources (Dodson-Lavelle, 2015, pp. 4, 47, 50; Harrington & Dunne, 2015, p. 627; Kabat-Zinn, 2011, pp. 286, 289). Although he still trains with Buddhist teachers and views his "patients as Buddhas," since "literally everything and everybody is already the Buddha," Kabat-Zinn stopped identifying as a Buddhist once he realized that he "would [not] have been able to do what I did in quite the same way if I was actually identifying myself as a Buddhist" (Kabat-Zinn, 2010, para. 4, 2011, p. 300). A non-Buddhist public identity made it possible for Kabat-Zinn to introduce Buddhist beliefs and practices into the cultural mainstream without raising worries about Buddhist evangelism.

In 1979, Kabat-Zinn founded the Stress Reduction and Relaxation Clinic, later renamed the Center for Mindfulness in Medicine, Health Care, and Society (CfM), with the signature program Mindfulness-Based Stress-Reduction (MBSR), at the University of Massachusetts Medical School. By the mid-2010s, CfM had enrolled

22,000 patients, certified 1000 instructors, spawned more than 700 MBSR programs in medical settings across more than 30 countries, and become a model for innumerable MBIs in hospitals, prisons, public schools, government, media, professional sports, and businesses (CfM, 2014a, para. 1; Wylie, 2015, p. 19). Kabat-Zinn envisioned MBSR as a way to:

> Take the heart of something as meaningful, as sacred if you will, as Buddha-dharma and bring it into the world in a way that doesn't dilute, profane or distort it, but at the same time is not locked into a culturally and tradition-bound framework that would make it absolutely impenetrable to the vast majority of people. (2000, p. 227)

The "particular techniques" taught in MBSR are "merely launching platforms" for "direct experience of the noumenous, the sacred, the Tao, God, the divine, Nature, silence, in all aspects of life," resulting in a "flourishing on this planet akin to a second, and this time global, Renaissance, for the benefit of all sentient beings and our world" (Kabat-Zinn, 1994a, p. 4, 2003, pp. 147–48; 2011, p. 281). As detailed elsewhere (Brown, 2016), Buddhist teachings infuse MBSR at every level: (1) development of program concept, (2) systematic communication of core Buddhist beliefs, (3) teacher prerequisites, training, and continuing education requirements, and (4) resources suggested to MBSR graduates.

To make MBSR acceptable to non-Buddhists, Kabat-Zinn downplayed its Buddhist foundations. In his own words, Kabat-Zinn "bent over backward" to select vocabulary that concealed his understanding of mindfulness as the "essence of the Buddha's teachings" (2011, p. 282). Melissa Myozen Blacker, who spent 20 years as a teacher and director of programs at CfM, recalls that "the MBSR course was partly based on the teachings of the four foundations of mindfulness found in the *Satipattana Sutta* … and we included this and other traditional Buddhist teachings in our teacher training." Yet, "for the longest time, we didn't say it was Buddhism at all. There was never any reference to Buddhism in the standard 8-week MBSR class; only in teacher training did we require retreats and learning about Buddhist psychology" (Wilks, Blacker, Boyce, Winston, & Goodman, 2015, p. 48). As scientific publications won credibility for MBSR, Kabat-Zinn gradually began to "articulate its origins and its essence" to health professionals, yet "not so much to the patients," whom he has intentionally continued to leave uninformed about the "dharma that underlies the curriculum" (2011, pp. 282–83).

Kabat-Zinn has claimed that the "dharma" is itself universal, rather than specifically Buddhist. What he seems to mean, however, is that dharmic assumptions are universally true (Davis, 2015, p. 47). This claim may be undercut by his choice of an "untranslated, Buddhist-associated Sanskrit word" (Helderman, 2016, p. 952). Jeff Wilson argues that "Dharma is itself a religious term, and even to define it as a universal thing is a theological statement" (2015). Indeed, Kabat-Zinn's intentional lack of transparency about the dharmic "essence" of MBSR with program participants calls into question the concept's universality.

In developing MBSR, Kabat-Zinn foregrounded the term "mindfulness" because of its potential to do "double-duty." For audiences unfamiliar with Buddhism, mindfulness sounds like a universal human capacity to regulate attention. But the term can also serve as a "place-holder for the entire dharma," an "umbrella term" that "subsumes all of the other elements of the Eightfold Noble Path" (2009, pp. xxviii–xxiv). The term can be traced etymologically to Pāli language Buddhist sacred texts, especially the *Satipatthāna Sutta*, or "The Discourse on the Establishing of Mindfulness." *Sammā sati*, often translated as "right mindfulness," comprises the seventh aspect of what is frequently translated as the "Noble Eightfold Path" to liberation from suffering, the fourth of the "Four Noble Truths" of Buddhism (Wilson, 2014, p. 16). When addressing Buddhist audiences, Kabat-Zinn cites "the words of the Buddha in his most explicit teaching on mindfulness, found in the *Mahasatipatthana Sutra*, or great sutra on mindfulness." It is the "direct path for the purification of beings, for the surmounting of sorrow and lamentation, for the disappearance of pain and grief, for the attainment of the true way, for the realization of liberation [Nirvana]—namely, the four foundations of mindfulness" (2009, p. xxix). Kabat-Zinn explains that his:

> Choice to have the word mindfulness does [sic] double-duty as a comprehensive but tacit umbrella term that included other essential aspects of dharma, was made as a potential skillful means to facilitate introducing what Nyanaponika Thera referred to as the heart of Buddhist meditation into the mainstream of medicine and more broadly, health care and wider society. (2009, pp. xxviii–xxix)

The flexibility of the term mindfulness offered a means, then, of introducing Buddhist concepts into the cultural mainstream.

Much as mindfulness serves as a euphemism for *Buddhadharma*, the term "stress" is a secular-sounding translation of the Buddhist concept of *dukkha*. The promise of "stress reduction" functions in MBSR as an "invitational framework" to:

> Dive right into the experience of *dukkha* in all its manifestations without ever mentioning *dukkha*; dive right into the ultimate sources of *dukkha* without ever mentioning the classical etiology, and yet able to investigate craving and clinging first-hand, propose investigating the possibility for alleviating if not extinguishing that distress or suffering (cessation), and explore, empirically, a possible pathway for doing so (the practice of mindfulness meditation writ large, inclusive of the ethical stance of *śīla*, the foundation of *samadhi*, and, of course, *prajñā*, wisdom—the eightfold noble path) without ever having to mention the Four Noble Truths, the Eightfold Noble Path, or *śīla*, *samadhi*, or *prajñā*. In this fashion, the Dharma can be self-revealing through skillful and ardent cultivation. (2011, p. 299, emphasis original)

Stress reduction is thus, in Kabat-Zinn's view, essentially *dukkha*-reduction.

The term mindfulness might be analyzed linguistically as an instance of synecdoche, a rhetorical trope in which a part of something refers to the whole (Chandler, 2002, p. 132). Avowedly secular MBI teachers make few, if any, overt references to Buddhism. But they do teach the term mindfulness. For instance, Goldie Hawn's MindUP curriculum insists that "to get the full benefit of MindUp lessons, children will need to know a specific vocabulary," chiefly the term mindfulness itself (Hawn Foundation, 2011, p. 40). The term functions as a sign that points toward a wider constellation of available meanings. Stephen Batchelor, meditation teacher and advocate of "Secular Buddhism," observes that "although doctors and therapists who employ mindfulness in a medical setting deliberately avoid any reference to Buddhism, you do not have to be a rocket scientist to figure out where it comes from. A Google search will tell you that mindfulness is a form of Buddhist meditation" (2012, p. 88). Individuals who experience benefits from a program designated as "mindfulness" may seek to go "deeper" by exploring additional "mindfulness" resources. As people discover associations between mindfulness and Buddhism, they may, by transitive inference reasoning, assign credit to Buddhism for positive experiences (Phillips, Wilson, & Halford, 2009; Waldmann, 2001). Thus, the term mindfulness itself, even when framed with secular language, can point practitioners toward Buddhism.

Ethical Dimensions of Mindfulness

Far from being an ethically neutral set of techniques, MBIs are founded upon Buddhist assumptions about the nature of reality and corresponding ideals for relationships among humans and indeed all sentient beings. CfM-trained MBI teacher Rebecca Crane explains that:

> Inherent within mindfulness teaching is the message that there are universal aspects to the experience of being human: centrally, that we all experience suffering, which ultimately comes from ignorance about ourselves and the nature of reality. Mindfulness practice leads us to see more clearly the ways we fuel our suffering and opens us to experiencing our connection with others. (Crane et al. 2012, p. 79)

Brooke Dodson-Lavelle, director of the Mind and Life Institute's Ethics, Education, and Human Development Initiative, analyzed MBSR alongside other purportedly "secular" meditation programs (Cognitively-Based Compassion Training, or CBCT, and Innate Compassion Training, or ICT). She concludes that despite the "universal rhetoric" and "normative generalizations" employed by all three programs, they are all "culturally and socially conditioned" and "very Buddhist," though reflecting different Buddhist traditions. Each "promotes a different diagnosis of suffering, an interpretation of its cause, an evaluation of judgment regarding the good, and a path for overcoming that suffering and/or realizing the good." The programs are "morally substantive as a consequence of the fact that they tell people, at least implicitly, stories about what they *ought* to be thinking, feeling, or doing." They are "ethically substantive as a consequence of the fact that they establish or encourage particular ways of conceptualizing the self, the good life, and the potential for transformation of the self towards a better kind of life" (2015, pp. 28, 161, 163). The foundational assumptions of each program shape their definitions and prescriptions of morality and ethics.

Buddhist Ethics Implicit in MBIs

The debate among mindfulness advocates is less about whether ethics should be included in the teaching of mindfulness, than whether its teaching should be explicit or implicit. Dodson-Lavelle identifies two competing Buddhist models of human nature: innativist, or discovery, and constructivist, or developmental. The debate "hinges on whether the qualities of awakening are innate to one's mind or whether they need to be cultivated" (2015, p. 28). In the former model, it is unnecessary to teach ethics explicitly because the practice of mindfulness itself enables participants to discover their own innate ethical tendencies (Cheung, forthcoming, p. 3; Lindahl, 2015a). Thus, Kabat-Zinn asserts that "mindfulness meditation writ large" is "inclusive of the ethical stance of *śīla*" (2011, p. 299). Margaret Cullen, one of the first 10 certified MBSR instructors, elaborates that the "intention of MBSR" is "much greater than simple stress reduction." It dispels "greed, hatred, and delusion" (the "three poisons," according to Buddhist thought) and has "elements of all of the *brahma vihāras*" (the four virtues, or "antidotes": loving-kindness, compassion, sympathetic joy, and equanimity, that the Buddha reputedly prescribed) "seamlessly integrated into it" (2011, p. 189). Mindfulness teacher Sharon Salzberg emphasizes that mindfulness "naturally leads us to greater loving-kindness" by diminishing "grasping, aversion and delusion" (2011, p. 177). By innativist reasoning, ethical qualities emerge through the practice of mindfulness, with or without explicit ethical instruction.

Many MBI teachers come from an innativist stance and reason that it is not only unnecessary to teach Buddhist ethics explicitly, it is disadvantageous because doing so may exclude potential beneficiaries. MBI teacher (of MBSR and Mindfulness-Based Cognitive Therapy, or MBCT) Jenny Wilks warns that "explicitly Buddhist ethics could potentially offend participants who are atheist, Christian, [or] Muslim" (Wilks in Cheung, forthcoming, p. 7). Omitting openly Buddhist instruction does not worry Wilks because "key Dharma teachings and practices are implicit … even if not explicit," making MBIs "more of a distillation than a dilution"—a form of "highly accessible Dharma" (2014, sect. 4 para. 5, sect. 5 para. 3, sect. 6 para. 3). Wilks elaborates that "although we wouldn't use the terminology of the three *lakkhanas* [marks of existence: *anicca*, or impermanence; *dukkha*, or suffering; and *anatta*, or no-self] when teaching MBPs [mindfulness-Based programs], through the practice people often do come to realize the changing and evanescent nature of their experiences" (2014, sect. 4 para. 8). Cullen notes that although it is "common to begin with breath awareness," MBIs progress to "bring awareness to other aspects of experience, such as thoughts and mental states in order to promote insights into no-self, impermanence and the reality of suffering" (2011, p. 192). Bob Stahl, Adjunct Senior Teacher for the CfM Oasis Institute, confirms that "without explicitly naming the 4 noble truths, 4 foundations of mindfulness, and 3 marks of existence, these teachings are embedded within MBSR classes and held within a field of loving-kindness" (2015, p. 2). Thus, MBSR and other secularly framed MBIs presume that mindfulness training can produce ethical benefits.

Reflecting constructivist assumptions that virtues need to be developed, some MBIs teach ethics more explicitly. One common approach is to incorporate "loving-kindness" meditations aimed at cultivating wholesome states of mind. As neuroscience researchers Thorsten Barnhofer and colleagues explain, "the term loving kindness or *metta*, in the Pali language, refers to unconditional regard and nonexclusive love for all beings and is one of the four main Buddhist virtues" (2010, p. 21).

Therapist Donald McCown notes that the "Brahmaviharas [the four virtues] have had a significant impact on the curriculum and pedagogy of the MBIs." In particular, *mettā*, variously translated as "loving-kindness," "friendliness," or "heartfulness," meditations instill a virtuous "attitude toward oneself, toward one's experience moment by moment, and toward others. Its emotional charge is powerful." McCown suggests that "if there is a source for an inherent ethical stance of the MBIs, this may well be it" (2013, p. 52). Although MBSR and MBCT manuals do not include *mettā* meditations, many MBI teachers (including Kabat-Zinn) do complement their teachings in this way. Meditations used in MBIs typically begin by speaking blessings over oneself: "May I be safe and protected from inner and outer harm. May I be happy and contented. May I be healthy and whole to whatever degree possible. May I experience ease of wellbeing." The "field of loving-kindness" expands first to loved ones and ultimately to "our state," "our country," "the entire world," "all animal life," "all plant life," "the entire biosphere," and "all sentient beings." "May all beings near and far … our planet and the whole universe" be "safe and protected and free from inner and outer harm," "happy and contented," "healthy and whole," and "experience ease of well-being" (Kabat-Zinn, n.d., 3.2). In the assessment of historian Jeff Wilson, *mettā* practitioners are:

> Not simply taught value-neutral awareness techniques—they are coached to cultivate profoundly universal feelings of compassion and love for all people and every living thing. This perspective on life is not only value laden but is also promoted as both improving the world and as key to one's own health and happiness. (2014, p. 172)

Even so, purportedly "secular" MBIs, such as Mindful Schools and Inner Kids, often do include *mettā* meditations (described as "heartfulness" or "friendly wishes") in their curricula (Bahnsen, 2013; Greenland, 2013, sect. 4). Although MBIs may be differentiated by whether they reflect innativist or constructivist assumptions about human nature, and thus whether they teach ethics implicitly or explicitly, many MBIs share an ethical concern.

Mindfulness Defined in Ethical Terms

Influential definitions of mindfulness include an ethical dimension. One of the most widely cited definitions is that popularized by Kabat-Zinn: "paying attention in a particular way: on purpose, in the present moment, and non-judgmentally" (1994b, p. 4). Amy Saltzman, a pioneer in teaching mindfulness to youth through her Still Quiet Place program, defines mindfulness as "paying attention, here and now, with kindness and curiosity" (2014, p. 2). Neither definition reduces mindfulness to bare attentional training. Rather, they indicate a particular ethical stance of *how* one should pay attention—nonjudgmentally, with kindness and curiosity—and this ethical stance comes from a Buddhist "way of seeing the world" (Dodson-Lavelle, 2015, p. 42). Psychologist Stephen Stratton notes that defining mindfulness as a "curious, nonjudgmental, and accepting orientation to present experiencing" reflects a "comprehensive life view," not just a "therapeutic technique" (2015, pp. 102–103). Buddhists differ about whether the goal of mindfulness should be non-judgmental acceptance or ethical discernment (Dreyfus, 2011, p. 51)—but either stance is an ethical one.

MBI training guides provide more details about the "foundational attitudes" that mindfulness teachers should cultivate. The CfM "Standards of Practice" guidelines list: "non-judging, patience, a beginner's mind, non-striving, acceptance or acknowledgement, and letting go or letting be" (Santorelli, 2014, p. 10). Such attitudes are, according to psychologist Steven Stanley, "related to core virtues found in early Buddhist texts, such as generosity, loving-kindness, empathetic joy and compassion" (2015, p. 99). Buddhist philosopher John Dunne explains that MBSR emphasizes the "letting go" of judgments of the good and bad or pleasant and unpleasant because such thoughts "seem especially relevant to oneself when they are highly charged or value-laden," and therefore "ensnare us all the more easily" in the attachments that cause suffering (2011, p. 8). As the Buddhist monk Bhikkhu Bodhi clarifies, stopping the causes of suffering requires recognizing humanity's "proclivity to certain unwholesome mental states called in Pali *kilesas*, usually translated 'defilements'" (1999). The foundational attitudes instilled by MBI teachers imply Buddhist-inflected value judgments about which states of mind are (un) wholesome.

Marketing materials for MBIs advertise ethical benefits. Indeed, part of the appeal of MBIs is that they appear to offer an inexpensive, secularized practice that instills the same moral and ethical virtues as religion. For example, Goldie Hawn's signature MindUP curriculum purportedly instills "empathy, compassion, patience, and generosity"—a list of virtues that Hawn derived from, but does not credit to, her training in Buddhist ethics (Hawn Foundation, 2011, pp. 11–12, 40–43, 57; Hawn, 2005, p. 436). The official MindUP website proclaims that the program enhances "empathy and kindness," "nurtures optimism and happiness" and "increases empathy and compassion" (The Hawn Foundation, 2016, para. 2, 4). Rebecca Calos, Director of Programs and Training for The Hawn Foundation, asserts that "awareness of the mind without judgment" helps children to become "more compassionate" and better able to express "kindness" to others—a conclusion that follows from Buddhist assumptions about the three poisons, four virtues, and interconnectedness of all beings (2012, para. 2, 4, 5). Although rooted in a Buddhist worldview, the program presents its virtues as "secular" and "universal"—an assumption interrogated below.

Transparency Compromised by Secular Framing

MBIs are commonly marketed as completely "secular" or, in sparse acknowledgement of Buddhist roots, as "secularized." It is rare, however, for program advocates to define the term "secular" or its presumed opposite, "religion," or to explain what they have removed or changed to make mindfulness secular. Marketers may rely on simple speech acts: the program in question is secular because it is declared to be so. Alternatively, promoters may vaunt empirically demonstrated or scientifically validated effects, given a common assumption that practices are either secular/

scientific or religious/spiritual, but not both. In point of fact, practices can be both secular and religious simultaneously, and concepts of the secular, the religious, the spiritual, and the scientific have often intermingled and co-constituted one another (Asad, 2003; Calhoun, Juergensmeyer, & Van Antwerpen, 2011; Jakobsen & Pellegrini, 2008; Lopez, 2008; Taylor, 2007).

The common idea that mindfulness is secular because it is not religious implies a narrow, Protestant-biased understanding of religion as reducible to verbal proclamations of beliefs. By this reasoning, secularizing a practice consists simply of removing overt linguistic references to transcendent beliefs. For example, mindfulness-in-education leader Patricia Jennings uses a *Dictionary.com* definition of religion as a "set of beliefs." Since mindfulness does not "require any belief," she concludes that it is not "inherently religious" (2016, p. 176). "Religion" may, however, be envisioned more broadly as encompassing not only belief statements, but also practices perceived as connecting individuals or communities with transcendent realities, aspiring toward salvation from ultimate problems, or cultivating spiritual awareness and virtues (Durkheim, 1984, p. 131; Smith, 2004, pp. 179–196; Tweed, 2006, p. 73). A complementary way of describing religion is to identify "creeds" (explanations of the meaning of human life or nature of reality), "codes" (rules for moral and ethical behavior), "cultuses" (rituals or repeated actions that instill or reinforce creeds and codes), and "communities" (formal or informal groups that share creeds, codes, and cultuses)—all of which can be seen in the contemporary mindfulness movement (Albanese, 2013, pp. 2–9). This is important because many people assume that a practice is nonreligious if one participates with the intention of accruing secular, defined as this-worldly, benefits. This view fails to account for the various channels through which participating in religious practices can transform initially secular intentions.

Removal of superficial linguistic or visual markers of "religion" is not the same thing as secularization. Patricia Jennings is one of the first MBI movement leaders to articulate "recommendations for best practices to ensure secularity" in public schools. Jennings suggests that teachers are on safe ground as long as they avoid such obviously religious markers as "using a bell from a religious tradition (such as a Tibetan bowl or cymbals used in Tibetan Buddhist rituals," "introducing names, words, or sounds that come from a religious or spiritual tradition … as a focus of attention," "use of *Sanskrit* names and identifying areas of the body associated with spiritual and religious significance (e.g., *chakras*)," or verbal cues that loving-kindness recitations transmit "any sort of spiritual or metaphysical energy" (2016, pp. 176–77). Removing such religious symbols (all of which are common in public-school mindfulness instruction) makes it more difficult for the casual observer to perceive religious associations. Jennings is explicitly not suggesting that "one should conceal the fact that such associations between practices and religious and spiritual traditions exist," but her recommendations do not probe the substantive difficulties of extricating mindfulness from Buddhist ethical foundations (p. 177).

Offering MBIs in secular settings heightens the importance of transparency about live associations of mindfulness with Buddhist ethics. This is because the risks of unforeseen ethical violations may be greater when mindfulness is taught in explicitly secular as opposed to Buddhist contexts. People may reasonably assume that programs offered in settings commonly recognized as secular—such as government-supported schools or hospitals—are themselves secular, or else the programs would not be there. When religious experts teach in the context of religious institutions, people expect instruction in how to perform religious rituals. When those in positions of social or legal power and authority—for instance, public-school teachers, doctors, psychological therapists, prison volunteers, or employers—offer explicitly secular services, individuals may have difficulty recognizing when health-promoting techniques bleed into religious cultivation (Cohen, 2006, pp. 114–135). Similarly, patients may assume that fee-based services offered by psychologists, doctors, nurses, or other professional therapists, as opposed to chaplains, are "medical" rather than "religious." Whereas consumers expect religious groups to offer free religious services as a strategy to recruit adherents, consumers expect to pay for nonreligious commodities necessary to their health. Consumers tend, moreover, to associate higher prices with higher-value goods and services. If medical insurance or school administrators cover costs, this enhances perceived medical/educational legitimacy.

Scientific Claims Imply Secularity

Assertions that MBIs are secular because scientifically validated warrant special care. This is because "science" conveys legitimating power in modern Western cultures. There is a long history of perceived conflict between "science" and "religion" in cultures influenced by the enlightenment, evolutionary biology, and scientific naturalism, and this history predisposes people to presume that scientifically validated practices are nonreligious (Lopez, 2008). Blurring this presumed binary, scientific research confirms that many religious and spiritual practices produce physical and mental health benefits (Aldwin, Park, Jeong, & Nath, 2014; Koenig, King & Carson, 2012).

Scientific publications reporting empirical benefits lend credibility to claims that mindfulness is secular. This creates an ethical responsibility to be honest about the strengths and weaknesses of the scientific evidence. Neuroscience researchers who are themselves sympathetic to mindfulness express caution about the inflated claims commonly made about the science supporting mindfulness (Britton, 2016; Kerr, 2014). As Dodson-Lavelle acknowledges:

> Existing data on the efficacy of mindfulness and compassion interventions in general are, frankly, not very strong. As a number of researchers have pointed out, studies of MBSR and related programs suffer from numerous methodological issues, including inconsistencies regarding the operationalization of 'mindfulness,' small sample sizes, a lack of active control groups, evidence that these programs are more effective than controls (when comparisons can be made), deficient use of valid measure and tools for assessment, and often little to no assessment of teacher competence or fidelity. (2015, p. 19)

One difficulty is that "there is no consensus on what the defining characteristics of a 'mindfulness practice' even *are* for *any* population" (Felver & Jennings, 2016, p. 3). Another issue is study quality. A systematic review of 18,753 citations excluded all but 47 trials with 3,515 participants, since others lacked the active control groups needed to rule out potential confounds. The meta-analysis concluded that mindfulness meditation programs show moderate evidence of improved anxiety and pain, but low evidence of improved stress/distress and mental health related quality of life. They also found insufficient evidence of any effect of meditation programs on positive mood, attention, substance use, eating habits, sleep, and weight. They found no evidence that meditation programs were better than any active treatment such as medication, exercise, or other behavioral therapies (Goyal et al., 2014). Some studies have even shown that while mindfulness participants self-report decreased stress, biological markers such as cortisol levels actually indicate increased stress (Creswell, Pacilio, Lindsay, & Brown, 2014; Schonert-Reichl et al., 2015). It is ethically problematic to make scientific claims about mindfulness that exceed the evidence, especially given the power of such claims to convince potential participants and sponsors that mindfulness is a fully secular intervention.

Intentional Lack of Transparency

Despite claiming to teach a completely secular technique, some of the leading MBI promoters envision secular mindfulness as propagating Buddhist ethics. The French Jesuit scholar Michel de Certeau draws an insightful distinction between "strategies" employed by those with access to institutional sources of power and "tactics" used by those on the margins (de Certeau, 1984, pp. xi–xxiv; Woodhead, 2014, p. 15). Until recently, most MBI leaders lacked institutional space to act strategically; instead, they developed tactics to introduce Buddhist ethical teachings covertly—through a process described by anthropologists Nurit Zaidman and colleagues as "camouflage," or carefully timed "concealing and gradual exposure" (Zaidman, Goldstein-Gidoni, & Nehemya, 2009, pp. 599, 616). Exhibiting what scholars call "code-switching" or "frontstage/backstage" behavior, these leaders describe their activities in one way for non-Buddhist audiences and in a very different way for Buddhist co-religionists (Gardner-Chloros, 2009; Goffman, 1959; Laird & Barnes, 2014, pp. 12, 19). For the latter, they refute charges of critics Ronald Purser and David Loy that MBIs reduce a transformative Buddhist ethical system to mere "McMindfulness" (Purser & Loy, 2013); Kabat-Zinn rebuts that MBIs promote the entire *Buddhadharma* (Kabat-Zinn, 2015, para. 6). When speaking to non-Buddhists, the tactics employed by MBI leaders include "disguise," "script," "Trojan horse," "stealth Buddhism," and "skillful means"—all terms used by MBI promoters themselves.

Instances of these tactics have been detailed elsewhere (Brown, 2016), but may be illustrated as follows. Daniel Goleman boasting of his efforts to code mindfulness as secular psychotherapy said that "the Dharma is so disguised that it could never be proven in court" (1985, p. 7). Actress and movie producer Goldie Hawn attests that she got Buddhist meditation "into the classroom under a different name" by writing a "script" that replaces the terms "Buddhism" and "meditation" with the euphemisms "neuroscience" and "Core Practice" (2013). Silicon Valley meditation teacher Kenneth Folk self-consciously employs "The Trojan Horse of Meditation" as a "stealth move" to "sneak" Buddhist "value systems" of "compassion and empathy" into profit-driven corporations (2013, para. 13–18). Kabat-Zinn disciple Trudy Goodman describes her approach as "Stealth Buddhism." Goodman's "secular" mindfulness classes, taught in "hospitals, and universities, and schools," admittedly "aren't that different from our Buddhist classes. They just use a different vocabulary." Goodman considers it "inevitable" that "anyone who practices sincerely, *whether they want it or not*" will shed the "fundamental illusion that we carry, about the 'I' as being permanent and existing in a real way" (2014, emphasis added). Kabat-Zinn describes MBSR as "skillful means for bringing the dharma into mainstream settings. It has never been about MBSR for its own sake" (2011, p. 281). Rather, MBSR and MBCT represent "secular Dharma-based portals" opening to those who would be deterred by a "more traditional Buddhist framework or vocabulary" (Williams & Kabat-Zinn, 2011, p. 12). Psychotherapist and religious studies scholar Ira Helderman observes that clinicians develop a variety of "innovative methods for maneuvering" between "religion" and "secular science or medicine." Some, like Kabat-Zinn, "incorporate actual Buddhist practices but *translate* them into items acceptable within scientific biomedical spheres" (2016, p. 942, emphasis original). Helderman asks of the translators: "Has the religious really been expunged or is it just in hiding?" (p. 952). He notes that these same "mindfulness practitioners also unveil and market the true Buddhist religious derivation of their modalities when public interest in Asian healing practices suggest that doing so would increase access to the healing marketplace rather than prevent it" (p. 950). Such practitioners envision mindfulness as one thing, namely Buddhism, but present it as something else, a (mostly) secular therapeutic technique—on the premise that mindfulness, however described, is inherently transformative.

Unintentional Lack of Transparency

It seems likely that most MBI advocates lack any intention to deceive. They are themselves convinced that mindfulness is fully secular and universal because its foundational assumptions and values seem to them self-evidently true and good; they themselves have experienced benefits from mindfulness, and scientific research seems to confirm this-worldly benefits. They may nevertheless unintentionally communicate more than a religiously neutral technique. This is because suppositions about the nature of reality can become so naturalized and believed so thoroughly that it is easy to infer that they are simply true and universal, rather than recognizing ideas as culturally conditioned and potentially conflicting with other worldviews.

Being convinced of the benefits of mindfulness can lead to an inadvertent conflation of Buddhist with universal ideals. For instance, describing the Eightfold Path as a "universal and causal law of nature, not unlike that of gravity" is, as Buddhist scholar Ronald Purser explains, "a faulty analogy … a category error," since Buddhist ideals, unlike natural laws, are "cultural artifacts" that reflect particular cultural norms (2015, p. 27). Mindfulness may seem merely to require "waking up" to "see things as they are." But this reflects the "myth of the given," that reality can be objectively presented and directly perceived (Forbes, 2015). Meditative experiences always require interpretations of their meaning, and interpretations are framed by worldviews. Although claiming to cultivate general human capacities and to promote universally shared values, MBIs offer culturally and religiously specific diagnoses and prescriptions for what is wrong with the world.

For example, the goal of attenuating desire and cultivating equanimity reflects a culturally specific ideal affect that values "low-arousal emotions like calm" (Lindahl, 2015b, p. 58). Believing that one has an unclouded view of reality can gloss hidden cultural constructs and the favoring of one set of lenses with which to view and interpret reality over another. This reasoning can justify upholding one culturally particular worldview as superior to others. This is not only a culturally arrogant position; it is precisely a *religious* attitude—a claim to special insight into the cause and solution for the ultimate problems that plague humanity.

Internal Grounds for Transparency

The benefits conveyed by mindfulness may seem to justify any intentional or unintentional lapses in transparency. For the sake of argument, assume for a moment that: (1) mindfulness alleviates suffering, (2) scientific research validates benefits, (3) MBIs can only continue in secular settings if mindfulness is presented as secular, (4) people are being deprived of the benefits of mindfulness because of biases against Buddhism or religion, and (5) individuals who would never knowingly visit a Buddhist center can gain an introduction to mindfulness and Buddhist ethics through MBIs, leading them to adopt a more accurate worldview, suffer less, behave more ethically, and come to be grateful for any unexpected religious transformations. By this train of reasoning, the benefits achieved through MBIs confirm that explicit communication of Buddhist ethics is inessential—and perhaps an undesirable obstacle to continuing and increasing cultural acceptance. Arguably, if people benefit from mindfulness, it does not matter whether they associate it with Buddhism or can articulate its ethical foundations.

This chapter takes the position that process matters. Confidence in the worth of mindfulness can create an ethical blind spot to implications of the processes through which mindfulness has been mainstreamed. Unethical processes may taint results, potentially resulting in more harm than good. The ethical grounds for transparency can be articulated within frameworks internal or external to Buddhism. The Noble Eightfold Path, specifically the aspects of right mindfulness, right intention, and right speech, is relevant precisely because MBIs are an outgrowth of Buddhist ethics (reflecting multiple, sometimes competing Buddhist schools). The goal here is not a comprehensive discussion, a task undertaken by those more qualified to do so in this volume and elsewhere, but more modestly to note Buddhist arguments for transparency.

Right Mindfulness

The term "mindfulness" is shorthand for a Buddhist value on "right mindfulness," *sammā sati*. Buddhist texts contrast right mindfulness with "wrong mindfulness," *micchā sati*. Buddhist advocates of transparency worry that mindfulness taught "only as meditative skills or strategies" without "an understanding of ethical action" results in wrong mindfulness, which can exacerbate suffering (Monteiro, Musten, & Compson, 2015, pp. 3, 6). Right mindfulness, in this view, must be "guided by intentions and motivations based on self-restraint, wholesome mental states, and ethical behaviors" (Purser & Loy, 2013, para. 9). Secularly framed MBIs, by contrast, are "refashioned into a banal, therapeutic, self-help technique" that can "reinforce" the "unwholesome roots of greed, ill will, and delusion." This amounts to a "Faustian bargain"—selling the very soul of mindfulness to enhance its cultural palatability (Purser & Loy, 2013, para. 6).

Right Intention

An argument for transparency can similarly be based on Buddhist understandings of "right intention," *sammā sankappa*. Meditation teacher Joseph Naft explains that "Right Intention depends on our understanding of the path and its practices and on our ability to actually do those practices" (2010, para. 2). Buddhist monk William Van Gordon and psychologist Mark Griffiths (2015) argue pointedly that "a central theme of Buddhist training is that individuals should approach Buddhist teachings with the 'right intention' (i.e. to develop spiritually) and of their own accord"—in contrast to "Kabat-Zinn's approach of thrusting (what he deems to be) Buddhism into the mainstream and teaching it to the unsuspecting masses (i.e. without their 'informed consent.')" (2015, para. 6). By this reasoning, Kabat-Zinn has an "ethical obligation" to make his agenda of mainstreaming *Buddhadharma* through MBSR "abundantly clear to participants" (para. 3). A central concern here is that mindfulness practice developed as a means to make progress along the Noble Eightfold Path. One cannot practice mindfulness with right intention if one does not understand what it can, and by original design should, facilitate.

Right Speech

Those arguing against transparency often frame MBIs as an epitome of skillful speech. For example, one commentator in an online discussion of Goldie Hawn's concealment of the Buddhist origins of mindfulness concludes that she is "trying to reach a bigger audience using skillful [sic] speech. Very Buddhist IMO [in my opinion]" (Tosh, 2012, para. 2). This position alludes to classical Buddhist texts that justify deception when employed to alleviate suffering. By contrast, the historian Jeff Wilson argues that exceptions to this dictum have only applied to Buddhas and advanced Bodhisattvas who are free from self-interest (Wilson, 2014, p. 90); proprietary, trademarked MBIs appear, by contrast, to be invested in the self-interested, commercial, therapeutic market. Sharpening the critique, Dodson-Lavelle calls attention to a Mindfulness in Education Network e-mail listserv on which "regular postings appear that either blatantly or suggestively describe ways in which program developers and implementers have 'masked' or 'hidden' the Buddhist roots of their mindfulness-Based education programs." Dodson-Lavelle elaborates that "the sense is that one needs to employ a secular rhetoric to gain access into educational institutions, and once one's 'foot is in the door,' so to speak, one is then free to teach whatever Buddhist teachings they deem appropriate" (2015, p. 132). The problem, then, is less that MBIs remove Buddhist terminology to make them accessible to broader audiences, but that the adoption of secular rhetoric is disingenuous and incomplete—Buddhist teachings *are* introduced in actual classes, despite secular curricular framing.

Certain MBI promoters have responded to religious controversy by revising their internet presence to obscure Buddhist associations, rather than opting to become more transparent about Buddhist sources and explain what exactly has been done to secularize programming. For example, in 2015, a school board member and parent in Cape Cod, Massachusetts called attention to institutional connections between Calmer Choice (Cultivating Awareness Living Mindfully Enhancing Resilience) and MBSR and Jon Kabat-Zinn, and cited statements by Kabat-Zinn linking MBSR with Buddhism. Prior to the controversy, Calmer Choice directors advertised the program as a "Mindfulness-Based Stress Reduction (MBSR) Program" that was "informed by the work of renowned Dr. Jon Kabat-Zinn" on its IRS Form 990-EZ (Calmer Choice, 2012, p. 2), Calmer Choice's official website (Calmer Choice, 2015d, para. 5, 2015e, para. 5); Facebook (2011a), Twitter (@mindful_youth, 2013), LinkedIn (Jensen, 2015), Disqus (@fionajensen, 2014), GuideStar (Calmer Choice, 2011b), and in interviews of Founder and Executive Director Fiona Jensen (Jensen, 2010, pp. 3, 10, 2013, p. 9). The formal prerequisites for Calmer Choice Instructor Training (as articulated by Director of School and Community-Based Programming Katie Medlar and Program Director Adria Kennedy, and taught at least as recently as the 2013–2014 school year) include "daily practice of formal and informal mindfulness" and "an 8-week Mindfulness-Based Stress Reduction Training course"; suggested readings include Kabat-Zinn's *Wherever You Go* and *Full Catastrophe Living* (Calmer Choice, 2015b, para. 7, 9, 2015c, sect. 3 para. 10).

The Calmer Choice website lists Jon Kabat-Zinn as an "Honorary Board" of Directors member (Calmer Choice, 2015a, para. 12).

In 2016, Calmer Choice responded to a legal memorandum (Broyles, 2016) by backing away from their previous efforts to market the program through emphasizing its associations with the better-known MBSR program and its "renowned" founder, Kabat-Zinn. In the thick of public controversy, Jensen insisted in a newspaper interview: "We don't teach MBSR, and our instructors aren't trained in MBSR" (Jensen in Legere, 2016a, Feb. 4, para. 14). In a subsequent interview (after the complaining school board member charged Calmer Choice with "scrubbing" its internet presence), Calmer Choice Board of Directors Chair David Troutman asserted that mentions of MBSR on the Calmer Choice website had been removed because "Calmer Choice does not teach MBSR" and the references had been "inadvertently added by volunteers"—although top administrators Jensen, Medlar, and Kennedy signed several of the internet documents making claims about MBSR and Kabat-Zinn (Troutman, in Legere, 2016b, Feb. 9, para. 7). It is unclear how much Calmer Choice has substantively changed their teacher training program, curriculum, or classroom practices. Rewriting promotional materials to obscure Buddhist associations and silence critics is not equivalent to secularization or honest speech.

There are Buddhist traditions that emphasize that skillful, or right, speech (*sammā vācā*) is honest and non-divisive. Influential Buddhist monk Bhante Gunaratana advises that skillful speech should always be truthful: if even silence may deceive, one must speak the whole truth, a consideration that supports full, as opposed to selective, disclosure of all that mindfulness entails (2001, p. 93). Meditation teacher Allan Lokos explains that "the pillar of skillful speech is to speak honestly, which means that we should even avoid telling little white lies. We need to be aware of dishonesty in the forms of exaggerating, minimizing, and self-aggrandizing. These forms of unskillful speech often arise from a fear that what we are is not good enough—and that is never true" (2008, para. 3). Although addressing individuals, Lokos's admonition may suggest a reason for the MBI movement to be more self-confident in forthrightly acknowledging what it actually is—without, for instance, exaggerating scientific evidence or minimizing Buddhist ethical foundations.

External Grounds for Transparency

Although non-Buddhists may be uninterested in Buddhist arguments for transparency, there are external grounds upon which there may be broader agreement: namely intellectual integrity, cultural diversity, and informed consent. It would be misleading to describe these principles as purely "secular," "universal," or as "Natural Laws," since, like Buddhist ideals, they have particular cultural histories. Nevertheless, as ideals that have relatively broad traction in many Western cultures, they can productively prompt reflection on the stakes of transparency.

Intellectual Integrity

The first of these principles, intellectual integrity, can be explained relatively briefly, using an analogy to plagiarism. The basic point is that one has an ethical, even if not a legal, obligation to acknowledge one's sources as a matter of honesty and respect for the authors' intellectual property rights. Some may counter that Buddhists "do not have a proprietary claim on mindfulness," but, as Lynette Monteiro, R. F. Musten, and Jane Compson express, "that begs the question of what model then underpins and guides the process of the MBIs" (2015, p. 12). Many Westerners consider "attribution" to be a "moral obligation." Thus, academic and professional institutions in the USA and Europe develop policies which stipulate that "one is permitted to copy another's words or ideas if and only if he attributes them to their original author" (Green, 2002, pp. 171, 175). Analogies may also be drawn to: (1) "theft law," which "prohibits the misappropriation of 'anything of value,'" including "intangible property" if it is "commodifiable" or "capable of being bought or sold"; (2) the "misappropriation doctrine" in "unfair competition" law, namely that "a commercial rival should not be allowed to profit unfairly from the costly investment and labor of one who produces information"; and (3) the legal doctrine of "moral rights," which includes (a) the "right of integrity," which "prevents others from destroying or altering an artist's work without the artist's permission," (b) the "right of disclosure," which "allows the artist the right to decide when a given work is completed and when, if ever, it will be displayed, performed, or published," and (c) the "right of attribution," which is "both positive and negative. An author or artist has the right both to be identified as the author of any work that she has created and to prevent the use of her name as the author of a work she did not create." Each of these analogies suggests that an originator of an idea is entitled to receive "credit" for that idea—in its entirety, without distorting modifications, and without the originator's reputation being used to legitimize the copy—especially when money is at stake (pp. 172, 204, 206, 219). MBIs may be faulted for taking, without adequate attribution, ideas developed by Asian Buddhists, modifying these ideas in ways that may be objectionable to some of their originators, and profiting financially (possibly at the expense of explicitly Buddhist market alternatives) through trademarked programs presented as innovations that embody the "essence" of ancient spiritual wisdom distilled into a modern, secular science.

Cultural Diversity

Mindfulness is often presented as a "values-neutral therapy" that will not conflict with the beliefs of those from any or no religious tradition. According to Buddhist mindfulness teacher Lynette Monteiro, this position is a "fallacy" (2015, p. 1). As a practicing therapist, Monteiro recognizes that "regardless of the intention to not impose extraneous values," therapists, as well as clients, inevitably bring implicit values to the therapeutic relationship (p. 4). MBIs are both "rooted in a spiritual tradition," specifically "Buddhism," and even when formulated as secularized interventions, remain "spiritually oriented and therefore imbued with values." Buddhist values, which cannot be assumed to be "universal," are "ever-present and exert a subtle influence on actions, speech and thoughts" (pp. 1, 2). Buddhist ethics are "contained, explicitly or implicitly, in the content of a mindfulness program" and also "modelled or embodied in the person of the MBI teacher." The "very act of teaching a philosophy derived from an Eastern spiritually oriented practice" risks conflict with the "individual values and faith traditions" of clients (pp. 3, 4). This may be problematic from a Buddhist perspective; Zen teacher Barbara O'Brien observes that right speech entails taking care not to "speak in a way that causes disharmony or enmity" (2016, para. 7). Mindfulness researcher Doug Oman raises a related concern that "dominant approaches to mindfulness" risk "unmindfulness of spiritual diversity" (2015, p. 36). Oman notes that "many MBSR instructors and writings reflect a Buddhist orientation" and that "middle-term and long-term" effects of participating in MBSR seem to include joining Buddhist organizations. Oman questions whether "breath-focused mindfulness meditation that emphasizes sensory awareness is truly belief neutral" given that "for many Christians, it is not breath meditation" but "meditation upon Scripture" that is valued (2012, p. 4, 2015, pp. 51–52). Oman thus identifies an "emerging compassion-related challenge: respecting cultural and religious diversity" (2015, p. 52). As Monteiro sees the challenge, demonstrating "actual respect for the client's values and ethics" lies not in silence about Buddhist ethics, but rather in transparent communication (2015, p. 5). Transparency offers clients an opportunity to evaluate how their own values match those of the therapist and, if they do not match, whether they want to adopt practices premised upon another religious or cultural system.

The diverse experiences of MBI participants falsify the alleged universality of MBI-promoted values. In Dodson-Lavelle's teaching experience, the universalist notion that "all beings want to be happy and avoid suffering" has "failed to resonate" with many participants (2015, pp. 17, 96–99, 162). Failure to recognize that MBIs reflect a "very Buddhist way of conceiving of suffering" tends to "flatten the experience of suffering," and it "delegitimizes participants' experiences by universalizing the experience of suffering and its causes" (pp. 160–61). Mindfulness teachers should not expect all clients to share a Buddhist perspective. Less than 1% of the US population identifies as Buddhist, compared with 71% Christian (Pew Research Center, 2015). Although there are other indications that some Americans of other or no religious affiliation (23% of adults) have adopted certain Buddhist-inspired beliefs and values, the compatibility of Buddhist and client views cannot be safely assumed.

Compassion Contested

One of the most commonly advertised benefits of mindfulness is that it makes people more compassionate. Implicitly, compassion is a universal, and therefore secular, value (Dodson-Lavelle, 2015, p. 168; Ozawa-de Silva, 2015, p. 1). On its face, denying that one values compassion would sound perverse. Assuming the goodness and universality of compassion obscures the cultural and religious specificity of: (1) how compassion is defined in Buddhist traditions, (2) the logic that connects mindfulness with compassion, and (3) conflicting understandings of compassion. To simplify, in Buddhism compassion (*karuna*) stems from the idea that life is suffering, and humans should want to alleviate that suffering. Mindfulness cultivates compassion by offering insight into reality, including the causes of suffering, the path to its relief, and the interconnectedness of all beings; thus, understanding one's own suffering makes one more aware of the suffering of others and, reciprocally, wanting others to be free from suffering relieves one's own suffering (Dodson-Lavelle, 2015).

Although many Buddhists and Christians agree in identifying "compassion" as a core value, the two perspectives define the term so differently that it is misleading to identify it as a "universal value." Buddhists and Christians begin with fundamentally different assumptions about the nature of life (suffering vs. good), what is wrong with the world (any attachment vs. only those attachments that lead to disobedience to God's laws), the quality of existence (impermanent vs. eternal), the nature of the self (no-self vs. uniquely created in God's image for enduring relationship with God), and the source of compassion (waking up to understand that everyone shares the same Buddha nature so that compassion for others relieves everyone's suffering including one's own vs. God's sacrificial love demonstrated by Jesus's willingness to embrace suffering and death, which inspires Christians to repent of disobedience to God, turn to Jesus for salvation, and sacrifice their own needs for other ontologically distinct "selves"). The key point here is that it is simplistic and distorting to assert that compassion is a universal value.

Professional Ethical Standards

Anyone motivated by compassion to alleviate the suffering of others might be well advised to respect others' freedom to choose their own cultural, religious, and spiritual resources. Even the Dalai Lama has recognized that "if you bring in Buddhist teachings in a context where the person has no Buddhist leanings, it raises sensitive issues of religion and spirituality" because "you are trying to change someone's basic outlook on life" (Dalai Lama in Kabat-Zinn & Davidson, 2011, p. 120). Professionals whose responsibilities include therapeutic relationships with patients or clients have more formal ethical duties. Doug Oman warns that many MBI teachers have failed to meet their "professional obligations to recognize, respect, and seek competency in addressing religious diversity," including "proactive respect for diverse traditions" (2012, p. 4). Oman notes that "the ethical codes of most human service professions require respect for religious diversity as one form of respect for cultural diversity" (2015, p. 52). For example, the Joint Commission on Accreditation of Healthcare Organizations, which oversees the accreditation of 19,000 US health care organizations, since 2004 has required health care teams to perform spiritual assessments that determine "the *patient's* denomination, beliefs, and what spiritual practices are important to the *patient*"—not the care provider (Warnock, 2009, p. 469, emphasis added). The Joint Commission standard for hospitals is that "the hospital respects, protects and promotes patient rights," including the patient's "cultural and personal values," and "accommodates the patient's right to religious and other spiritual services" (2016, sect. RI.0.01.01. EP6,9). The *Code of Ethics for Nurses with Interpretive Statements* (2001) specifies that "an individual's lifestyle, value system, and religious beliefs should be considered in planning healthcare with and for each patient" (Warnock, 2009, p. 476). Nurse Carla Warnock argues that health care providers should at a minimum "respect and value each individual as a whole, including their culture and any religion or faith they may practice," and urges that the principles of "informed consent" be followed in implementing any "spiritual interventions" (2009, 477).

Cassandra Vieten and Shelley Scammell delineate guidelines for psychotherapists and mental health professionals in a handbook on *Spiritual & Religious Competencies in Clinical Practice*. First in the list of 16 competencies identified is that "psychologists demonstrate empathy, respect, and appreciation for clients from diverse spiritual, religious, or secular backgrounds and affiliations." Additionally, "psychologists are aware of how their own spiritual or religious background and beliefs may influence their clinical practice and their attitudes, perceptions, and assumptions about the nature of psychological processes" (2015, p. xi.). Vieten and Scammell explain that "people typically aren't aware of their own biases," yet "we each hold implicit biases that have been conditioned by our upbringing, region, class, and culture and by the media" (p. 23). They analogize that "worldviews function like sunglasses. They filter our perceptions" (p. 37). The therapist may perceive "a 'truth' about life that's a given" whereas the "client holds a completely different truth" (p. 38). The American Psychological Association's *Ethical Principles for Psychologists and Code of Conduct* states that "psychologists are aware of and respect cultural, individual, and role differences, including those based on age, gender, gender identity, race, ethnicity, culture, national origin, religion, sexual orientation, disability, language, and socioeconomic status" (2010, p. 4). Based on these principles, Vieten and Scammell conclude that "it's unethical to force, recommend, or even encourage religious or spiritual practices in a hospital, clinic, or health care setting" (p. 116). Any "proselytizing or presenting your own spiritual or religious worldview in the context of therapy, even when done with the best of intentions, is never appropriate" (p. 117). It is important, moreover, to "become aware of your biases and know that you may also have implicit conditioning that you aren't aware of in relation to religious or spiritual issues" (p. 131). Therapists have an affirmative responsibility, then, to make intentional efforts to recognize their own biases and to actively respect the potentially divergent perspectives of their clients.

It is therefore ironic that this same handbook promotes mindfulness meditation for therapists and their clients, apparently taking its universality as a given. Vieten and Scammell assert that "mindful awareness … allows us to see things as they actually are more clearly." The text advises its readers: "Right now, take ten full breaths while keeping your attention on your breathing. Actually stop reading and try it" (p. 127). The authors continue: "We highly recommend that you engage in some sort of mindfulness training … cultivating a mindful stance as a therapist will increase your ability to conduct effective therapy with all of your clients, including those with diverse religious and spiritual backgrounds and beliefs" (p. 129). The authors admit, moreover, that "some of the books we most often recommend" to clients include "Rick Hanson and Richard Mendius's *Buddha's Brain* (2009)," an explicitly Buddhist guide to mindfulness meditation (p. 152). Vieten and Scammell's promotion of mindfulness exemplifies the ethical blind spot created by confidence in its benefits. The authors assume that mindfulness, by contrast to other religious and spiritual perspectives or practices, offers an unobstructed window onto reality that is universally helpful in any therapeutic situation.

Cultural Appropriation and Cultural Imperialism

The MBI movement risks inadvertent cultural appropriation and cultural imperialism: in extracting, and potentially distorting, cultural resources from a socially less privileged group of cultural "others" and imposing those resources on still less privileged "others," for the primary benefit of the socially dominant group (King, 1999, p. 2; Purser, 2015, p. 24). Middle to upper class European Americans have played a primary role in adapting and marketing mindfulness, using financial and social capital to develop, fund, administer, and teach MBIs. In advertising mindfulness as secular and universal, MBI leaders often claim to extricate the mindfulness technique from the so-called "cultural baggage" of Asian Buddhism (Williams & Kabat-Zinn, 2011, p. 14). The adoption of secular rhetoric to make mindfulness acceptable in the public square is "capable of violence," and can be a "deliberate imposition," an "agent of socialization for a competing worldview," and an "aspect of colonizing assimilation" (Delaney, Miller, & Bisono, 2007; Dueck & Reimer, 2009, p. 220; Stratton, 2015, p. 103; Walsh & Shapiro, 2006, p. 228). Universalist rhetoric privileges the perspectives of mindfulness promoters, many of whom are white and economically privileged, as "objective and representative of reality," "standing outside of culture, and as the universal model of humans" (DiAngelo, 2011, p. 59; Ng & Purser, 2015, para. 4). Film studies theorist Richard Dyer defines hegemony as the "expression of the interests and world-views of a particular social group or class so expressed as to pass for the interest and world-view of the whole of society" (1993, pp. 93–94). In the case of MBIs, the interests and worldviews of socially privileged European American Buddhists hegemonically pass for universal truths and values needed by all of society.

There are two dangers here: the first involves the relationship between the MBI movement and Asian Buddhists. Religious studies scholar Jane Iwamura argues that socially powerful groups often achieve "hegemonic strength through channels that appear benign on their surface" (2011, pp. 7, 115). Positive orientalist stereotypes, for instance of Asians as possessing more wisdom and spiritual insight, can most easily "go unchallenged and unseen" (p. 5). Making matters worse, "the particular way in which Americans write themselves into the story is not a benign, nonideological act; rather, it constructs a modernized cultural patriarchy in which Anglo-

Americans reimagine themselves as the protectors, innovators, and guardians of Asian religions and culture and wrest the authority to define these traditions from others" (p. 21). Lauding the wisdom of Asian Buddhists for developing mindfulness, yet insisting that Asian Buddhists lack proprietary rights, has the effect of licensing appropriation and redefinition to serve the interests of MBI leaders.

The second danger involves the relationship between the MBI movement and those denoted as its special beneficiaries. Iwamura uses the term "Virtual Orientalism" to describe American interactions with Asian cultures that involve racialization and cultural stereotyping, or the blunting of distinctions among individuals (Iwamura, 2011, pp. 6–7). Iwamura's analysis may be extended to interpret mindfulness programs targeted at nonwhite populations as participating in dual racialization and cultural stereotyping of both Asian Buddhists and American people of color, and as implying a cultural evolution narrative. MBI leaders often vaunt their benevolence in bestowing the benefits of mindfulness on people of color and lower social class. For example, CfM director Saki Santorelli boasts that:

> We embedded an MBSR Clinic into a large community health center caring for under-served, underrepresented populations in Worcester, Massachusetts, providing access via free childcare and transportation. Participants included African Americans; Latinos from central, south, and Caribbean-rim countries; and native and immigrant Caucasians, all with income levels below the national poverty line. We have taught mindfulness to prison inmates and correctional staff in prisons across Massachusetts. Mindfulness is being taught to diverse populations of school-age children in the cities of Oakland, Baltimore, New York, Minneapolis, and Los Angeles—to name a few. (2016, p. 2)

Implicitly, MBIs can carry a hefty financial price tag. An 8-week MBSR class taught at CfM headquarters runs between $545 for someone with a household income below $40,000 up to $725 if one's household income reaches $50,000 (CfM, 2014b, para. 3). Offering free or reduced-priced access to mindfulness training thus extends opportunities to those who are otherwise disenfranchised.

Financial accessibility is, however, only one factor, or there would be no need to note the racial and ethnic composition of the groups served. Such references may suggest that people of color or recent immigrant status are more in need of mindfulness because they are naturally less able to self-regulate. In support of this interpretation, mindfulness-in-schools programs are disproportionately targeted toward "inner-city schools" with large populations of African-American and Latino children. Promotional videos typically feature such schools as being transformed by mindfulness into oases of non-stressful academic achievement, kindness, and optimism. For example, the film *Room to Breathe* portrays a white woman, Mindful Schools Executive Director of Programs Megan Cowan, teaching mindfulness to African-American and Latino children in a San Francisco public middle school after overcoming the so-called "defiance" of students who failed to share Cowan's academic and social goals (Long, 2012). Implicitly, disadvantaged children have caused their own problems, and it is their responsibility to muster interior resources to become successful neoliberal subjects in an educational and social environment structured by racism and poverty (Ng & Purser, 2015, para. 8; Reveley, 2016, p. 497). As American Studies scholar, education policy analyst, and mindfulness advocate Funie Hsu has argued, students may receive the message that they alone, rather than systemic social injustices, are to blame for their suffering. Hsu finds it particularly worrisome that mindful school programs target low-income "students of color, especially black and brown boys" in a manner that "mystifies the structure of social oppression" and perpetuates "racial disciplining based on negative stereotypes" (Hsu, 2014, sect. 4, para. 7–9). Such a perspective condescends to racial and ethnic others as having unenlightened cultural practices. Mindfulness missionaries might be criticized for failing to respect the students' own cultural and religious strategies for confronting systemic injustices, instead imposing a white authority figure's preferred contemplative tradition in order to promote her goals of study and competitive individualism, regardless of the students' own goals or priorities. Yet many of those targeted by MBIs already have deeply cherished religious traditions and spiritual resources that they consider efficacious in coping with life's challenges. Indeed, African-American and Latino communities are statistically more religiously active—and predominantly Christian—than the non-Hispanic, white American populations who generally administer MBI programs (Kosmin & Keysar, 2009).

The language used to frame mindfulness-in-schools programs suggests reformer anxiety to protect society—and the reformers' own children—from the consequences of "un-mindful" misbehavior. For instance, clinical psychologist Patricia Broderick's *Learning to Breathe* mindfulness curriculum is marketed as an antidote to "disruptive behavior in the classroom, poor academic performance, [and] out-of-control emotions" that might provoke "acting out by taking drugs, displaying violent behavior or acting in by becoming more depressed" (2013, para. 1, 3). A clinical study linked from the Mindful Schools website collected self-report survey data from Baltimore City "low-income, minority" public-middle-school students, "99.7% African-American, and 99% eligible for free lunch"; the study purports to show the utility of mindfulness in reducing "trauma-associated symptoms among vulnerable urban middle school students" (Mindful Schools, 2016, note 29; Sibinga, Webb, Ghazarian, & Ellen, 2016, p. 1). Implicit in such curricula and study designs is an obliquely racial narrative, in which students of color are more "vulnerable" to losing control, and a tangentially religious narrative in which Christianity has failed America's children—the nation's future. "Secularized" Buddhism offers hope for salvation as mindfulness rescues children, especially minority children who are portrayed as threats to themselves and to those around them, and thus rescues America's future through the "bridge figure of the child" (Iwamura, 2011, 20).

Informed Consent

The term "informed consent" has its origins in health care tort law. It was coined in 1957 in the medical malpractice case of *Salgo v. Leland Stanford Jr. University*; the patient awoke from a medical procedure paralyzed, having consented to the procedure without being informed that paralysis was a known, though rare, risk (Faden & Beauchamp, 1986, p. 125). The World Medical Association *Declaration of Lisbon on the Rights of the Patient* affirms that patients have the "right to give or withhold consent to any diagnostic procedure or therapy—even if refusing treatment is life-threatening (World Medical Association, 1981/2015, p. 2). The principle of informed consent is broadly applicable not only to health care but also to other situations in which a person's rights of personal autonomy and self-determination are at stake. The basic idea is that service-providers have an affirmative ethical obligation to give clients access to full and accurate information needed to make the decisions they want to make. Providers should facilitate the process by which individuals are empowered to base decisions on their own "personal values, desires, and beliefs, to act with substantial autonomy." Informed decision-making requires understanding both short- and long-term consequences of decisions and extends not only to medical risks and benefits, but also to "long-range goals and values," including religious commitments (Faden & Beauchamp, 1986, pp. 302, 307).

Ethical theorists Ruth Faden and Tom Beauchamp articulate criteria that must be met for informed consent to be achieved. These are: "(1) a patient or subject must *agree* to an intervention based on an *understanding* of (usually disclosed) relevant *information*, (2) consent must *not be controlled* by influences that would engineer the outcome, and (3) the consent must involve the intentional giving of *permission* for an intervention" (1986, p. 54, emphasis original). Faden and Beauchamp emphasize several aspects of the informed consent process. Patients must understand the nature of proffered interventions; for an act to be "intentional, it must correspond to the actor's conception of the act in question" (Beauchamp, 2010, p. 66). The actor must also understand the "foreseeable consequences and possible outcomes that might follow as a result of performing and not performing the action." The provider's "manipulative underdisclosure of pertinent information" to influence a decision violates these ethical principles (Faden & Beauchamp, 1986, pp. 300, 8).

Applying the principles of informed consent to MBIs, mindfulness instructors have an affirmative ethical obligation to supply full and accurate information needed for participants to give truly informed consent. Clients must understand the nature of mindfulness meditation, including its origins and ongoing associations with Buddhism, and be made aware of any alternative treatments that might be more suitable. Clients must also understand the potential for adverse effects and religious effects of participating in programs that are marketed as safe and secular. Mindfulness researcher Willoughby Britton, an Assistant Professor of Psychiatry and Human Behavior at Brown University, urges that informed consent must include "thorough and honest disclosure" of the "nature, probability and magnitude of both benefits and harms," which, given differing potentials of MBIs for various participants with diverse conditions, often requires "face-to-face consultation that is tailored to each participant" (2016, p. 106). Any lack of transparency on the part of providers for the purpose of encouraging participation—even if motivated by a compassionate desire to relieve suffering—is unethical. Psychologists and Buddhists Edo Shonin, William Van Gordon, and Mark Griffiths argue that "there is a need and duty to make service-users (and the wider scientific community) fully aware of the underlying intentions of MBIs and/or of the extent to which it can realistically be said that MBIs are actually grounded in traditional Buddhist practice" (2013, p. 3). Ronald Purser similarly suggests that "one reason why Kabat-Zinn and his MBSR teachers are so adamant that ethics remain 'implicit' in their curriculum is that it is part of this camouflage strategy." MBSR participants "believe they are receiving medically and scientifically based therapies, when in reality they are gradually being introduced to religious practices, without full disclosure or informed consent." The intentionally cultivated "dual identities" of mindfulness "may have legal implications in terms of an evasion of professional accountability and a potential violation of informed consent laws." Purser concludes that this sort of "stealth Buddhism" is "an ethical issue" of "truth in advertising" (2015, pp. 25–26).

Adverse Effects

MBI providers have an ethical responsibility to volunteer full information about what might happen when people practice mindfulness meditation, including the potential for unexpected or adverse effects. Certain of the same Buddhist teachings that encourage meditation also predict difficult experiences. According to Britton, varied experiences with meditation are "well documented in Buddhist texts" (Britton, 2014, para. 22). Mind and Life Institute Research Associate Chris Kaplan gives the example of a *sutta*, a canonical discourse attributed to the Buddha or one of his disciples, "where monks go crazy and commit suicide after doing contemplation on death" (Kaplan in Rocha, 2014, para. 28). Certain modern Buddhist meditation teachers interpret the classical texts as advising that experiential knowledge of suffering, or *dukkha ñanas*, are an inevitable stage in the path toward enlightenment. Psychologist and Buddhist meditation teacher Ron Crouch thus reasons from his reading of Buddhist texts and from his experiences teaching meditation that it is an ethical obligation of instructors to "tell students up front about the negative effects of meditation" so that they can make "an informed choice about whether to proceed or not"; failure to do so is, in Crouch's view, "just dangerous" (Crouch, 2011, para. 22). In considering the relevance of such warnings about meditation practiced in overtly Buddhist contexts to secularly framed MBIs, it is important to keep two factors in mind. First, prominent MBI leaders intend for MBIs to function as portals to deeper meditation experiences. Second, some MBI participants do, through this exposure, find their way to explicitly Buddhist meditation.

It is not only Buddhists who warn of potentially negative experiences from meditation. As early as 1977, the American Psychiatric Association (APA) issued a position statement calling for "well-controlled studies" that include evaluation of "contraindications, and dangers of meditative techniques" (p. 6). As meditation has become more popular, adverse effects have been noted with sufficient frequency that the APA *Diagnostic and Statistical Manual of Mental Disorders* (DSM) added to its 1994 edition the diagnostic category of "Religious and Spiritual Problems" to account for meditative and other spiritual experiences that resemble mental illness (Farias & Wikholm, 2015, loc. 2201; Vieten & Scammell, 2015, p. 65).

Most scientific studies of mindfulness meditation, whether in Buddhist or MBI contexts, do not look for adverse effects. Britton explains that varied effects are "not well documented in the scientific literature because nobody is asking about them" (Britton, 2014, para. 22). According to Miguel Farias, Director of Studies in Psychological Research at the University of Oxford, "it's difficult to tell how common [negative] experiences are, because mindfulness researchers have failed to measure them, and may even have discouraged participants from reporting them by attributing the blame to them" (Farias in Foster, 2016, para. 12). Psychologist Stephen Stratton urges that "adequate informed consent will be helped by future research into the negative effects related to mindfulness and contemplative practices" (2015, p. 113).

Despite the lack of systematic study, there is a growing body of empirical evidence of adverse effects from mindfulness and other forms of meditation. Reporting on 17 primary publications and five literature reviews of reported meditation side effects, psychologist Kathleen Lustyk and colleagues identify potential risks to mental, physical, and spiritual health, and recommend participant screening procedures, research safety guidelines, and standards for researcher training (Lustyk, Chawla, Nolan, & Marlatt, 2009). After reviewing 75 scientific articles on meditation, including mindfulness, psychotherapists Alberto Perez-de-Albeniz and Jeremy Holmes concluded that "meditation is not free from side effects, even for long-term meditators or experienced teachers. Nor is it free of contraindications" (2000, p. 55). Psychiatrist John Craven advises that meditation is contraindicated for patients with a "history of psychotic episodes of dissociative disorder," "schizoid personality traits," "hypochondriacal or somatization disorders," or who are otherwise "likely to be overwhelmed and decompensate with the loosening of cognitive controls on the awareness of inner experience" (1989, p. 651). It is not only psychologically disturbed patients who report negative effects; it is just that they may be less capable of managing them. Craven reports that the most frequent negative effects of meditation are "nausea, dizziness, uncomfortable kinesthetic sensations and mild dissociation," as well as "feelings of guilt," anxiety-provoking "powerful affective experiences," "fear and anxiety," "grandiosity, elation," "bragging about experiences," as well as "psychosis-like symptoms, suicide and destructive behaviour" (p. 651). Other researchers have reported "difficult thoughts or feelings" (Lomas, Cartwright, Edginton, & Ridge, 2014, p. 201), "depersonalization and derealization" (Epstein & Lieff, 1981, pp. 137–38), "anxieties, intense ecstasies and moments of depersonalization" (Dunne, 2011, p. 15), "fragmentation of the self which can manifest itself as dissociation, grandiosity, terror, or delusion" (Blanton, 2011, p. 143), acute psychotic episodes, agitation, weeping, screaming, paranoia, bizarre behavior, and suicide attempts (Walsh & Roche, 1979, p. 1085). One meditator interviewed by Mind and Life Institute Research Associate Tomas Rocha recounted: "I had a vision of death with a scythe and a hood, and the thought 'Kill yourself' over and over again" (Rocha, 2014, para. 2). Negative effects of meditation thus range from mildly uncomfortable to life-threatening.

The "Varieties of Contemplative Experience" (VCE) study led by Willoughby Britton and Jared Lindahl (2017) recruited Western (85 percent from the U.S.) meditators (n = 60) in the Theravāda, Zen, and Tibetan Buddhist traditions who reported experiences described as "challenging, difficult, distressing, functionally impairing, and/or requiring additional support." Catalogued experiences include: fear, anxiety, panic, or paranoia (reported by 82 percent of respondents); depression, dysphoria, or grief (57 percent); change in worldview (48 percent); delusional, irrational, or paranormal beliefs (47 percent); physical pain (47 percent); re-experiencing of traumatic memories (43 percent); rage, anger, or aggression (30 percent); agitation or irritability (23 percent); and suicidality (18 percent). Symptom duration ranged from days to more than ten years, with a median of 1–3 years; most subjects (73 percent) indicated a moderate to severe level of impairment, and 17 percent required inpatient hospitalization. Although the study did not address MBIs and excluded children, respondents reported "challenging or difficult experiences under similar conditions" as MBIs: "in the context of daily practice [28 percent]; while meditating less than 1 hour per day [25 percent], or within the first 50 hours of practice [18 percent]; and with an aim of health, well-being or stress-reduction." Practitioners encountered difficulties with practices "not dissimilar from the primary components" of MBIs, such as "mindfulness of breathing" (Lindahl, Fisher, Cooper, Rosen, & Britton, 2017).

Adverse effects have been reported for both short-term and long-term meditators, in both MBI and Buddhist contexts. Psychiatrists Mark Epstein and Jonathan Lieff have observed through their clinical work with hundreds of meditators that even the "early stages of meditation practice" can produce "explosive experiences," some of which are "pathological" (1981, pp. 138, 144). Psychotherapists Ilan Kutz and colleagues assessed 20 participants in a 10-week MBI who were also receiving psychotherapy. These introductory, secularly framed meditation classes were for some "difficult and disquieting," provoking feelings of "agitation and restlessness," "pain-fear-anger," loneliness, sadness, emptiness, "feelings of defenselessness, which in turn produced unpleasant affective experiences, such as fear, anger, apprehension and despair," sometimes "accompanied by sobbing during the meditation session" (1985, pp. 215–16). Four of twenty subjects reported a "dramatic unveiling" of latent memories of "incest, rejection, and abandonment" in "intense, vivid forms" (p. 215). Psychologist Deane Shapiro assessed 27 long-term meditators following a Vipassana retreat; 17 (63%) reported at least one adverse effect, and two (7%) "suffered profound adverse effects … of such intensity that they stopped meditating." Reported experiences include: boredom and pain, confusion, depression, severe shaking, feeling more judgmental of others, increased negative emotions, more emotional pain, increased fears and anxiety, disorientation, feeling spaced out, decreased attentional clarity, less motivation in life, feeling more uncomfortable in the real world, "loss of self," and "egolessness which brought deep terror and insecurity." Even meditators with the most extensive experience were no less likely to report adverse effects. Shapiro concludes by urging "the critical importance of being sensitive to the adverse influences in short, as well as long term meditators" and of not allowing Buddhist "belief systems" to predispose meditation enthusiasts to see "growth where there may in fact be harm occurring" (1992a, pp. 62, 64–65, 66). The risks of adverse effects pertain to both beginning and advanced meditators.

When presented as a secular, universal intervention, equally safe and appropriate for anyone, the risks of negative experiences from mindfulness practice may be heightened. Jenny Wilks, who teaches both Buddhist and secularly framed mindfulness, warns that "secular mindfulness teachers may not be aware of the kinds of things that can come up for people practicing meditation—both problematic spiritual emergencies and profound insights—and won't know how to guide people with these" (2014, sect. 3 para. 5). The term "spiritual emergencies" was coined by Stanislov and Christina Grof in 1989 as a classification for acute psychospiritual crises that they observed to be commonly induced by meditation or other intense experiences (Grof & Grof, 1989). Psychologists Miguel Farias and Catherine Wikholm describe meditation as a "Buddha Pill" in that it affects individuals differently and can bring about unwanted or unexpected side-effects (2015, loc. 3352). They ask, "Is meditation then a Buddha pill? No, it isn't in the sense that it does not constitute an easy or certain cure." But, they also answer, "yes, in the sense that, like medication, meditation can produce changes in us both physiologically and psychologically, and that it can affect all of us differently. Like swallowing a pill, it can bring about unwanted or unexpected side-effects in some individuals, which may be temporary, or more long-lasting" (loc. 3356).

Some MBI leaders are more careful than others to inform participants about the risks of adverse effects. MBSR training offered through the CfM does, to its credit, identify "Screening Criteria for Exclusion from the Stress Reduction Program": "suicidality," "psychosis," "PTSD," "depression or other major psychiatric diagnosis," "social anxiety," and substance "addiction." Participants sign an informed consent form only after an interviewer explains one-on-one that risks include "feelings of sadness, anger, fear," and that a "history of trauma, abuse, significant recent loss or major life changes, or addiction to substances may heighten these reactions" (Blacker et al., 2015, pp. 37–38; Santorelli, 2014, pp. 6–7). Such screening procedures do not prevent adverse effects, but they do at least reduce the likelihood that those with histories of severe psychological disorders will enroll. Other MBIs, including school-based programs, may not make similar disclosures. For example, Calmer Choice promotes itself as a "universal prevention program" that is designed to stop "violence, suicide, and self-destructive behaviors in young people" (Calmer Choice, 2015e, para. 2, 2016, para. 3). Such advertising raises ethical questions given that other mindfulness programs (including MBSR, which is a prerequisite for Calmer Choice instructors; Calmer Choice, 2015b, para. 7) recognize suicidality and serious emotional problems as exclusionary criteria, and given that children (especially those who have suffered trauma at home) may be especially susceptible and ill-prepared to respond to the challenges of meditation (Sibinga, Webb, Ghazarian, & Ellen, 2016).

Mindfulness teachers, including instructors of secularly framed MBIs, should disclose information about the risks of meditation. Once informed, individuals may conclude that the potential benefits of meditation outweigh the potential harms, but they need to be made aware of both in order to make informed decisions about whether to begin or continue meditating. Transparency about the Buddhist foundations of mindfulness is directly relevant to transparency about the potential for unexpected or adverse effects because certain of the same Buddhist teachings that encourage mindfulness also predict difficult experiences. Moreover, MBIs are often intended to be, and/or in effect become, doorways to overtly Buddhist meditation. Thus, adverse effects and religious effects should be considered in tandem.

Religious Effects

Ethical obligations to disclose potential effects of mindfulness extend to religious effects. It is no secret among mindfulness teachers that secular mindfulness can be a doorway to religion and spirituality, including Buddhism. Thupten Jingpa, translator for the Dalai Lama, reflects that: "one of the interesting things about mindfulness, is that the initial emphasis on the secularization of the language really makes it less threatening to many people. It offers a very, very, skillful route to get to that experience, and then as people's experience deepens, there is no denying the fact that it does open to deeper spirituality" (Shonin & Van Gordon, 2016, p. 280). A number of Buddhist meditation teachers have published accounts of witnessing an increase in the number of people taking explicitly Buddhist classes or coming on Buddhist retreats after being introduced to mindfulness through an MBI (Goodman, 2014; Blacker in Wilks et al., 2015, p. 54; Britton, 2011, para. 37; Kabat-Zinn, 2010, para. 32; Wilks, 2014, sect. 4 para. 4). For example, Stephen Batchelor notes that "on every Buddhist meditation course I lead these days, there will usually be one or two participants who have been drawn to the retreat because they want to deepen their practice of 'secular mindfulness'" (2012, p. 88). Batchelor suggests that an "unintended consequence" of even an 8-week secular MBSR course can be that it opens for participants "unexpected doors into other areas of their life, some of which might be regarded as the traditional domains of religion" (pp. 88–89). As one MBSR graduate attested, "I took an 8 week Mindfulness-Based Stress Reduction Course 2 years ago without knowing anything about Buddhism ... That program spurred my curiosity and here I am learning all about the Four Noble Truths" (JKH, 2015). Mindfulness teacher Barry Boyce suggests that a "natural outgrowth of the mindfulness movement is that there are more candidates who might want to get involved with more rigorous training in the various Buddhist traditions" (Wilks et al., 2015, p. 54). Pediatrician and mindfulness teacher Dzung Vo explains how public-school mindfulness programs play a role in this movement. In Vo's "experience working with mindfulness with children and youth, a lot of the benefit is not immediate, obvious, or concrete. So much of it is about planting seeds, and I sometimes see the flowers bloom many months later." School programs prepare youth to be "open and interested in exploring mindfulness more deeply" when given opportunities outside the school context. Thus, school programs can be "skillful means, and ways of opening more 'dharma doors'" (2013, para. 1–2, 5). The "skillfulness" of using secular language to open dharma doors might be questioned from a Buddhist ethical framework (as suggested above); from a non-Buddhist framework, disclosure of potential religious and spiritual effects is essential for informed consent.

Social science research confirms anecdotal observations of a correlation between secularly framed MBIs and religious and spiritual experiences. Psychologist Jeffrey

Greeson and colleagues conducted quantitative survey research on 600 MBSR participants (2011, $n = 279$; 2015, $n = 322$). Most participants enrolled wanting improved mental health (90%), help managing stress (89%), and improved physical health (61%); half (50%) agreed that "exploring or deepening my sense of spirituality" motivated enrollment (2011). After 8 weeks, 54% reported that the course had deepened their spirituality, including personal faith, meaning, and sense of engagement and closeness with some form of higher power or interconnectedness with all things—aspects of spirituality that overlap with religion (2011). The authors conclude that mental health benefits from MBSR can be attributed to increases in daily spiritual experiences (2011, 2015). Other studies similarly correlate MBSR participation with increased spirituality scale scores (Astin, 1997; Carmody & Kristeller, 2008).

Psychological studies, employing interview and survey methodologies, indicate that mindfulness practice draws some participants toward Buddhism. Psychologist Timothy Lomas and colleagues conducted in-depth interviews of 30 meditators, most of whom first tried meditation for secular reasons, such as stress management. But, the authors conclude, "meditation became their gateway to subsequent interest in Buddhism," and over time "meditation and Buddhism had become inextricably linked" (Lomas, Cartwright, Edginton, & Ridge, 2014, p. 201). Psychologist Dean Shapiro used written surveys to study Vipassana retreat participants before and after (1 month and 6 month intervals) their retreat experience; questions explored reasons participants first started meditating, length of meditation experience, and current intentions and religious identifications. Shapiro found that intentions of mindfulness practitioners changed over time, shifting along a continuum from self-regulation, to self-exploration, to self-liberation (from the "egoic self," understood in Buddhist terms). Longer-term meditators were less likely to be religious "Nones" or monotheists and more likely to identify as Buddhist or with "All" religions (1992b, p. 34). Many people assume that one's initial intentions in participating in a practice determine whether the practice is for that person "secular" or "religious." Psychologist Shauna Shapiro and colleagues clarify that "intentions" are "dynamic and evolving, which allows them to change and develop with deepening practice" (Shapiro, Carlson, Astin, & Freedman, 2006, p. 376). This helps explain empirical findings of a transition from secular to Buddhist motivations.

The presumed distinction between "secular" and "Buddhist" mindfulness may be so fragile as to dissolve upon examination. As historian Anne Harrington and philosopher John Dunne put it, "therapeutic mindfulness today sits on an unstable knife edge between spirituality and secularism, therapeutics, and popular culture" (2015, p. 630). Farias and Wikholm argue that it is a "common myth" that "we can practise meditation as a purely scientific technique with no religious or spiritual leanings." They base this conclusion on research showing that:

> Meditation leads us to become more spiritual, and that this increase in spirituality is partly responsible for the practice's positive effects. So, even if we set out to ignore meditation's spiritual roots, those roots may nonetheless envelop us, to a greater or lesser degree. Overall, it is unclear whether secular models of mindfulness meditation are fully secular. (2015, loc. 3293)

Psychologist Stephen Stratton similarly concludes that the "distinction between the secular and the religious and/or spiritual when it comes to meditation in general and mindfulness in particular" may be "simplistic" (2015, p. 113). Marketing mindfulness as secular, implicitly defined as resulting in empirically validated effects, may both veil and heighten religious effects by inducing participation by those who might otherwise object to joining in a Buddhist practice.

There are ethical implications of the blurring of secular and spiritual mindfulness. Stratton asks: "Can the potential for religious-spiritual effects be ethically omitted from a description of this therapeutic technique?" He answers that "such an omission seems difficult to defend" (2015, p. 105). According to Stratton, "a more culturally aware perspective might suggest that religious-spiritual dimensions are always potentially present, even in overtly secular processes. Reflecting ethically, it seems more reasonable to consider the degree of religious-spiritual influence, not its presence or absence. It is unwise to assume that no religious-spiritual process is engaged when using secularized meditational practices in applied or research settings" (p. 113). Stratton notes that some Christian groups, particularly "Fundamentalist and Evangelical Christians" may avoid "any meditation beyond explicitly Christian prayer-based forms" for "religious-spiritual reasons" and that "counselors and researchers need to remain aware of the influence of these cultural dynamics for ethical practice. Awareness of this multicultural influence strongly suggests the need for religious-spiritual assessment for those who are introduced to therapeutic meditative practices in counseling" (p. 106). Stratton urges "increased attention to informed consent for meditational and prayer-based practices. It seems realistic to provide education about religious-spiritual effects that may arise while participating in interventions that include meditational practices, even when secularized" (p. 113). In the absence of such disclosures, consent to participate in mindfulness cannot be described as informed.

Encouraging mindfulness practice by advertising secular benefits may be ethically problematic if there is reason to expect that doing so might lead people to embrace ideas (about the ultimate nature of life and of the self or of the cause and solution for suffering) and goals (such as relinquishing attachments and dispelling illusions) that some people might reject if they understood them up front. Some participants or guardians who have signed formal consent forms may not have done so had they been given more information about the history of mindfulness meditation and its current cultural and religious associations.

Coercion

When mindfulness is presented as a secular, universal intervention beneficial to everyone, informed consent processes may be bypassed entirely. Employers may mandate participation, much as they would require attendance at other workshops designed to enhance productivity (Foster, 2016, para. 18). Prisoners may be indirectly pressured by offers of privileged treatment—accommodations in a quieter wing of the building and specially prepared vegetarian meals—in exchange for their willingness to participate in meditation retreats (Bowen, Bergman, & Witkiewitz, 2015, 1458). Goldie Hawn has stated that it is her goal to see MindUP or similar programs "absolutely mandated in every state … that's our mission." (2011, para. 67). Public-school students are not asked whether they want to opt out of math class; anecdotal evidence suggests that school administrators do not always make it easy for parents to opt their children out of mindfulness, giving the reason that it is a secular enrichment activity—and implying that no one rational would abstain for religious reasons. Certain school mindfulness programs are designed to permeate the entire school day, to be a "lifestyle" or "way of teaching and being," permeating the "overall school culture," rather than a self-contained curriculum such as math (Brown, 2015, para. 4; Calmer Choice, 2015e, para. 7). When mindfulness activities are scattered throughout the day—a few minutes of meditation several times daily, accompanied by frequent reminders to maintain a mindful attitude at all times—opting out is practically impossible without withdrawing from social institutions altogether.

Many MBIs are offered in public institutions that serve vulnerable populations from diverse cultural and religious backgrounds. In such settings, promoting mindfulness as a secular, universal intervention may be culturally and religiously disrespectful, divisive, and coercive. For example, public-school students are a "'captive' audience," in a vulnerable position because of compulsory attendance, the impressionability of youth, and the institutional authority of teachers (Justice William O. Douglas in *Engel v. Vitale*, 1962, para. 11). School children, like other vulnerable populations, such as prisoners, employees in economically precarious working environments, those who are ill enough to need hospital or hospice services, and particular racial and ethnic minorities, merit special protection of autonomy (National Commission, 1979). This is because vulnerable populations might feel undue pressure to accept offered services although they lack substantial understanding of those services or their potential effects both short- and long-term (Miller, 1983, p. 11). Yet, these are the very groups targeted by a number of MBIs.

Differentials in power and knowledge inherent to the educational, medical, prison, and corporate systems give those in privileged positions an affirmative ethical obligation to investigate religious dimensions of interventions, volunteer information about potential conflicts between interventions and prior religious convictions or practices, and avoid direct or indirect religious indoctrination. The risks of undue coercion are intensified when mindfulness is sponsored by those in positions of social authority who command respect, trust, and/or obedience. Hierarchical relationships, for instance therapist–patient, employer–employee, and teacher–student, encourage social inferiors, namely patients, employees, and students, to trust information given by social superiors, namely their therapists, employers, or teachers. Group instruction, especially on institutional grounds, can exert an indirect, coercive pressure to conform to what the instructor (or sponsoring authority) says to do and peers can be observed as doing. Even if participation is voluntary, individuals may feel pressured to participate. Despite the existence of opt-out provisions, it can be socially costly for social inferiors to appear to question their superiors' wisdom or to deviate from the behavior of their peers.

Conclusion

Many Americans, scholars included, tend to base their evaluations of MBIs on the starting assumption that they are fully secular. To illustrate, philosopher Andreas Schmidt defends MBIs against charges that they "constitute an illegitimate promotion of a particular worldview or way of life." Schmidt's argument pivots on his presuppositions that MBIs are devoid of (1) metaphysical assumptions, (2) ethical standards, or (3) contested values. He asserts without evidence that "while MBIs in healthcare and schools draw on and resemble traditional Buddhist meditative practices in various ways, they do not make any metaphysical or religious assumptions and are specifically designed to be secular" (2016, p. 451). Furthermore, MBIs are:

> Not committed to substantive ethical standards about what is good, bad, right or wrong. While such practices often include compassion exercises, I think the ability to be compassionate and mindful of those around one should again be considered a general moral and social *skill* rather than a particular, contentious ethical viewpoint. (p. 452, emphasis original)

If these premises are incorrect, then Schmidt's ethical reflections instead suggest that MBIs violate philosophical principles of "liberal neutrality": that "public policies should not aim to promote particular conceptions of the good" (p. 452). Although Schmidt concludes that "MBIs should avoid strong ethical commitments," this chapter has made a case that the embeddedness in MBIs of metaphysical assumptions, ethical standards, and contested values (such as compassion) instead indicates the need for transparency about implicit ethical commitments (p. 450).

None of this analysis is meant to argue against offering optional MBIs—provided that participation is truly voluntary and based upon fully informed consent. In public institutions such as schools where social authorities have power to influence culturally and religiously diverse populations, lunch-time or after-hours programs avoid much of the risk of coercion (*Good News Club v. Milford Central School*, 2001). The key here is transparency: about the origins and live associations of mindfulness with Buddhist ethics, and the potential for adverse and/or religious effects—even when initial motivations for practice appear purely secular. Training programs for MBI teachers should address the responsibility of teachers to be transparent about these issues, as well as to disclose any personal affiliations with Buddhist concepts, values, practices, or communities. Mindfulness programs have been able to "reap the benefits of being perceived as a secular therapy" (Lindahl, 2015b, p. 61), but the cost has often been a lack of transparency about goals and/or potential outcomes. There are ethical grounds, both internal and external to Buddhism, for reconceiving of transparency as an essential element of MBIs in secular contexts.

References

@fionajensen. (2014). Comment on RWJF Culture of Health Blog, Fighting off those waves of stress. *Disqus*. Retrieved April 23, 2016 from https://disqus.com/home/discussion/rwjfcultureofhealthblog/fighting_off_those_waves_of_stress/#comment-1606728745

@mindful_youth. (2013, January 25 [joined]). Calmer Choice. *Twitter*. Retrieved April 23, 2016 from http://www.tweetrecord.com/mindful_youth

Albanese, C. (2013). *America, religions and religion* (5th ed.). Boston: Wadsworth.

Aldwin, C., Park, C., Jeong, Y., & Nath, R. (2014). Differing pathways between religiousness, spirituality, and health: A self-regulation perspective. *Psychology of Religion and Spirituality, 6*(1), 9–21.

American Psychiatric Association Task Force on Meditation. (1977). Position statement on meditation. *American Journal of Psychiatry, 134*, 6.

American Psychological Association. (2010). *Ethical principles of psychologists and code of conduct*. Retrieved April 26, 2016 from http://www.apa.org/ethics/code/principles.pdf

Asad, T. (2003). *Formations of the secular: Christianity, Islam, modernity*. Stanford, CA: Stanford University Press.

Astin, J. A. (1997). Stress reduction through mindfulness meditation: Effects on psychological symptomatology, sense of control, and spiritual experiences. *Psychotherapy and Psychosomatics, 66*, 97–106.

Bahnsen, M. (2013). Healthy habits of mind. *Persona Film*. Retrieved April 26, 2016 from http://www.mindfulschools.org/resources/healthy-habits-of-mind/

Barnhofer, T., Chittka, T., Nightingale, H., Visser, C., & Crane, C. (2010). State effects of two forms of meditation on prefrontal EEG asymmetry in previously depressed individuals. *Mindfulness, 1*(1), 21–27.

Batchelor, S. (2012). A secular Buddhism. *Journal of Global Buddhism, 13*, 88–89.

Blacker, M., Meleo-Meyer, F., Kabat-Zinn, J., Koerbel, L., & Santorelli, S. (2015). *Authorized curriculum guide for mindfulness-based stress reduction*. Worcester, MA: Center for Mindfulness.

Beauchamp, T. L. (2010). Autonomy and consent. In F. G. Miller & A. Wertheimer (Eds.), *The ethics of consent: Theory and practice* (pp. 55–78). New York: Oxford University Press.

Blanton, P. G. (2011). The other mindful practice: Centering prayer and psychotherapy. *Pastoral Psychology, 60*, 133–147.

Bodhi, B. (1999; November 30, 2013). The Noble Eightfold Path: The way to the end of suffering. *Access to Insight* (Legacy Edition). Retrieved February 7, 2017 from http://www.accesstoinsight.org/lib/authors/bodhi/waytoend.html

Bowen, S., Bergman, A. L., & Witkiewitz, K. (2015). Engagement in Buddhist meditation practices among non-Buddhists: Associations with religious identity and practice. *Mindfulness, 6*(6), 1456–1461.

Britton, W. B. (2011). *The dark night project*. Interview by V. Horn. Buddhist Geeks 232. Retrieved April 11, 2016 [removed by October 21, 2016] from http://www.buddhistgeeks.com/2011/09/bg-232-the-dark-night-project/

Britton, W. B. (2014, April 25). *Meditation nation*. Interview by L. Heuman. Tricycle. Retrieved April 8, 2016 from http://tricycle.org/trikedaily/meditation-nation/

Britton, W. B. (2016). Scientific literacy as a foundational competency for teachers of mindfulness-based interventions. In D. McCown, D. Reibel, & M. S. Micozzi (Eds.), *Resources for teaching mindfulness: A cross-cultural and international handbook* (pp. 93–119). New York: Springer.

Broderick, P. (2013). *Learning to breathe: A mindfulness curriculum for adolescents to cultivate emotion regulation, attention, and performance*. Oakland, CA: New Harbinger Publications. Retrieved April 12, 2016 from https://www.newharbinger.com/learning-breathe

Brown, A. (2015, November 23). A way of teaching and being. *Mindful Schools*. Retrieved April 21, 2016 from http://www.mindfulschools.org/implementation-stories/a-way-of-teaching-and-being/

Brown, C. G. (2016). Can "secular" mindfulness be separated from religion? In R. E. Purser, D. Forbes, & A. Burke (Eds.), *Handbook of mindfulness: Culture, context, and social engagement* (pp. 75–94). New York: Springer.

Broyles, D. R. (2016, February 2). *Legal and practical concerns regarding the district's Calmer Choice mindfulness curriculum.* Retrieved April 23, 2016 from http://www.nclplaw.org/wp-content/uploads/2011/12/DYRSD-Legal-Opinion-Memorandum-2-2-161.pdf

Calhoun, C., Juergensmeyer, M., & Van Antwerpen, J. (2011). *Rethinking secularism.* New York: Oxford University Press.

Calmer Choice. (2011a [timeline begins]; revised 2016). About. *Facebook.* Retrieved January 25, 2016 [pre-revision] and April 23, 2016 [post-revision] from https://www.facebook.com/CalmerChoice/info/?tab=page_info

Calmer Choice. (2011b [year IRS granted 50s(c)(3) status]; revised 2016). Profile. *GuideStar.* Retrieved February 25, 2016 [pre-revision] and April 23, 2016 [post-revision] from https://www.guidestar.org/profile/27-2836997

Calmer Choice. (2012). *IRS Form 990-EZ.* Retrieved April 23, 2016 from http://990s.foundation-center.org/990_pdf_archive/272/272836997/272836997_201212_990EZ.pdf

Calmer Choice. (2015a). *Board of directors.* Retrieved April 23, 2016 from http://www.calmer-choice.org/board-of-directors/

Calmer Choice. (2015b; revised 2017). *Instructor training.* Retrieved April 23, 2016 [pre-revision] and February 7, 2017 [post-revision] from http://calmerchoicenews.weebly.com/instructor-training.html

Calmer Choice. (2015c). *Participating schools.* Retrieved April 23, 2016 from http://www.calmer-choice.org/participating-schools/

Calmer Choice. (2015d; removed 2016). Resources. *Calmer Choice.* Retrieved November 27, 2015 [pre-removal] from http://www.calmerchoice.org/resources/

Calmer Choice. (2015e; revised 2016). School-based programs [re-titled School programs]. *Calmer Choice.* Retrieved November 27, 2015 [pre-revision] and April 23, 2016 [post-revision] from http://www.calmerchoice.org/school-programs/

Calmer Choice. (2016). Cultivating awareness, living mindfully, enhancing resilience. *1440 Foundation.* Retrieved April 28, 2016 from http://1440.org/who-we-support/calmer-choice/

Calos, R. (2012, November 27). Social and emotional learning empowers children. *Scientific American: Streams of consciousness.* Retrieved April 26, 2016 from http://blogs.scientificamerican.com/streams-of-consciousness/social-and-emotional-learning-empowers-children/

Carmody, R., & Kristeller, M. (2008). Mindfulness, spirituality, and health-related symptoms. *Journal of Psychosomatic Research, 64*(4), 393–403.

CfM [Center for Mindfulness in Medicine, Health Care, and Society]. (2014a). *History of MBSR.* Retrieved April 25, 2016 from http://www.umassmed.edu/cfm/stress-reduction/history-of-mbsr/

CfM [Center for Mindfulness in Medicine, Health Care, and Society]. (2014b). *Tuition and payment plans.* Retrieved April 12, 2016 from http://www.umassmed.edu/cfm/stress-reduction/mbsr-8-week/tuition--payment-plans/

Chandler, D. (2002). *Semiotics: The basics.* New York: Routledge.

Cheung, K. (forthcoming). Implicit and explicit ethics in mindfulness-based programs in a broader context. In R. Purser, S. Stanley & N. Singh (Eds.), *Ethical foundations of mindfulness.* New York: Springer.

Cohen, M. H. (2006). *Healing at the borderland of medicine and religion.* Chapel Hill: University of North Carolina Press.

Crane, R. S., Kuyken, W., Williams, J. M. G., Hastings, R. P., Cooper, L., & Fennell, M. J. V. (2012). Competence in teaching mindfulness-based courses: Concepts, development and assessment. *Mindfulness, 3,* 76–84.

Craven, J. (1989). Meditation and psychotherapy. *Canadian Journal of Psychiatry, 34*(7), 648–653.

Creswell, J. D., Pacilio, L. E., Lindsay, E. K., & Brown, K. W. (2014). Brief mindfulness meditation training alters psychological and neuroendocrine responses to social evaluative stress. *Psychoneuroendocrinology, 44,* 1–12.

Crouch, R. (2011, June 12). The dark night. *Aloha Dharma.* Retrieved April 26, 2016 from https://alohadharma.com/page/3/

Cullen, M. (2011). Mindfulness-based interventions: An emerging phenomenon. *Mindfulness*, *2*(3), 186–193.

Davis, J. H. (2015). Facing up to the question of ethics in mindfulness-based interventions. *Mindfulness*, *6*(1), 46–48.

de Certeau, M. (1984). *The practice of everyday life* (Trans. S. F. Rendall). Berkeley, CA: University of California Press.

Delaney, H. D., Miller, W. R., & Bisono, A. M. (2007). Religiosity and spirituality among psychologists: A survey of clinician members of the American Psychological Association. *Professional Psychology: Research and Practice*, *38*, 538–546.

DiAngelo, R. (2011). White fragility. *International Journal of Critical Pedagogy*, *3*(3), 54–70.

Dodson-Lavelle, B. (2015). Against one method: Toward a critical-constructive approach to the adaptation and implementation of Buddhist-based contemplative programs in the United States. Ph.D. dissertation, Emory University.

Dreyfus, G. (2011). Is mindfulness present-centered and non-judgmental? A discussion of the cognitive dimensions of mindfulness. *Contemporary Buddhism*, *12*(1), 41–54.

Dueck, A., & Reimer, K. (2009). *A peaceable psychology: Christian therapy in a world of many cultures*. Grand Rapids, MI: Brazos Press.

Dunne, J. (2011). Toward an understanding of nondual mindfulness. *Contemporary Buddhism*, *12*(1), 71–88.

Durkheim, É. (1984). *The division of labor in society* (reprint ed.). New York: Simon & Schuster.

Dyer, R. (1993). *The matter of images: Essays on representations*. New York: Routledge.

Engel v. Vitale. (1962). 370 U.S. 421. Retrieved April 25, 2016 from http://caselaw.findlaw.com/us-supreme-court/370/421.html

Epstein, M. D., & Lieff, J. D. (1981). Psychiatric complications of meditation practice. *The Journal of Transpersonal Psychology*, *13*(2), 137–147.

Faden, R. R. & Beauchamp, T. L., with King, N. M. P. (1986). *A history and theory of informed consent*. New York: Oxford University Press.

Farias, M., & Wikholm, C. (2015). *The Buddha pill: Can meditation change you?* London: Watkins.

Felver, J. C., & Jennings, P. A. (2016). Applications of mindfulness-based interventions in school settings: An introduction. *Mindfulness*, *7*, 1–4.

Folk, K. (2013). *The Trojan horse of meditation*. Interview by V. Horn, E. Horn, & K. S. Bearer. BG296. Retrieved January 2, 2016 [removed by February 7, 2017] from www.buddhistgeeks.com/2013/09/bg-296-the-trojan-horse-of-meditation/

Forbes, D. (2015, June). *Critical integral urban education: From neoliberal to transformational?* Paper presented at Mindfulness & Compassion: The Art and Science of Contemplative Practice Conference, San Francisco State University, CA.

Foster, D. (2016, January 23). Is mindfulness making us ill? *The Guardian*. Retrieved April 21, 2016 from http://www.theguardian.com/lifeandstyle/2016/jan/23/is-mindfulness-making-us-ill

Gardner-Chloros, P. G. (2009). *Code-switching*. New York: Cambridge University Press.

Goffman, E. (1959). *The presentation of self in everyday life*. Garden City, NY: Doubleday.

Goleman, D. (1985, summer). *Inquiring Mind*, *2*(1), 7.

Good News Club v. Milford Central School. (2001). 533 U.S. 98. Retrieved April 25, 2016 from http://caselaw.findlaw.com/us-supreme-court/533/98.html

Goodman, T. (2014). *Stealth Buddhism*. Interview by V. Horn & E. Horn. BG331. Retrieved April 5, 2016 [removed by December 19, 2016] from www.buddhistgeeks.com/2014/08/bg-331-stealth-buddhism/

Goyal, M., Singh, S., Sibinga, E. M. S., Gould, N. F., Rowland-Seymour, A., Sharma, R., … Haythornthwaite, J. A. (2014). Meditation programs for psychological stress and well-being: A systematic review and meta-analysis. *JAMA Internal Medicine*, *174*(3), 357–368.

Green, S. P. (2002). Plagiarism, norms, and the limits of theft law: Some observations on the use of criminal sanctions in enforcing intellectual property rights. *Hastings Law Journal*, *54*(1), 167–242.

Greenland, S. K. (2013). *The inner kids program*. Retrieved April 26, 2016 from http://www. susankaisergreenland.com/inner-kids-program.html

Greeson, J. M., Smoski, M. J., Suarez, E. C., Brantley, J. G., Ekblad, A. G., Lynch, T. R., & Wolever, R. Q. (2015). Decreased symptoms of depression after Mindfulness-Based Stress Reduction: Potential moderating effects of religiosity, spirituality, trait mindfulness, sex, and age. *The Journal of Alternative and Complementary Medicine*, *2*(3), 166–174.

Greeson, J. M., Webber, D. M., Smoski, M. J., Brantley, J. G., Ekblad, A. G., Suarez, E. C., & Wolever, R. Q. (2011). Changes in spirituality partly explain health-related quality of life outcomes after Mindfulness-Based Stress Reduction. *Journal of Behavioral Medicine*, *34*(6), 508–518.

Grof, S., & Grof, C. (1989). *Spiritual emergency: When personal transformation becomes a crisis*. Los Angeles, CA: J. P. Tarcher.

Gunaratana, B. H. (2001). *Eight mindful steps to happiness: Walking the Buddha's path*. Boston: Wisdom.

Harrington, A., & Dunne, J. D. (2015). When mindfulness is therapy: Ethical qualms, historical perspectives. *American Psychologist*, *70*(7), 621–631.

Hawn, G. (2011, April 20). Goldie Hawn talks "MindUP" and her mission to bring children happiness. Interview by M. Schnall. *Huffington Post*. Retrieved January 4, 2016 from http://www. huffingtonpost.com/marianne-schnall/goldie-hawn-mindup_b_850226.html

Hawn, G. (2013). *Address for Heart-Mind 2013*. The Dalai Lama Center for Peace-Education. Retrieved January 2, 2016 from https://www.youtube.com/watch?v=7pLhwGLYvJU

Hawn, G. (2005). A lotus grows in the mud. New York: Putnam.

Helderman, I. P. (2016). Drawing the boundaries between "religion" and "secular" in psychotherapists' approaches to Buddhist traditions in the United States. *Journal of the American Academy of Religion*, *84*(4), 937–972.

Hsu, F. (2014, October 14). Four Noble Truths: Part 4. *Buddhist Peace Fellowship*. Retrieved April 24, 2016 from http://www.buddhistpeacefellowship.org/systemic-youth-suffering-the-twelve-fold-social-path-of-transformation/

Iwamura, J. N. (2011). *Virtual orientalism: Asian religions and American popular culture*. New York: Oxford University Press.

Jakobsen, J. R., & Pellegrini, A. (Eds.). (2008). *Secularisms*. Durham: Duke University Press.

Jennings, P. (2016). Mindfulness-based programs and the American public school system: Recommendations for best practices to ensure secularity. *Mindfulness*, *7*, 176–178.

Jensen, F. (2010, fall). *De-stressing at school*. Retrieved April 23, 2016 from http://ase.tufts.edu/ occupationalTherapy/documents/notes-fall2010.pdf

Jensen, F. (2013, April 21). A lifeline for teens. *Mindful, 9*.

Jensen, F. (2015; revised 2016). Profile. *LinkedIn*. Retrieved December 12, 2015 [pre-revision] and April 23, 2016 [post-revision] from https://www.linkedin.com/in/fiona-jensen-532a1625

JKH. (2015, May 15). Comment on R. K. Payne, What's ethics got to do with it? The misguided debate about mindfulness and morality (May 14, 2015). *Tricycle*. Retrieved January 4, 2016 from http://www.tricycle.com/blog/whats-ethics-got-do-it

Kabat-Zinn, J. (1994a). *Catalyzing movement towards a more contemplative/sacred-appreciating/ non-dualistic society*. The Contemplative Mind in Society Meeting of the Working Group, Sponsored by The Nathan Cummings Foundation & Fetzer Institute (September 29-October 2). Retrieved April 26, 2016 from http://www.contemplativemind.org/admin/wp-content/ uploads/2012/09/kabat-zinn.pdf

Kabat-Zinn, J. (1994b). *Wherever you go, there you are: Mindfulness meditation in everyday life*. New York: Hyperion.

Kabat-Zinn, J. (2000). Indra's net at work: The mainstreaming of Dharma practice in society. In G. Watson, S. Batchelor, & G. Claxton (Eds.), *The psychology of awakening: Buddhism, science, and our day-to-day lives* (pp. 225–249). York Beach, ME: Weiser.

Kabat-Zinn, J. (2003). Mindfulness-based interventions in context: Past, present, and future. *Clinical Psychology: Science and Practice*, *10*(2), 144–156.

Kabat-Zinn, J. (2009). Forward. In F. Didonna (Ed.), *Clinical handbook of mindfulness* (pp. xxv–xxxii). New York: Springer.

Kabat-Zinn, J. (2010, October 7). *Mindfulness and the cessation of suffering. An exclusive new interview with mindfulnless pioneer Jon Kabat-Zinn.* Interview by Danny Fisher. Lion's Roar: Buddhist Wisdom for Our Time. Retrieved August 21, 2017 from http://www.lionsroar.com/mindfulness-and-the-cessation-of-suffering-an-exclusive-new-interview-with-mindfulness-pioneer-jon-kabat-zinn/

Kabat-Zinn, J. (2011). Some reflections on the origins of MBSR, skillful means and the trouble with maps. *Contemporary Buddhism, 12*(1), 281–306.

Kabat-Zinn, J. (2015, May 18). *This is not McMindfulness by any stretch of the imagination. Interview by E. Shonin. The Psychologist.* Retrieved August 21, 2017, from https://thepsychologist.bps.org.uk/not-mcmindfulness-any-stretch-imagination

Kabat-Zinn, J. (n.d.). *Guided mindfulness meditation.* Series 1–3. Retrieved January 4, 2016 from http://www.mindfulnesscds.com/

Kabat-Zinn, J., Davidson, R. J., (Eds.), with Houshmand, Z. (2011). *The mind's own physician: A scientific dialogue with the Dalai Lama on the healing power of meditation.* Oakland, CA: New Harbinger Publications.

Kerr, C. (2014, October 1). Don't believe the hype. Interview by L. Heuman. *Tricycle.* Retrieved April 8, 2016 from http://tricycle.org/trikedaily/dont-believe-hype/

King, R. (1999). *Orientalism and religion: Postcolonial theory, India and 'The Mystic East'.* New York: Routledge.

Koenig, H., King, D., & Carson, V. B. (Eds.). (2012). *Handbook of religion and health* (2nd ed.). New York: Oxford University Press.

Kosmin, B. A. & Keysar, A. (2009). *The American religious identification survey (ARIS 2008): Summary report.* Hartford, CT: Trinity College. Retrieved April 2, 2016 from http://commons.trincoll.edu/aris/files/2011/08/ARIS_Report_2008.pdf

Kutz, I., Leserman, J., Dorrington, C., Morrison, C. H., Borysenko, J. Z., & Benson, H. (1985). Meditation as an adjunct to psychotherapy: An outcome study. *Psychotherapy and Psychosomatics, 43*(1), 209–218.

Laird, L. D. & Barnes, L. L. (2014, October). *Stealth religion in the borderland: Undercover healers in the hospital.* Paper presented at Conference on the Hospital: Interface between Secularity and Religion, Boston University, MA.

Legere, C. (2016a, February 4). D-Y parents rally support for Calmer Choice. *Cape Cod Times.* Retrieved April 23, 2016 from http://www.capecodtimes.com/article/20160204/NEWS/160209811

Legere, C. (2016b, February 9). *Calmer Choice director says MBSR program not taught in schools.* Retrieved April 23, 2016 from http://www.capecodtimes.com/article/20160209/NEWS/160209486

Lindahl, J. (2015a). *Two theoretical approaches to mindfulness and compassion: Evaluating the merits and the weaknesses of the discovery model and the developmental model.* Presentation at Mindfulness and Compassion: The Art and Science of Contemplative Practice Conference, San Francisco State University.

Lindahl, J. (2015b). Why right mindfulness might not be right for mindfulness. *Mindfulness, 6*(1), 57–62.

Lindahl, J. R., Fisher, N. E., Cooper, D. J., Rosen, R. K., & Willoughby B. Britton, W. B. (2017). The varieties of contemplative experience: A mixed-methods study of meditation-related challenges in Western Buddhists. *PLOS ONE 12*(5): e0176239, 1–38.

Lokos, A. (2008, winter). Skillful speech. *Tricycle.* Retrieved April 3, 2016 from http://www.tricycle.com/precepts/skillful-speech

Lomas, T., Cartwright, T., Edginton, T., & Ridge, D. (2014). A religion of wellbeing? The appeal of Buddhism to men in London, United Kingdom. *Psychology of Religion and Spirituality, 6*(3), 198–207.

Long, R. (2012). *Room to breathe.* San Francisco, CA: Video Project.

Lopez, D. S., Jr. (2008). *Buddhism and science: A guide for the perplexed*. Chicago: University of Chicago Press.

Lustyk, M., Chawla, N., Nolan, R., & Marlatt, G. (2009). Mindfulness meditation research: Issues of participant screening, safety procedures, and researcher training. *Advances in Mind-Body Medicine, 24*, 20–30.

McCown, D. (2013). *The ethical space of mindfulness in clinical practice: An explanatory essay*. London: Jessica Kingsley Publishers.

Miller, J. C., III. (1983, October 14). *FTC policy statement on deception*. Retrieved April 25, 2016 from https://www.ftc.gov/system/files/documents/public_statements/410531/831014deceptionstmt.pdf

Mindful Schools. (2016). Research on mindfulness. *Mindful Schools*. Retrieved April 24, 2016 from http://www.mindfulschools.org/about-mindfulness/research/

Monteiro, L. (2015, November). *Ethics and secular mindfulness programs: Sila as victim of the fallacy of values-neutral therapy*. Paper presented at the American Academy of Religion, Atlanta, GA.

Monteiro, L., Musten, R. F., & Compson, J. (2015). Traditional and Contemporary Mindfulness: finding the middle path in the tangle of concerns. *Mindfulness, 6*, 1–13.

Naft, J. (2010, March 29). Right intention. Inner frontier: Cultivating spiritual presence. Retrieved April 3, 2016 from http://www.innerfrontier.org/InnerWork/Archive/2010/20100329_Right_Intention.htm

National Commission for the Protection of Human Subjects in Biomedical and Behavioral Research. (1979, April 18). *The Belmont Report*. Retrieved April 25, 2016 from http://www.hhs.gov/ohrp/regulations-and-policy/belmont-report/index.html

Ng, E. & Purser, R. (2015, October 2). White privilege and the mindfulness movement. *Buddhist Peace Fellowship*. Retrieved January 4, 2016 from http://www.buddhistpeacefellowship.org/white-privilege-the-mindfulness-movement/

O'Brien, B. (2016). Right speech: The Buddha's words. *About religion*. Retrieved April 26, 2016 from http://buddhism.about.com/od/theeightfoldpath/a/rightspeech.htm

Oman, D. (2012). Shall the twain meet? Buddhist meditation, science, and diversity. *PsycCRITIQUES, 57*(30), 1–7.

Oman, D. (2015). Cultivating compassion through holistic mindfulness: Evidence for effective intervention. In T. G. Plante (Ed.), *The psychology of compassion and cruelty: Understanding the emotional, spiritual, and religious influences*. Santa Barbara, CA: Praeger.

Ozawa-de Silva, B. (2015, November). *Contemplative science, secular ethics and the Lojong tradition: A case study*. Paper presented at the American Academy of Religion, Atlanta, GA.

Perez-De-Albeniz, A., & Holmes, J. (2000). Meditation: Concepts, effects and uses in therapy. *International Journal of Psychotherapy, 5*(1), 49–58.

Pew Research Center. (2015, November 3). *U.S. public becoming less religious*. Retrieved April 11, 2016 from http://www.pewforum.org/files/2015/11/201.11.03_RLS_II_full_report.pdf

Phillips, S., Wilson, W. H., & Halford, G. S. (2009, December 11). What do transitive inference and class inclusion have in common? Categorical (co)products and cognitive development. *PLoS Computational Biology, 5*(12), e1000599.

Purser, R. (2015). Clearing the muddled path of traditional and contemporary mindfulness: A response to Monteiro, Musten, and Compson. *Mindfulness, 6*(1), 23–45.

Purser, R. & Loy, D. (2013, July 1). Beyond McMindfulness. *Huffington Post*. Retrieved January 5, 2016 from http://www.huffingtonpost.com/ron-purser/beyond-mcmindfulness_b_3519289.html

Reveley, J. (2016). Neoliberal meditations: How mindfulness training medicalizes education and responsibilizes young people. *Policy Futures in Education, 14*(4), 497–511.

Rocha, T. (2014, June 25). The dark knight of the soul. *The Atlantic*. Retrieved April 25, 2016 from http://www.theatlantic.com/health/archive/2014/06/the-dark-knight-of-the-souls/372766/

Saltzman, A. (2014). *A Still Quiet Place: A mindfulness program for teaching children and adolescents to ease stress and difficult emotions*. Oakland, CA: New Harbinger Publications.

Salzberg, S. (2011). Mindfulness and loving-kindness. *Contemporary Buddhism, 12*(1), 177–182.

Santorelli, S. F. (Ed.). (2014). *Mindfulness-Based Stress Reduction (MBSR): Standards of practice*. Worcester, MA: CFM.

Santorelli, S. F. (2016, spring). Does mindfulness belong in public schools?: Two views: Yes—mindfulness is a secular practice that benefits students. *Tricycle*, 66–67.

Schmidt, A. T. (2016). The ethics and politics of mindfulness-based interventions. *Journal of Medical Ethics*, *42*, 450–454.

Schonert-Reichl, K. A., Oberle, E., Lawlor, M. S., Abbott, D., Thomson, K., Oberlander, T. F., & Diamond, A. (2015). Enhancing cognitive and social–emotional development through a simple-to-administer mindfulness-based school program for elementary school children: A randomized controlled trial. *Developmental Psychology*, *5*(1), 52–66.

Shapiro, D. H., Jr. (1992a). Adverse effects of meditation: A preliminary investigation of long-term meditators. *International Journal of Psychosomatics*, *39*(1–4), 62–67.

Shapiro, D. H., Jr. (1992b). A preliminary study of long-term meditators: Goals, effects, religious orientation, cognitions. *The Journal of Transpersonal Psychology*, *24*(1), 23–39.

Shapiro, S. L., Carlson, L. E., Astin, J. A., & Freedman, B. (2006). Mechanisms of mindfulness. *Journal of Clinical Psychology*, *62*(3), 373–386.

Shonin, E., & Van Gordon, W. (2016). Thupten Jingpa on compassion and mindfulness. *Mindfulness*, *7*(1), 279–283.

Shonin, E., Van Gordon, W., & Griffths, M. (2013). Mindfulness-based interventions: Towards mindful clinical integration. *Frontiers in Psychology*, *4*(194), 1–4.

Sibinga, E. M. S., Webb, L., Ghazarian, S. R., & Ellen, J. M. (2016). School-based mindfulness instruction: An RCT. *Pediatrics*, *137*(1), e20152532.

Smith, J. Z. (2004). *Relating religion: Essays in the study of religion*. Chicago: University of Chicago Press.

Stahl, B.. (2015, February 28). *The heart of the Dhamma; Central elements of MBSR: The essence of the Dhamma*. Center for Mindfulness Secure Online Forum (pp. 1–2).

Stanley, S. (2015). Sīla and Sati: An exploration of ethics and mindfulness in Pāli Buddhism and their implications for secular mindfulness-based applications. In E. Shonin, W. Van Gordon, & N. N. Singh (Eds.), *Buddhist foundations of mindfulness* (pp. 89–113). Cham: Springer.

Stratton, S. P. (2015). Mindfulness and contemplation: Secular and religious traditions in Western context. *Counseling and Values*, *60*(1), 100–118.

Taylor, C. (2007). *A secular age*. Cambridge, MA: Harvard University Press.

The Hawn Foundation. (2011). *MindUP curriculum: Brain-focused strategies for learning—and living, Grades pre-k-2*. New York: Scholastic.

The Hawn Foundation (2016). *MindUP™*. The Hawn Foundation. Retrieved April 26, 2016 [removed by October 24, 2016] from http://thehawnfoundation.org/mindup/

The Joint Commission. (2016, January). *The Joint Commission comprehensive accreditation manual for hospitals*. Oakbrook Terrace, IL: The Joint Commission.

Tosh. (2012, January). *Goldie Hawn's unoriginal book*. NewBuddhist.com. Retrieved April 9, 2016 from http://newbuddhist.com/discussion/13742/goldie-hawns-unoriginal-book

Tweed, T. A. (2006). *Crossing and dwelling: A theory of religion*. Cambridge, MA: Harvard University Press.

Van Gordon, W. & Griffiths, M. D. (2015, July). For mindful teaching of mindfulness. *The Psychologist*. Retrieved March 31, 2016 from thepsychologist.bps.org.uk/volume-28/july-2015/mindful-teaching-mindfulness

Vieten, C., & Scammell, S. (2015). *Spiritual and religious competencies in clinical practice*. Oakland, CA: New Harbinger Publications.

Vo, D. (2013, November 12). Comment on F. Hsu, The heart of mindfulness: A response to the New York Times. *Buddhist Peace Fellowship*. Retrieved April 27, 2016 from http://www.buddhistpeacefellowship.org/the-heart-of-mindfulness-a-response-to-the-new-york-times/

Waldmann, M. R. (2001). Predictive versus diagnostic causal learning: Evidence from an overshadowing paradigm. *Psychonomic Bulletin and Review*, *8*(3), 600–608.

Walsh, R., & Roche, L. (1979). Precipitation of acute psychotic episodes by intensive medita-tion in individuals with a history of schizophrenia. *American Journal of Psychiatry, 136*(8), 1085–1086.

Walsh, R., & Shapiro, S. L. (2006). The meeting of meditative disciplines and Western psychology. *American Psychologist, 61*, 227–239.

Warnock, C. J. P. (2009). Who pays for providing spiritual care in healthcare settings? The ethical dilemma of taxpayers funding holistic healthcare and the First Amendment requirement for separation of church and state. *Journal of Religion and Health, 48*, 468–481.

Wilks, J. (2014, September 8). Secular mindfulness: Potential and pitfalls. *Insight Journal.* Retrieved January 4, 2016 from http://www.bcbsdharma.org/2014-10-8-insight-journal/

Wilks, J., Blacker, M. M., Boyce, B., Winston, D., & Goodman, T. (2015, spring). The mindfulness movement: What does it mean for Buddhism? *Buddhadharma: The Practitioner's Quarterly,* 46–55.

Williams, J. M. G., & Kabat-Zinn, J. (2011). Mindfulness: Diverse perspectives on its meaning, origins, and multiple applications at the intersection of science and Dharma. *Contemporary Buddhism, 12*(1), 1–18.

Wilson, J. (2014). *Mindful America: Meditation and the mutual transformation of Buddhism and American culture.* New York: Oxford University Press.

Wilson, J. (2015, December 4). *Buddhist practice beyond religion.* Mindfulness Inc.: Lecture at Smith College, Northampton, MA. Retrieved August 21, 2017 from http://www.smith.edu/buddhism/videos.php

Woodhead, L. (2014). Tactical and strategic religion. In N. M. Dessing, N. Jeldtoft, J. S. Nielsen, & L. Woodhead (Eds.), *Everyday lived Islam in Europe* (pp. 9–22). Farnham: Ashgate.

World Medical Association (1981/2015). *Declaration of Lisbon on the rights of the patient.* Lisbon: World Medical Assembly.

Wylie, M. S. (2015). The mindfulness explosion. *Psychotherapy Networker, 39*(1), 19–45.

Zaidman, N., Goldstein-Gidoni, O., & Nehemya, I. (2009). From temples to organizations: The introduction and packaging of spirituality. *Organization, 16*(4), 597–621.

Chapter 4
Professional Ethics and Personal Values in Mindfulness-Based Programs: A Secular Psychological Perspective

Ruth Baer and Laura M. Nagy

In Buddhist traditions, where most mindfulness practices have their roots, mindfulness training is accompanied by explicit instruction in ethical conduct (Monteiro, Musten, & Compson, 2015). In contemporary discussions of mindfulness, the most commonly cited of the Buddhist teachings on ethical conduct are the eightfold path and the five precepts. The former is described as a path to the cessation of suffering and includes eight elements: three representing ethical behavior (right speech, right action, and right livelihood), two representing wisdom (right view, right intention), and three representing mental or meditative development (right effort, right concentration, and right mindfulness). The term *right* signifies that each element of the path leads to reduced suffering for self and others (Amaro, 2015; Monteiro et al., 2015); for example, *right livelihood* means earning one's living in a way that is benevolent and causes no harm. Ethical behavior in the Buddhist traditions is further described in the five precepts: to refrain from killing, lying, stealing, sexual misconduct, and the misuse of intoxicants. These are sometimes expressed in more general terms (e.g., non-harmful speech) and are understood as methods of training that facilitate one's own awakening and the well-being of others, rather than as commandments from a higher authority (Amaro, 2015).

In developing the curricula for contemporary Western mindfulness-based programs (MBPs) in mainstream secular contexts, pioneers such as Jon Kabat-Zinn (1982) and Marsha Linehan (1993) adapted a variety of meditation practices from Buddhist traditions but did not include explicit instruction in the eightfold path, the five ethical precepts, or other Buddhist teachings. This was intentional and has several advantages. For cultural and legal reasons, mindfulness training can be provided in a wider range of contemporary Western settings if the programs are

R. Baer, PhD (✉) • L.M. Nagy
Department of Psychology, University of Kentucky,
115 Kastle Hall, Lexington, KY 40506-0044, USA
e-mail: rbaer@uky.edu; lauramsmart@gmail.com

© Springer International Publishing AG 2017   87
L.M. Monteiro et al. (eds.), *Practitioner's Guide to Ethics and Mindfulness-Based Interventions*, Mindfulness in Behavioral Health,
DOI 10.1007/978-3-319-64924-5_4

genuinely secular. In addition, many codes of professional ethics for providers of health care and mental health services require respect for participants' right of self-determination and respect for diversity in multiple domains, including religion and culture, among others. Adherence to these ethical standards typically means that health care and mental health professionals must be careful not to impose moral frameworks or religious beliefs on patients, clients, students, or other participants. Helping participants to clarify their own values and behave in values-congruent ways is more consistent with professional ethical codes and is an important element of many MBPs. Psychological research on working with values in MBPs is discussed later in this chapter.

MBPs have exploded in popularity and are now available in a variety of mainstream environments, including medical and mental health settings, schools, workplaces, prisons, and the military. Numerous reviews of the literature (Chiesa, Calati, & Serretti, 2011; Eberth & Sedlmeier, 2012; Khoury, Sharma, Rush, & Fournier, 2015; Khoury et al., 2013; Tang, Hölzel, & Posner, 2015) have shown that MBPs have many benefits. Strong evidence supports their efficacy for reducing anxiety, depression, and stress and for helping people cope with illness and pain. Some studies show that MBPs increase positive moods and cultivate compassion for self and others. MBPs may also improve some forms of attention and memory and they appear to have measurable effects on the brain. Although the research base is stronger for some outcomes than for others, the efficacy of MBPs seems reasonably clear. However, concerns have been expressed about the relationship between contemporary MBPs and the ancient Buddhist traditions from which many mindfulness practices originate. Many of these concerns involve ethical issues, and they come from diverse perspectives, with some authors suggesting that contemporary MBPs are too close to their Buddhist roots while others argue that too much of the Buddhism has been stripped away (Baer, 2015).

For example, some authors have expressed the view that, because mindfulness has its roots in Buddhism, MBPs are inherently spiritual (Monteiro, 2016) or even Buddhist (Purser, 2015), and that claims of secularity are misleading and may violate professional ethical standards related to truthful communication and informed consent (Purser, 2015; Van Gordon & Griffiths, 2015). That is, if a program is Buddhist-based, professional ethics codes may require this to be communicated clearly in descriptive material and informed consent documents. Failure to do so may lead to accusations of *stealth Buddhism* (Purser, 2015) and may violate laws as well as ethical standards. These issues arose in the case of the Calmer Choice program, a public-school-based MBP in the USA, where the constitution prohibits religious programs in government-funded settings (Jennings, 2016). Calmer Choice was challenged by the National Center for Law and Policy, which argued that the program is Buddhist in orientation and violates the constitutional prohibition against government establishment of religion. Other legal experts disagreed. According to the Cape Cod Times (February 4, 2016), an attorney for the American Civil Liberties Union expressed the following opinion:

Many mindfulness and yoga programs in schools are considered secular, nonreligious activities and do not violate the Establishment Clause...Simply because an activity or concept may be similar to that in one or many religions does not make it religious; otherwise, for example, schools would not be able to teach students to be kind to each other. Here, the school system has a secular purpose in using the Calmer Choice program, and there is no indication the town is endorsing any religion. This is not an Establishment Clause violation.

The legal challenge to Calmer Choice was dropped before the case went to court and the program remains in place. Although this case was never adjudicated, the circumstances suggest that mindfulness-based programs in American public schools, or other government-funded settings, may be subject to legal challenge if they are perceived as religiously based. American courts are likely to examine whether such programs have the effect of advancing religion or creating an excessive entanglement between government and religion (Lindahl, 2015; Witte, 2005). The inclusion in the curriculum of explicit instruction in a Buddhist ethical framework, such as the eightfold path or the five precepts, might make it more difficult to argue that a program is suitable for a secular setting.

On the other hand, some authors have noted that in Buddhist traditions, mindfulness is intended to facilitate the growth of insight, wisdom, and virtue over a lifetime (Davidson, 2016), rather than symptom reduction or improved well-being in the shorter term, and have raised concerns about the extent to which contemporary MBPs have "dissociated a practice from the ethical framework for which it was originally developed" (Harrington & Dunne, 2015, p. 621). According to this perspective, the absence of explicitly taught ethics in MBPs might contribute to the use of mindfulness for harmful purposes. A commonly cited example is the provision of mindfulness training within businesses or corporations, whose profit-driven activities might cause harm to the environment, the economy, or their employees' well-being. Some authors have suggested that without explicit instruction in ethics, mindfulness training might promote employees' acquiescence with unethical business practices or passive acceptance of oppressive working conditions (Purser, 2015).

In response to these concerns, MBPs have been developed that include explicit teaching of Buddhist foundations, including the eightfold path, the five ethical precepts, and conceptions of impermanence and nonself. Known as second-generation MBPs (Margolin, Beitel, Schuman-Olivier, & Avants, 2006; Margolin et al., 2007; Shonin, Van Gordon, Dunn, Singh, & Griffiths, 2014), these programs have been shown in several studies to have significant effects on psychological functioning. However, there is no evidence that they are more effective than MBPs that do not include explicit Buddhist-based training. Moreover, participants' willingness to resist unethical business practices or oppressive working conditions is rarely assessed. In a worksite study of one of the second-generation MBPs, middle managers reported that the program helped them to be "less preoccupied with their own agenda and entitlements" and "better able to align themselves with corporate strategy" (Shonin & Van Gordon, 2015). Shonin et al. (2014) suggested that:

Via the meditation-induced understanding that there is not a self that exists inherently, independently, or as a permanent entity, employees can begin to dismantle their emphasis on the
"I," the "me," and the "mine," and can better synchronize their own interests with those of
the organizations. (p. 819)

The authors did not comment on the ethical practices or working conditions of
the businesses in which the participants were employed. It is unclear whether or
how the explicitly Buddhist-based elements of the training would have influenced
participants' responses to an ethically problematic work environment.

This worksite study showed significant reductions in distress and improvements
in job satisfaction and performance. Accordingly, we acknowledge that explicitly
Buddhist-based MBPs may be useful and effective in some environments. However,
we argue that for legal, ethical, and cultural reasons, secular MBPs are essential for
many settings. We also argue that the adaptation of mindfulness practices from
Buddhist traditions into contemporary MBPs for mainstream settings does not lead
to a form of mindfulness that is devoid of ethics; rather, mindfulness becomes integrated into contexts and systems that have their own ethical standards (Crane, 2016).
In the health care and mental health fields, these standards are articulated in codes
of ethics that guide the conduct of professionals in the delivery of their services,
including MBPs. In addition, psychological research and practice are increasingly
concerned with the role of personal values in mental health. The recent psychological literature describes a variety of methods for identifying personal values and
strengthening values-consistent behavior.

In the remainder of this chapter, we elaborate on professional ethics and personal
values as two ways of addressing ethical issues related to MBPs. We argue that these
two perspectives can work together to serve the interests and well-being of people
seeking help through MBPs, as well as the teachers, therapists, and other professionals who provide the MBPs. We then conclude with a brief discussion of challenges facing the young but maturing field of mindfulness teaching as it develops its
own standards of ethics and integrity.

Professional Ethics

In the following sections, we provide an overview of professional ethics codes for
the health care and mental health fields and make three general points. First, current
professional ethics codes are grounded in a long tradition that spans many centuries
and reflects values held by many cultures around the world. Second, contemporary
ethics codes for psychology and related professions articulate principles and standards that are both entirely secular and generally consistent with the ethical teachings of the eightfold path and the five precepts. Third, professional ethics codes
support the health care and mental health professions as fields that are neither religious, necessarily spiritual, nor values-neutral. That is, when responsibly integrated
into the health care and mental health fields, mindfulness-based training can be both
entirely secular and firmly rooted in ethical values.

Background: Professional Ethics in Psychology

Most professions that serve the public are underpinned by codes of ethics. Such codes serve several purposes (Fisher, 2016). They educate and socialize students, trainees, and members of the profession by clarifying mutual expectations for professional behavior. They provide guidance for resolving ethical dilemmas that arise in professional work. A well-articulated ethics code demonstrates to the public that the profession has a consensus on acceptable professional conduct and clear standards for acting in consumers' interests. When consumers have complaints about professional services, an ethics code assists the courts, licensing boards, and other agencies empowered to evaluate professional behavior and, if necessary, impose consequences for ethical violations. Finally, a profession that shows convincingly that it can regulate itself with an ethics code may be less susceptible to regulation by external authorities, who might make rules that seem unreasonable to members of the profession (Fisher, 2016).

The health care and mental health professions, including medicine, psychology, social work, and others, are governed by long-standing and continually evolving codes of ethics. The first ethics code for psychologists was developed by the American Psychological Association (APA), beginning in 1947, when the professional activity of psychologists, which previously had focused primarily on research, was expanding to include provision of mental health services. The APA's code was developed using the critical incident method. APA members were invited to send in descriptions of ethically challenging situations they had encountered in their work and to comment on the issues involved. A committee reviewed over 1000 incidents and extracted ethical themes. Most of these were concerned with psychologists' relationships with and responsibilities to others, including clients or patients, students, research participants, and other professionals. A series of drafts of the proposed ethics code was provided to the APA membership for comment. After several revisions, the first version of the code was published in 1953 (Fisher, 2016).

APA's ethics code is frequently updated, with ten revisions published since 1953. The revision process continues to be based on the experiences and perspectives of APA members and reflects the evolving roles of psychologists in society; these include therapy or counseling, teaching, supervision, consultation, administration, program development and evaluation, and research (Fisher, 2016). The current version of the code (APA 2002, 2010) has separate sections for aspirational principles and enforceable standards of conduct. The five aspirational principles intended to "guide and inspire psychologists toward the very highest ethical ideals of the profession" (APA, 2002, p. 3) are:

Beneficence and nonmaleficence: Psychologists strive to benefit the people with whom they work and to avoid causing harm. They protect the rights and welfare of all who might be affected by their work. They guard against personal, financial, social, organizational, or political factors that might lead to misuse of their influence.

Fidelity and responsibility: Psychologists strive to establish relationships of trust with the individuals and groups with whom they work and with their communities and society.

Integrity: Psychologists strive to be honest, truthful, and accurate in all aspects of their work. They keep their promises and do not "steal, cheat, or engage in fraud, subterfuge, or intentional misrepresentation of fact" (p. 3).

Justice: Psychologists strive for fairness in all aspects of their work, including equal access and quality of services for all.

Respect for rights and dignity: Psychologists recognize people's rights to privacy, confidentiality, and self-determination. They respect diversity based on age, gender, gender identity, race, ethnicity, culture, national origin, religion, sexual orientation, disability, language, and socioeconomic status. They strive to eliminate bias based on any of these factors from their work.

Because they are defined as aspirational, the five general principles of APA's ethics code do not provide a basis for disciplinary bodies to impose sanctions on psychologists charged with ethical violations. In contrast, the standards of conduct are enforceable and cover a variety of specific issues relevant to the practice of psychology, including confidentiality, informed consent, conflict of interest, advertising, record keeping, fees, and many others. Some of the standards of conduct do not require specific behavior, but instead describe issues to be considered in managing potentially challenging situations. For example, multiple relationships (e.g., providing professional services to a neighbor or relative) are not firmly prohibited, but should be avoided if they are likely to impair the psychologist's objectivity, competence, or effectiveness, or if they pose a risk of harm or exploitation to the client. For other standards, specific behaviors are required or proscribed. For example, psychologists must obtain informed consent before conducting a psychological evaluation. They are prohibited from making false statements about their credentials or their services and from engaging in sexual intimacies with clients.

Historical Roots of Psychological Ethics Codes

Although psychology is a relatively young profession, the APA's ethics code follows a centuries-long tradition of medical ethics codes from many parts of the world. According to Sinclair (2012), the field of medicine has the longest documented history of ethics codes of any profession. The oldest known code of medical ethics is found in the *Code of Hammurabi* from the Babylonian empire (eighteenth century BCE); it includes nine laws related to the practice of medicine, as well as numerous laws covering other matters. Two other medical ethics codes have survived from before the common era. The *Ayurvedic Instruction*, from India in the sixth century BCE, provides instructions to medical students on ethical medical practice. The *Hippocratic Oath*, from Greece (fourth century BCE), is part of a larger work called the *Hippocratic Corpus* and describes ethical responsibilities of physicians to those they serve. The *Corpus* has been studied for centuries by physicians in many parts of the world. Modified versions of the Hippocratic Oath are still used today in many medical schools as part of a ritual for graduating students.

Medical ethics codes from within the common era include *Advice to a Physician* (from Persia, 950), whose first chapter is devoted entirely to medical ethics; the *Seventeen Rules of Enjuin* (1500), written for Japanese medical students and based on Buddhist thought and the Shinto tradition; the *Five Commandments and Ten Requirements* (1617), the most comprehensive description of medical ethics in China from before the twentieth century; and *A Physician's Ethical Duties* (1770), also from Persia. More recent codes include the *Medical Code of Ethics of the American Medical Association* (1847) and the *Nuremburg Code of Ethics in Medical Research* (1946); the latter was developed in response to the atrocities of medical experimentation with prisoners in concentration camps during World War II.

As the first ethics code for psychologists, the APA's code served as a model for related professions (forensic psychiatry, psychiatric nursing, pastoral counseling, psychoanalysis, marriage and family therapy, school counseling, substance abuse counseling, etc.) and for ethics codes in other countries. Many adopted the organizational structure of the APA's code, with separate sections for aspirational principles and enforceable standards of conduct. Others adopted a "moral framework format" (Sinclair, 2012, p. 16) in which the entire code is organized around core ethical principles. One example is the British Psychological Society's (2009) ethics code, which articulates four core principles: respect, competence, responsibility, and integrity. Subsumed under each principle is a statement of values to guide ethical reasoning and a set of behavioral standards describing the conduct expected of the Society's members. For example, the principle of respect is defined by valuing the dignity and worth of all persons; specific behavioral standards are related to privacy and confidentiality, informed consent, respect for individual and cultural differences, and self-determination. The principle of integrity is defined by the values of honesty, accuracy, clarity, and fairness; the behavioral standards govern all forms of professional communication, avoidance of exploitation and conflict of interest, maintenance of personal boundaries (no sexual or romantic relationships with clients, students, or junior colleagues), and avoidance of all forms of harassment.

Commonalities Among Historical and Current Ethics Codes

The *Universal Declaration of Ethical Principles for Psychologists* (2008) was developed by a joint committee of the International Union of Psychological Science and the International Association of Applied Psychology (Gauthier, Pettifor, & Ferrero, 2010). Based on a six-year study of psychological ethics codes from around the world, it describes ethical principles that are common to most codes and believed to be based on widely shared human values. The *Universal Declaration* is aspirational only and provides values related to each core principle but no enforceable

Table 4.1 Core principles and related values of the *Universal Declaration of Ethical Principles for Psychologists*

Core principle	Related values
I. Respect for the dignity of persons and peoples	• Respect for the unique worth and inherent dignity of all human beings • Respecting diversity, customs, and beliefs • Free and informed consent • Privacy and confidentiality • Fairness and justice
II. Competent caring for the well-being of persons and peoples	• Active concern for well-being • Taking care not to do harm • Maximizing benefits and minimizing harm • Correcting or offsetting harm • Developing and maintaining competence • Self-knowledge • Respect for the ability of persons and peoples to care for themselves and others
III. Integrity	• Honesty • Truthfulness and openness • Avoiding incomplete disclosure • Maximizing impartiality and minimizing biases • Avoiding conflicts of interest
IV. Professional and scientific responsibilities to society	• Increasing knowledge in ways that promote the well-being of society and all its members • Using psychological knowledge for beneficial purposes and preventing it from being misused • Conducting its affairs in a way that promotes the well-being of society and all its members • Adequately training its members in their ethical responsibilities and required competencies • Developing ethical awareness and sensitivity • Being as self-correcting as possible

standards of conduct, which are expected to vary across cultures. A central objective of the *Universal Declaration* is to provide a moral framework that psychological organizations anywhere in the world can use to develop or evaluate their own ethics codes. Its four core principles are very similar to those of the British Psychological Society, the Canadian Code of Ethics for Psychologists, and several others; they also overlap substantially with the five aspirational principles of the APA's code. The core principles and related values of the *Universal Declaration* are shown in Table 4.1.

To examine commonalities among the historical ethics codes described earlier and to compare them with contemporary codes, Sinclair (2012) organized elements of the historical codes into categories based on the four principles of the *Universal Declaration*. This work, summarized in Table 4.2, shows considerable consistency across history and cultures in ethical principles for the medical and psychological professions. A notable exception is the *Code of Hammurabi*, which, according to Sinclair (2012), has little in common with the four principles of the *Universal*

Table 4.2 (continued)

Ethical codes	Respect for dignity	Competent caring for well-being	Integrity	Professional and scientific responsibilities
The Seventeen Rules of Enjuin Japan, 1500	You should rescue even such people as you dislike or hate. You should not tell what you have learned from the time you enter a woman's room.	You should be delighted if, after treating a patient without success, the patient receives medicine from another physician and is cured.	You should not exhibit avarice, and you must not strain to become famous.	(None)
The Five Commandments and Ten Requirements China, 1617	Physicians should be ever ready to respond to any calls of patients, high or low, rich or poor. They should treat them equally. The secret diseases of female patients…should not be revealed to anybody…	A physician or surgeon must first know the principles of the learned. He must study all the ancient standard medical books ceaselessly day and night, and understand them thoroughly so that the principles enlighten his eyes and are impressed on his heart.	If the case improves, drugs may be sent, but physicians should not visit them again for lewd reward.	(None)
A Physician's Ethical Duties Persia, 1770	He must not be proud of his class or family and must not regard others with contempt. A physician…must protect the patient's secrets and not betray them	He must never be tenacious in his opinion, and continue in his fault or mistake, but, if it possible, he is to consult with proficient physicians and ascertain the facts.	Practice medicine with integrity… Do not replace precious herbal materials provided by the family of patients with inferior ones. A physician…must not hold his students or his patients under his obligation.	He must not withhold medical knowledge; he should teach it to everyone in medicine without discrimination between poor and rich, noble or slave.
Medical Code of Ethics of the American Medical Association USA, 1847	…such professional services should always be cheerfully and freely accorded. …none of the privacies of personal and domestic life… should ever be divulged…	Every case committed to the charge of a physician should be treated with attention, steadiness, and humanity. Consultations should be promoted in difficult cases…	…unnecessary visits are to be avoided as they…render him liable to be suspected of interested motives.	As good citizens, it is the duty of physicians to be ever vigilant for the welfare of the community, and to bear their part in sustaining its institutions and burdens.

Table 4.2 Elements of medical ethics codes across centuries and cultures and their relationships to the four principles of the *Universal Declaration of Ethical Principles for Psychologists* (Sinclair, 2012)

Ethical codes	Respect for dignity	Competent caring for well-being	Integrity	Professional and scientific responsibilities
Code of Hammurabi Babylonian empire Eighteenth century BCE	If a physician…saves the eye, he shall receive ten shekels… If the patient be a freed man, he receives five shekels…If he be a slave, his owner shall give the physician two shekels	(None)	(None)	(None)
Ayurvedic Instruction India, sixth century BCE	It is the duty of all good physicians to treat…all Brahmins, spiritual guides, paupers, friends, neighbors, devotees, orphans, and people who come from a distance as if they are his own friends.	You should, with your whole heart, strive to bring about the cure of those that are ill. There is no end to medical science, hence, heedfully devote yourself to it.	You shall speak words that are… truthful, beneficial, and properly weighed and measured. You should give up… deception, falsehood…and other reprehensible conduct.	You should always seek, whether standing or sitting, the good of all living creatures.
Hippocratic Oath Greece, fourth century BCE	Whatever houses I may visit, I will come for the benefit of the sick, remaining free of all intentional injustice…	I will keep them from harm… I will apply dietetic measures for the benefit of the sick according to my ability and judgment…	Whatever houses I might visit, I will come for the benefit of the sick, remaining free of… all mischief, and in particular of sexual relations with both male and female persons, be they free or slaves.	…to give a share of precepts and oral instruction and all the other learning to my sons and the sons of him who has instructed me, and to pupils who have…taken an oath according to the medical law.
Advice to a Physician Persia, 950	A physician should respect confidences and respect the patient's secrets. In protecting a patient's secrets, he must be more insistent than the patient himself.	A medical student should be constantly present in the hospital so as to study disease processes and complications under the learned professor and proficient physicians.	A physician is to prudently treat his patients with food and medicine out of good and spiritual motives, not for the sake of gain.	Be kind to the children of your teachers and if one of them wants to study medicine you are to teach him without any remuneration.

(continued)

Declaration and indicates that not everyone was considered of equal worth in the society of the time. The remaining comparisons show that contemporary psychological ethics codes, as reflected in the principles of the *Universal Declaration*, are rooted in traditions that extend at least 26 centuries into the past and come from many parts of the world. Common values include concern for well-being, professional competence, maximizing benefit and minimizing harm, confidentiality, avoiding conflicts of interest, and truthfulness.

Professional Ethics and Buddhist Ethics

Contemporary ethics codes provide a "common morality" (Knapp & VandeCreek, 2006, p. 4) among professionals whose religious and spiritual backgrounds, moral beliefs, and philosophies are likely to be diverse. The APA acknowledges this diversity among psychologists by making its code entirely secular and applicable "only to psychologists' activities that are part of their scientific, educational, or professional roles as psychologists" and not to "purely private conduct of psychologists" (APA, 2002, p. 2). This respect for the religious and cultural diversity of the psychologists themselves parallels the code's requirement to respect the diversity of people with whom psychologists work. That is, neither psychologists nor their clients are required to adopt an ethical framework based on a particular religious or spiritual tradition.

Even so, substantial commonality between the APA's code and the ethical teachings described in the eightfold path and the five precepts is evident. The entire code can be seen as an attempt to ensure that the practice of psychology, in its many manifestations, is a form of right livelihood; i.e., a way of earning a living that is benevolent and minimizes harm. In both general and specific ways, much of the code deals with right action and/or right speech. The aspiration to do no harm is central to the ethics code and is expressed in many of the standards of conduct; for example, psychologists are prohibited from engaging in discrimination, harassment, and exploitation. Following a controversy about psychologists' involvement in military interrogations of post-9/11 detainees, they are also prohibited from activities that would "justify or defend violating human rights" (APA, 2010, p. 4, 2015).

The general principle of integrity and numerous related standards require psychologists to be truthful and to refrain from stealing (or taking things not given, Goldstein & Kornfield, 2001); for example, psychologists must not make false or deceptive statements about their credentials, fees, services, or other aspects of their work. They may not use bait-and-switch tactics (i.e., luring clients with an initial low fee and then unexpectedly raising their rates), and must not submit false information to insurance companies to increase reimbursements. The code explicitly prohibits sexual intimacies with clients, clients' relatives or significant others, students, and supervisees. Misuse of intoxicants is not explicitly mentioned, but psychologists are required to refrain from undertaking professional activities when personal problems (such as substance misuse) could interfere with their ability to work competently.

The APA's code also includes standards related to preventing harm when working in organizations. Fisher (2016) notes that organizations often hire psychologists to meet the organization's goals, rather than the employees' goals. For example, an organization might hire a psychologist to develop a screening test to identify applicants likely to be competent and productive in particular positions. If the psychologist follows the ethical standards for test construction and use, i.e., develops a test that meets adequate standards for reliability, validity, and culture-fairness and explains the nature and purpose of the test to applicants, there is no conflict with the ethics code. On the other hand, if a business wishing to let go of senior employees as a cost-cutting strategy asks a psychologist to develop a test that would be difficult for older employees to pass, this would violate the principle of justice and the ethical standards related to unfair discrimination, test construction, and use of assessments (Fisher, 2016). The psychologist in this situation is ethically obligated to refuse to design or administer such an instrument.

Ethical Professional Services and Values-Neutrality

Several authors have noted that psychological practice is not a values-neutral enterprise (Hathaway, 2011; Monteiro, 2016); indeed, values pervade the process in a variety of ways. In addition to the professional ethics codes, which imbue the process with widely shared values (benevolence, non-harming, respect, integrity, responsibility, competence), individual psychologists have their own values, as do their clients, students, and other participants. Despite the inescapable and complex influences of these sets of values on professional work, the delivery of psychological services sometimes appears to be values-neutral. This paradox is attributable to elements of the ethics codes that require professionals to respect the right of self-determination and the diverse perspectives of their clients in a wide range of domains, including domains in which professionals and clients may hold very different views.

For example, if a client in psychotherapy discloses that she is accidentally pregnant and considering an abortion, the ethical therapist may help the client explore her thoughts and feelings on the matter and the possible impact of this decision (either way) on her mental health, but must maintain an evenhanded openness that honors the client's right to make her own decision about whether to continue the pregnancy, regardless of the therapist's personal or religious beliefs about the morality of abortion. The same applies to clients with problems related to sexual orientation, divorce, end-of-life questions for the terminally ill, and other potentially controversial matters, and to clients who express racist, sexist, political, or other opinions that the therapist finds objectionable.

Maintaining this stance of apparent neutrality regarding specific issues that arise in treatment does not require professionals to give up their religious, spiritual, or other values; however, professionals are more likely to work competently with diversity in these areas if they are aware of their own beliefs and values and their potential impact on their work (Vieten et al., 2013). For example, a therapist who is clearly in touch with her belief that homosexual behavior is immoral may have better awareness of her responses to an adolescent client reporting same-sex attraction; similarly, a self-aware therapist who supports legal abortion may be better able to monitor his responses to a client who finds purpose in life by picketing abortion clinics. Self-awareness and reflection are essential if therapists are to make sound decisions about how to work ethically with clients who present them with difficult conflicts between their personal values and their professional obligation to respect their clients' values.

The stance of apparent neutrality about clients' values has limits. Respect for clients' autonomy and diversity does not require unqualified endorsement of moral relativism, which holds that all standards of conduct are equally valid (Knapp & VandeCreek, 2007). For example, if a client expresses an intention to commit an act of violence (e.g., to assault or kill someone, or to set off an explosion in a public place), the therapist must take steps to prevent it, and if unable to dissuade the client is legally required (in most of the USA) to warn the intended victim (if identifiable) and to inform the police. That is, the therapist is not required to respect the client's intention to commit violence, even if this intention is based on a religious, moral, or philosophical belief system to which the client is deeply committed. Similarly, a therapist working with parents who use abusive forms of punishment with their children must try to help the parents modify their disciplinary strategies and, if unable to do so, may have to notify child protection authorities, even if the parents believe their disciplinary methods to be normative within their culture.

In these difficult situations, respectful dialogue may enable skilled professionals to help their clients find non-harmful ways of achieving their goals while respecting their belief systems and cultural norms. However, when abuse is clearly occurring, or when violent harm is imminent, the principles of benevolence and non-malevolence temporarily supersede respect for clients' autonomy. Knapp and VandeCreek (2007) describe this stance as a form of *soft universalism*: a middle position between ethical absolutism, which holds that there is one universally valid ethical code, and moral relativism. Soft universalism assumes that many values are widely endorsed, but that cultures and societies differ on how they are expressed. Soft universalism underlies the Universal Declaration of Ethical Principles for Psychologists described earlier, which articulates core principles and related values, but includes no specific standards of conduct, because the latter "will vary with different religious, social, and political beliefs and conditions" (Pettifor, 2004, p. 265).

Professional Ethics for Spiritually Oriented Interventions

Spiritually oriented interventions are difficult to define. Hathaway (2011) notes that some authors use this term for interventions that include clearly religious elements such as references to scripture, religious imagery, or prayer (Richards

& Bergin, 2005). Other authors describe meditation, exploration of meaning and purpose, kindness, forgiveness, and gratitude as spiritual practices or tools (Plante, 2009). Kapuscinski and Masters (2010) suggest that a focus on God or the transcendent distinguishes spirituality from constructs such as meaning, purpose, and wisdom; from this perspective, interventions that work explicitly with these concepts are not necessarily spiritual. Kristeller (2011) states that within contemporary therapeutic contexts, "a wholly secular practice of meditation has developed" (p. 197), while noting that "the spiritual foundation has never been too far away" (p. 198).

In the mindfulness literature, a variety of views is evident. Monteiro (2016) notes that the Buddhist roots of mindfulness mean that MBIs can be considered "a class of spiritually oriented approaches" (p. 216). Vieten and Scammell (2015) state that many mindfulness and yoga programs are "largely secularized" but may include elements with "quasi-spiritual undertones" such as the ringing of bells and prayers of compassion (p. 114). The developers of MBCT (Segal, Williams, & Teasdale, 2013) do not discuss spirituality; however, in an adaptation of MBCT for the general public, Williams and Penman (2011) state that meditation and mindfulness are not a religion and can be practiced by people of any religion as well as by atheists and agnostics. Linehan (2015), the developer of dialectical behavior therapy (DBT), states that mindfulness can be taught and practiced in either a secular or a spiritual way; accordingly, the mindfulness skills in DBT are "purposely provided in a secular format" (p. 151) while guidelines for optional discussion of mindfulness as a spiritual practice are provided for therapists whose clients are interested in this perspective.

Clearly, MBPs are not always conceptualized as spiritually oriented; however, when they are, professional ethics for spiritually oriented interventions should be considered (Vieten & Scammell, 2015). Several mental health disciplines have begun to discuss spiritual and religious competencies and ethical guidelines for providers of spiritually oriented programs, including psychology, psychiatry (Campbell, Stuck, & Frinks, 2012; Verhagen & Cox, 2010), social work (Sheridan, 2009), and counseling (Young, Cashwell, Wiggins-Frame, & Belaire, 2002). Division 36 of APA (the Society for Psychology of Religion and Spirituality) developed a set of preliminary practice guidelines for clinical work with religious and spiritual issues (Hathaway, 2011; Hathaway & Ripley, 2009). These include obtaining informed consent for the use of spiritually oriented methods, accommodating clients' spiritual or religious traditions in helpful ways, and setting spiritual or religious treatment goals only if they are functionally relevant to the clients' concerns, among many others. Awareness of contraindications for spiritually oriented methods is also recommended; these might include psychotic symptoms, substantial personality pathology, and bizarre or idiosyncratic expressions of religion or spirituality. If iatrogenic effects become evident, spiritually oriented methods should be discontinued.

Personal Values

In the discussion of ethics in MBPs, personal values are important for two reasons. First, in secular settings, where teaching a particular ethical framework may be problematic, a promising alternative is to help participants to clarify their own values and strengthen their values-consistent behavior (Davis, 2015). Second, in addition to the values reflected in the ethics codes, professionals bring their own values to their work. The personal values of mindfulness-based teachers are likely to be generally consistent with ethics codes (benevolence, non-harming, integrity, etc.); however, values conflicts can arise around specific issues or circumstances and self-awareness is essential to navigating these situations skillfully. The following sections discuss psychological theories and research about personal values and the methods used in MBPs for working with values. Most of the literature on values in MBPs examines benefits to clinical or general populations; however, a few studies suggest that working with values also improves clinical skills and attitudes in mental health professionals.

Working with Values in MBPs

Among the evidence-based programs in which mindfulness skills are central, acceptance and commitment therapy (ACT; Hayes, Strosahl, & Wilson, 2012) provides the most comprehensive theoretical formulations about values and mental health, as well as methods for helping participants identify their values and behave in accordance with them. Values in ACT, therefore, are described in detail in the next section, followed by discussion of values-based methods in other MBPs.

ACT is based on a comprehensive theory of human functioning that integrates mindfulness- and acceptance-based processes with personally chosen values and values-consistent behavior (known as committed action). The mindfulness and acceptance processes in ACT are similar to those described in other MBPs and include flexible attention to the present moment, acceptance of present-moment experiences, defusion from thoughts (similar to decentering in MBCT), and a transcendent sense of self (recognition that thoughts and feelings are transitory events that do not define the person who is experiencing them). In ACT, values are conceptualized as essential to good psychological health because they intrinsically motivate behavior that leads to a deep sense of meaning, vitality, and engagement. The goal of ACT is to help clients develop lives that feel rich and satisfying—though not painless or easy—by the clients' own standards (Hayes et al., 2012).

In helping clients to identify their values, ACT therapists typically encourage the exploration of several domains that are important in many people's lives. Domains are suggested, rather than prescribed, to help clients focus on what may be most important to them. Commonly discussed domains include relationships (with family or friends), work (career, education, or running a household), community involvement (working for worthy causes, participating in community activities), spirituality (church involvement, communing with nature, or other practices identified by the client), and self-development (learning new skills, taking care of one's health, engaging in satisfying leisure activities). The importance of choosing one's own values, rather than those prescribed by authority figures or societal norms, is emphasized.

Discussion of values in ACT also includes qualities or characteristics that clients would like to embody in the domains that are most important to them. In the work domain, for example, clients may aspire to be creative, competent, or productive. In the relationship domain, they may wish to be loving, kind, supportive, assertive, or strong. Values are distinguished from goals, in that goals can be completed (e.g., learn a new software program, teach coworkers to use it), whereas the underlying values (to be competent and helpful at work) continue over the longer term. Upon completion of specific goals, other ways to be competent and helpful will present themselves.

Behaving in accordance with values can be stressful and difficult. Unpleasant thoughts and emotions may arise and these may become obstacles to committed action. Mindful awareness is conceptualized as a way to help clients work constructively with internal obstacles to values-consistent behavior. For example, a person who values helpfulness at work, but is anxious about speaking in groups might practice contributing to discussion with mindful acceptance of the unpleasant sensations (racing heart, sweating), rather than keeping quiet in meetings to avoid the stress of speaking up. The goal of ACT is not to decrease anxiety in meetings, though this may occur with consistent practice. Rather, the goal is to help the client develop a life that feels satisfying and meaningful, even when it is distressing or painful.

ACT has developed several tools to help clients explore their values. The Valued Living Questionnaire (Wilson, Sandoz, Flynn, Slater, & DuFrene, 2010), which is often used as a structured interview (Wilson & DuFrene, 2008), asks clients to consider 12 potentially valued domains: marriage, parenting, other family, friends, work, education, recreation, spirituality, community life, physical self-care (diet, exercise, sleep), the environment, and aesthetics (art, literature, music, beauty). Clients are urged to remember that not everyone values all of the domains; for example, some prefer not to marry or raise children, others may have little interest in community activities or spirituality. Discussion centers on the self-rated importance of each area, the client's actions in each area, and their satisfaction with their level of action. Clients who discover that they have been focusing on areas of low priority while neglecting domains they identify as important are helped to redirect their energies in more satisfying ways. Mindful compassion provides a helpful way of relating to the pain and regret associated with realizing that one's priorities may have been misplaced.

ACT also uses experiential exercises to help clients identify important values. Clients may be asked to write a brief epitaph for their own future tombstone that captures how they would like to be remembered; e.g., "He participated in life and helped his fellow human beings" (Hayes et al., 2012, p. 306). Alternatively, they might write a short speech they would like someone to give at a birthday party in their honor; for example, "John always puts the needs of his children first, guiding them with love, patience, and respect" or "Through her tireless volunteer work, Camille has helped to make our world a safer and cleaner place for all living beings" (Fleming & Kocovski, 2013, p. 32). Such exercises are followed by discussion of behaviors consistent with these values, especially behavioral changes needed to address values-behavior discrepancies. Mindfulness skills that may be helpful in working with barriers to committed action, such as pessimistic or self-critical thoughts ("This will never work," "I've wasted too much time"), and negative emotions (anxiety, sadness) are also practiced.

Many studies have shown that ACT leads to significant increases in self-reported psychological flexibility, defined as the ability to fully contact the present moment and behave in values-consistent ways in the presence of difficult thoughts and feelings (Hayes, Luoma, Bond, Masuda, & Lillis, 2006; Ruiz, 2010). Treatment outcome studies have not examined the effects of values work independently of the other components of ACT; however, laboratory studies suggest that even brief consideration of personal values leads to reliable changes in behavior. For example, in a study of pain tolerance using the cold pressor task (immersing a hand in very cold water), Branstetter-Rost, Cushing, and Douleh (2009) asked one group to imagine tolerating the pain for the sake of a highly ranked personal value (e.g., swimming in icy water to rescue a loved one), whereas a second group was coached in how to practice mindful acceptance of the pain with no reference to personal values, and a third group received no instructions for tolerating the pain. The values group tolerated the pain for significantly longer than the acceptance and no-instructions groups (means of 156, 69, and 36 s, respectively, $p < 0.001$). Several other laboratory studies have reported similar findings (Levin, Hildebrandt, Lillis, & Hayes, 2012).

Most treatment outcome studies of ACT are conducted with clinical populations or other volunteers; however, a small literature suggests that ACT is also helpful for improving professional skills in mental health clinicians. For example, Hayes et al. (2004) randomly assigned substance abuse counselors to an ACT-based training, multicultural training, or psychoeducation, and found that at 6-month follow-up, the ACT group showed significantly lower frequency of stigmatizing thoughts about their clients as well as reduced burnout. Clarke, Taylor, Lancaster, and Remington (2015) found that both ACT and psychoeducation, delivered in workshop format over two days, led to significant reductions in stigmatizing attitudes and improvements in therapist–client relationships in a large group of clinicians working with people with personality disorders.

Working with values has been incorporated into other evidence-based MBPs. During a sitting meditation in the final session of MBCT (Segal et al., 2013), participants are invited to contemplate a personal value (such as caring for themselves or spending more time with their children) that provides a reason to maintain their meditation practice. They write the values that come to mind on cards to keep with them. Mindfulness-based relapse prevention (Bowen, Chawla, & Marlatt, 2011) includes discussion of reasons to stay sober; these typically reflect important values such as working responsibly at a job, caring for a child, or relating to a spouse. Dialectical behavior therapy (DBT; Linehan, 2015) includes exploration of values as part of building a life that feels satisfying and meaningful. Although potential values are suggested to help clients consider possibilities (e.g., healthy relationships, productive work, contributing to the community), clients are strongly encouraged to identify values that are truly their own. Acceptance-based behavior therapy (Roemer, Orsillo, & Salters-Pednault, 2008), which integrates elements of ACT, MBCT, and DBT, uses writing exercises to help clients explore what they value in a variety of domains and includes goal setting and behavior change methods for increasing values-consistent behavior. Mindfulness-based eating awareness training (Kristeller, Wolever, & Sheets, 2014) helps participants consider the time and energy they spend thinking obsessively about food, eating, and weight, rather than work, school, family, or friends, and encourages them to increase their involvement in these valued activities.

Even when explicit values work is not part of the curriculum, participation in MBPs may implicitly cultivate awareness of personal values. Kabat-Zinn (2005) notes that mindfulness facilitates awareness of "the whispered longings" of one's own heart (p. 22). Although this point is not elaborated, these whisperings may reflect what participants value most deeply. Carmody, Baer, Lykins, and Olendzki (2009) found significant increases in a measure of purpose in life in participants in mindfulness-based stress reduction (MBSR). Following the eight-week course, participants reported a stronger sense of meaning, goal-directedness, and clarity about what they value. The recently proposed mindfulness-to-meaning theory (Garland, Farb, Goldin, & Fredrickson, 2015) also suggests that mindfulness training leads to increased purposeful engagement with life. Additional study of this promising theory is needed.

The Importance of Self-Chosen Values

Several theories of optimal human functioning emphasize the importance of autonomy: the ability to make one's own decisions and evaluate oneself by one's personal standards, rather than relying on approval from others. For example, self-determination theory (Ryan & Deci, 2000) identifies autonomy as one of three basic needs (along with competence and relatedness) that are essential for psychological health and life satisfaction. Ryff's (1989) comprehensive theory of psychological well-being also includes autonomy as a critical element of healthy functioning. The self-concordance model (Sheldon & Elliott, 1999) states that psychological well-being is enhanced when people pursue goals that reflect their authentic personal interests and values rather than goals prescribed by others (Gillet, Lafreniere, Vallerand, Huart, & Fouquereau, 2014; Sheldon, 2002). Similarly, self-affirmation theory (Steele, 1999) posits that affirmation of personal values protects against stressors by expanding participants' views of themselves and facilitating perspective on what is most important. All of these theories have strong empirical support.

In laboratory studies, participants asked to contemplate a self-identified personal value consistently show better outcomes than those who contemplate a value that is less important to them. Dependent variables have included helpful behavior, academic performance, health-related behavior, and cardiovascular functioning (see Cohen & Sherman, 2014, for a review).

There is no guarantee that self-identified values will be consistent with any particular ethical framework. However, clinical experience, especially with ACT, suggests that when clients are encouraged to think carefully about their deepest aspirations, most choose prosocial values, such as meaningful work, loving relationships, and contributions to a community (Hayes et al., 2012). When this does not happen, e.g., a client says that he values making a lot of money, further discussion about why money is important is likely to reveal prosocial underlying values, such as providing security or opportunities for one's family. The prevailing tendency to identify prosocial values is believed to reflect universal human requirements for biological survival, social interaction, and the welfare of groups (Schwartz & Bilsky, 1987, 1990). That is, individuals and societies are more likely to thrive if people take care of themselves, help each other, and work for the benefit of the group.

These universal needs do not invariably prevent harmful behavior or disagreements about what will cause harm. Experience suggests that a few clients identify values that are not prosocial, e.g., becoming wealthy to enjoy a materialistic lifestyle, rather than to benefit others. Some clients may identify prosocial values but choose to enact them in ways with that conflict with the therapist's personal values. For example, in advance of an important election, a client may decide to act on his value of community involvement by volunteering for the campaign of the therapist's non-preferred candidate. Another client may act on her value of generosity by donating money to an organization whose goals the therapist finds reprehensible. As noted earlier, adherence to professional ethical standards generally means that the therapist must not attempt to persuade these clients to do otherwise. Exceptions are made only when necessary to prevent specific types of harm.

Cultivating the Core Values of Kindness and Compassion

Kabat-Zinn (2005) and Segal et al. (2013) note that MBSR and mindfulness-based cognitive therapy (MBCT) are offered with a spirit of gentle compassion, friendliness, kindness, and warm hospitality. Segal et al. (2013) describe this attitude as fundamental, noting that without it, a mindfulness course "loses one of its foundational features" (p. 137). The personal mindfulness practice to which most teachers are committed is believed to cultivate their ability to embody these qualities in their teaching. This creates a warm and friendly atmosphere in their mindfulness courses, which encourages participants to experiment with treating themselves more kindly and compassionately.

Indeed, several studies have shown that mindfulness training leads to increases in empathy and compassion in clinical or community samples (Birnie et al., 2010; Condon et al., 2013; Keng et al., 2012; Kuyken et al., 2010) and in health care professionals and therapists in training (Gokhan, Meehan, & Peters, 2010; Shapiro, Brown, & Biegel, 2007; Shapiro, Schwartz, & Bonner, 1998). These findings are consistent with definitions of mindfulness that emphasize qualities of attention such as acceptance, nonjudgment, openness, friendliness, and kindness. For example, Feldman (2001) states that "true mindfulness is imbued with warmth, compassion, and interest" (p. 173). Grossman (2015) described these qualities as *virtuous* and suggested that, because mindfulness training involves consistent practice of these qualities, it cultivates an inherently ethical stance toward self and others.

Conclusions

As MBPs become more widely available around the world, the diversity of people who participate in them is likely to increase. Programs offered in secular settings must be able to accommodate participants from a wide range of religious, spiritual, and cultural backgrounds. Whether deeply committed to a particular faith or espousing no religion at all, participants must feel assured that their beliefs and values will be respected (Crane, 2016). Moreover, as the demand for MBPs expands, the diversity of people seeking professional training in how to provide them will also increase. Training that requires participation in overtly Buddhist practices or relies heavily on Buddhist frameworks or belief systems may create barriers to teachers from other traditions. For these reasons, while acknowledging that explicitly Buddhist-based programs may be beneficial in some settings, we have argued that mindfulness-based training will be more widely accessible if genuinely secular MBPs, with secular foundational ethics, are available.

This chapter has discussed two related approaches to ensuring that mainstream MBPs have strong ethical foundations that can be widely endorsed by people with diverse cultures and beliefs systems. First, codes of ethics for the health care and mental health professions are based on principles and values that have been recognized for centuries, in many parts of the world, as essential to the work of those who serve the unwell. While entirely secular, current ethics codes provide a shared set of principles and behavioral standards that are generally consistent with core ethical teachings from the Buddhist tradition. Of course, ethics codes do not ensure that all professionals will always behave ethically—no ethical framework can accomplish that. However, the organizational structures associated with professional ethics codes encourage ethical conduct in a variety of ways. Training and continuing education programs that keep professionals' knowledge up-to-date probably prevent many ethical violations. Boards and committees empowered to receive and investigate complaints can require remedial training, extra supervision, or other courses of action for professionals found to have committed ethical violations.

Second, when respect for diversity and self-determination makes it untenable to teach a particular ethical framework to participants in a secular program, well developed and empirically supported methods for helping participants to clarify their own values and behave consistently with them are available. Although self-identified values may not always be consistent with a particular ethical framework, theory, research, and clinical experience suggest that most people, when encouraged to think deeply about their most important aspirations, identify prosocial values. On the rare occasions when participants are causing harm, or seem likely to do so, professional ethics codes and legal standards support professionals in guiding clients toward less harmful behavior, within limits. When participants' values conflict with those of their teachers or therapists, awareness of their own values may help professionals navigate these difficult situations skillfully. The regular practice of mindfulness, to which most teachers of MBPs are committed, probably enhances clarity about their personal values while cultivating the ethical qualities of kindness and compassion.

This chapter has discussed professional ethics from the perspective of psychology and related professions. An important issue in the mindfulness-based field is that teachers of MBPs have a wide range of professional affiliations. Although many belong to the medical, mental health, or teaching professions, some do not. This means that as a group, teachers of MBPs follow a variety of ethics codes, and some may have no training in a code that addresses the ethical difficulties that teachers of MBPs are likely to encounter. Lack of familiarity with or commitment to a particular ethics code could impair the ability of mindfulness teachers to work skillfully with ethically challenging situations. It remains unclear whether mindfulness teachers should have their own professional ethics code or should adopt an existing code from one of the mental health or health care professions. Efforts to work with this critical issue are currently underway through professional discussion, the development of good practice guidelines for teachers of MBPs and their trainers, and through the articulation of professional training pathways that include training in ethics (e.g., http://mbct.com/training/mbct-training-pathway/).

Mindfulness teaching is a much younger profession than psychology. Crane (2016) suggests that this new field must develop its own form of professional integrity, and in doing so, it must prioritize two key concerns: the interests of the public to whom mindfulness courses are offered, and the quality of the training and support for teachers' work. We argue that ethics codes are essential to the protection of the public and therefore must be central to the development of this new field and to the training of teachers; we also emphasize that clarity about personal values, which is probably cultivated through regular mindfulness practice, contributes to the wise and compassionate application of the standards provided by the ethics codes. We hope that understanding of professional ethics and personal values, and how they work together, will be of help to this promising new field as it develops into a mature profession.

References

Amaro, A. (2015). A holistic mindfulness. *Mindfulness, 6*, 63–73.

American Psychological Association. (2002). Ethical principles of psychologists and code of conduct. *American Psychologist, 57*, 1060–1073.

American Psychological Association. (2010). 2010 Amendments to the 2002 'Ethical principles of psychologists and code of conduct'. *American Psychologist, 65*, 493.

American Psychological Association. (2015). *Report to the special committee of the Board of Directors of the American Psychological Association: Independent review relating to the APA Ethics Guidelines, national security interrogations, and torture.* Retrieved from http://www.apa.org/independent-review/APA-FINAL-report-7.2.15.pdf

Baer, R. A. (2015). Ethics, values, virtues, and character strengths in mindfulness-based interventions: A psychological science perspective. *Mindfulness, 6*, 956–969.

Bowen, S., Chawla, N., & Marlatt, A. (2011). *Mindfulness-based relapse prevention for addictive behavior: A clinician's guide.* New York, NY: Guilford Press.

Branstetter-Rost, A., Cushing, C., & Douleh, T. (2009). Personal values and pain tolerance: Does a values intervention add to acceptance? *The Journal of Pain, 10*, 887–892.

Birnie, K., Speca, M., & Carlson, L. D. (2010). Exploring self-compassion and empathy in the context of mindfulness-based stress reduction (MBSR). Stress and Health, 26, 359–371.

British Psychological Society. (2009). *Code of ethics and conduct: Guidance published by the Ethics Committee of the British Psychological Society.* Leicester.

Campbell, N., Stuck, C., & Frinks, L. (2012). Spirituality training in residency: Changing the culture of a program. *Academic Psychiatry, 36*, 56–59.

Carmody, J., Baer, R. A., Lykins, E., & Olendzki, N. (2009). An empirical study of the mechanisms of mindfulness in a mindfulness-based stress reduction program. *Journal of Clinical Psychology, 65*, 613–626.

Chiesa, A., Calati, R., & Serretti, A. (2011). Does mindfulness training improve cognitive abilities? A systematic review of neuropsychological findings. *Clinical Psychology Review, 31*, 449–464.

Clarke, S., Taylor, G., Lancaster, J., & Remington, B. (2015). Acceptance and commitment therapy-based self-management versus psychoeducation training for staff caring for clients with a personality disorder: A randomized controlled trial. *Journal of Personality Disorders, 29*, 163–176.

Cohen, G. L., & Sherman, D. K. (2014). The psychology of change: Self-affirmation and social psychological intervention. *Annual Review of Psychology, 65*, 333–371.

Condon, P., Desbordes, G., Miller, W., & Desteno, D. (2013). Meditation increased compassionate responses to suffering. Psychological Science, 24, 2125–2127.

Crane, R. (2016). Implementing mindfulness in the mainstream: Making the path by walking it. *Mindfulness.* https://doi.org/10.1007/s12671-016-0632-7

Davidson, R. J. (2016). Mindfulness-based cognitive therapy and the prevention of depressive relapse: Measures, mechanisms, and mediators. *JAMA Psychiatry, 73*, 547–548.

Davis, J. H. (2015). Facing up to the question of ethics in mindfulness-based intervention. *Mindfulness, 6*, 46–48.

Eberth, J., & Sedlmeier, P. (2012). The effects of mindfulness meditation: A meta-analysis. *Mindfulness, 3*, 174–189.

Feldman, C. (2001). The Buddhist path to simplicity. London: Thorsons.

Fisher, C. (2016). *Decoding the ethics code: A practical guide for psychologists* (4th ed.). Los Angeles, CA: Sage.

Fleming, J. E., & Kocovski, N. L. (2013). *The mindfulness and acceptance workbook for social anxiety and shyness.* Oakland, CA: New Harbinger.

Garland, E., Farb, N., Goldin, P., & Fredrickson, B. (2015). Mindfulness broadens awareness and builds eudaimonic meaning: A process model of mindful positive emotion regulation. *Psychological Inquiry, 26*, 293–314.

Gauthier, J., Pettifor, J., & Ferrero, A. (2010). The Universal Declaration of Ethical Principles for Psychologists: A culture-sensitive model for creating and reviewing a code of ethics. *Ethics and Behavior, 20*, 179–196.

Gillet, N., Lafreniere, M., Vallerand, R., Huart, I., & Fouquereau, E. (2014). The effects of autonomous and controlled regulation of performance-approach goals on well-being: A process model. *British Journal of Social Psychology, 53*, 154–174.

Gokhan, N., Meehan, E. F., & Peters, K. (2010). The value of mindfulness-based methods in teaching at a clinical field placement. *Psychological Reports, 106*, 455–466.

Goldstein, J., & Kornfield, J. (2001). *Seeking the heart of wisdom: The path of insight meditation.* Boston: Shambhala.

Grossman, P. (2015). Mindfulness: awareness informed by an embodied ethic. Mindfulness, 6, 17–22.

Harrington, A., & Dunne, J. D. (2015). When mindfulness is therapy: Ethical qualms, historical perspectives. *American Psychologist, 70*, 621–631.

Hathaway, W. L. (2011). Ethical guidelines for using spiritually oriented interventions. In J. D. Aten, M. R. McMinn, & E. L. Worthington (Eds.), *Spiritually oriented interventions for counseling and psychotherapy.* Washington, DC: American Psychological Association.

Hathaway, W. L., & Ripley, J. S. (2009). Ethical concerns around spirituality and religion in clinical practice. In J. D. Aten & M. M. Leach (Eds.), *Spirituality and the therapeutic process: A comprehensive resource from intake to termination* (pp. 25–52). Washington, DC: American Psychological Association.

Hayes, S. C., Bissett, R., Roget, N., Padilla, M., Kohlenberg, B., Fisher, G., … Niccolls, R. (2004). The impact of acceptance and commitment training and multicultural training on the stigmatizing attitudes and professional burnout of substance abuse counselors. *Behavior Therapy, 35*, 821–825.

Hayes, S. C., Luoma, J. B., Bond, F. W., Masuda, A., & Lillis, J. (2006). Acceptance and commitment therapy: Model, processes, and outcomes. *Behaviour Research and Therapy, 44*, 1–25.

Hayes, S. C., Strosahl, K. D., & Wilson, K. G. (2012). *Acceptance and commitment therapy: The process and practice of mindful change* (2nd ed.). New York, NY: Guilford Press.

Jennings, P. A. (2016). Mindfulness-based programs and the American public school system: Recommendations for best practices to ensure secularity. *Mindfulness, 7*, 176–178.

Kabat-Zinn, J. (1982). An outpatient program in behavioral medicine for chronic pain patients based on the practice of mindfulness meditation: Theoretical considerations and preliminary results. *General Hospital Psychiatry, 4*, 33–47.

Kabat-Zinn, J. (2005). Coming to our senses: Healing ourselves and the world through mindfulness. New York: Hyperion.

Kapuscinski, A., & Masters, K. (2010). The current status of measures of spirituality: A critical review of scale development. *Psychology of Religion and Spirituality, 2*, 191–205.

Keng, S., Smoski, M., Robins, C., Ekblad, A., & Brantley, J. (2012). Mechanisms of change in mindfulness-based stress reduction: self-compassion and mindfulness as mediators of intervention outcomes. Journal of Cognitive Psychotherapy, 26, 270–280.

Kuyken, W., Watkins, E., Holden, E., White, K., Taylor, R., Byford, S., et al. (2010). How does mindfulness-based cognitive therapy work? Behaviour Research and Therapy, 48, 1105–1112.

Khoury, B., Lecomte, T., Fortin, G., Masse, M., Therien, P., Bouchard, V., … Hofmann, S. G. (2013). Mindfulness-based therapy: A comprehensive meta-analysis. *Clinical Psychology Review, 33*, 763–771.

Khoury, B., Sharma, M., Rush, S. E., & Fournier, C. (2015). Mindfulness-based stress reduction for healthy individuals: A meta-analysis. *Journal of Psychosomatic Research, 78*, 519–528.

Knapp, S. J., & VandeCreek, L. D. (2006). *Practical ethics for psychologist: A positive approach.* Washington, DC: American Psychological Association.

Knapp, S. J., & VandeCreek, L. D. (2007). When values of different cultures conflict: Ethical decision making in a multicultural context. *Professional Psychology: Research and Practice, 38*, 660–666.

Kristeller, J. (2011). Spirituality and meditation. In J. Aten, M. McMinn, & E. Worthington (Eds.), *Spiritually oriented interventions for counseling and psychotherapy* (pp. 197–227). Washington, DC: American Psychological Association.

Kristeller, J., Wolever, R., & Sheets, V. (2014). Mindfulness-based eating awareness training (MB-EAT) for binge eating: A randomized clinical trial. *Mindfulness, 5*, 282–297.

Legere, C. (2016, February 4). D-Y parents rally support for Calmer Choice. *Cape Cod Times*. Retrieved October 13, 2016, from http://www.capecodtimes.com/article/20160204/NEWS/160209811

Levin, M., Hildebrandt, M., Lillis, J., & Hayes, S. C. (2012). The impact of treatment components suggested by the psychological flexibility model: A meta-analysis of laboratory-based component studies. *Behavior Therapy, 43*, 741–756.

Lindahl, J. R. (2015). Why right mindfulness might not be right for mindfulness. *Mindfulness, 6*, 57–62.

Linehan, M. M. (1993). *Cognitive-behavioral treatment of borderline personality disorder*. New York, NY: Guilford Press.

Linehan, M. M. (2015). *DBT skills training manual* (2nd ed.). New York, NY: Guilford Press.

Margolin, A., Beitel, M., Schuman-Olivier, Z., & Avants, S. K. (2006). A controlled study of a spirituality-focused intervention for increasing motivation for HIV prevention among drug users. *AIDS Education and Prevention, 18*, 311–322.

Margolin, A., Schuman-Olivier, Z., Beitel, M., Arnold, R., Fulwiler, C., & Avants, S. (2007). A preliminary study of spiritual self-schema (3-S+) therapy for reducing impulsivity in HIV-positive drug users. *Journal of Clinical Psychology, 63*, 979–999.

Monteiro, L. M. (2016). Implicit ethics and mindfulness: Subtle assumptions that MBIs are values-neutral. *International Journal of Psychotherapy, 20*, 210–224.

Monteiro, L. M., Musten, R. F., & Compson, J. (2015). Traditional and contemporary mindfulness: Finding the middle path in the tangle of concerns. *Mindfulness, 6*, 1–13.

Pettifor, J. (2004). Professional ethics across national boundaries. *European Psychologist, 9*, 264–272.

Plante, T. G. (2009). *Spiritual practices in psychotherapy: Thirteen tools for enhancing psychological health*. Washington, DC: American Psychological Association.

Purser, R. (2015). Clearing the muddled path of traditional and contemporary mindfulness: A response to Monteiro, Musten, and Compson. *Mindfulness, 6*, 23–45.

Richards, P. S., & Bergin, A. E. (2005). *A spiritual strategy for counseling and psychotherapy* (2nd ed.). Washington, DC: American Psychological Association.

Roemer, L., Orsillo, S. M., & Salters-Pednault, K. (2008). Efficacy of an acceptance-based behavior therapy for generalized anxiety disorder: Evaluation in a randomized controlled trial. *Journal of Consulting and Clinical Psychology, 76*, 1083–1089.

Ruiz, F. J. (2010). A review of acceptance and commitment therapy (ACT) empirical evidence: Correlational, experimental psychopathology, component and outcome studies. *International Journal of Psychology and Psychological Therapy, 10*, 125–162.

Ryan, R. M., & Deci, E. D. (2000). Self-determination theory and the facilitation of intrinsic motivation, social development, and well-being. *American Psychologist, 55*, 68–78.

Ryff, C. D. (1989). Happiness is everything, or is it? Explorations on the meaning of psychological well-being. *Journal of Personality and Social Psychology, 57*, 1069–1081.

Schwartz, S. H., & Bilsky, W. (1987). Toward a psychological structure of human values. *Journal of Personality and Social Psychology, 53*, 550–562.

Schwartz, S. H., & Bilsky, W. (1990). Toward a theory of universal content and structure of values: Extensions and cross-cultural replications. *Journal of Personality and Social Psychology, 58*, 878–891.

Segal, Z. V., Williams, J. M. G., & Teasdale, J. D. (2013). *Mindfulness-based cognitive therapy for depression: A new approach to preventing relapse* (2nd ed.). New York, NY: Guilford Press.

Shapiro, S. L., Brown, K. W., & Biegel, G. M. (2007). Teaching self-care to caregivers: Effects of mindfulness-based stress reduction on the mental health of therapists in training. *Training and Education in Professional Psychology, 1*, 105–115.

Shapiro, S. L., Schwartz, G. E., & Bonner, G. (1998). Effects of mindfulness-based stress reduction on medical and premedical students. *Journal of Behavioral Medicine, 21*, 581–599.

Sheldon, K. M. (2002). The self-concordance model of healthy goal striving: When personal goals correctly represent the person. In E. Deci & R. Ryan (Eds.), *Handbook of self-determination research* (pp. 65–86). Rochester, NY: University of Rochester Press.

Sheldon, K. M., & Elliott, A. (1999). Goal striving, need satisfaction, and longitudinal well-being: The self-concordance model. *Journal of Personality and Social Psychology, 76*, 482–497.

Sheridan, M. J. (2009). Ethical issues in the use of spiritually based interventions in social work practice: What are we doing and why. *Journal of Religion and Spirituality in Social Work: Social Thought, 28*, 99–126.

Shonin, E., & Van Gordon, W. (2015). Managers' experiences of Meditation Awareness Training. *Mindfulness, 6*, 899–909.

Shonin, E., Van Gordon, W., Dunn, T., Singh, N., & Griffiths, M. (2014). Meditation awareness training (MAT) for work-related well-being and job performance: A randomized controlled trial. *International Journal of Mental Health and Addiction, 12*, 806–823.

Sinclair, C. (2012). Ethical principles, values, and codes for psychologists: An historical journey. In M. M. Leach, M. J. Stevens, G. Lindsay, A. Ferrero, & Y. Korkut (Eds.), *The Oxford handbook of international psychological ethics* (pp. 3–18). Oxford: Oxford University Press.

Steele, C. M. (1999). The psychology of self-affirmation: Sustaining the integrity of the self. In R. F. Baumeister (Ed.), *The self in social psychology* (pp. 372–390). New York, NY: Psychology Press.

Tang, Y., Hölzel, B. K., & Posner, M. I. (2015). The neuroscience of mindfulness meditation. *Nature Reviews Neuroscience, 16*, 213–225.

Van Gordon, W., & Griffiths, M. D. (2015). For mindful teaching of mindfulness. *The Psychologist, 28*(7), 514.

Verhagen, P. J., & Cox, J. L. (2010). Multicultural education and training in religion and spirituality. In P. Verhagen, H. van Praag, J. Lopez-Ibor, J. Cox, & D. Moussaoui (Eds.), *Religion and psychiatry: Beyond boundaries* (pp. 587–610). Chichester: Wiley.

Vieten, C., & Scammell, S. (2015). *Spiritual and religious competencies in clinical practice: Guidelines for psychotherapists and mental health professionals.* Oakland, CA: New Harbinger.

Vieten, C., Scammell, S., Pilato, R., Ammondson, I., Pargement, K., & Lukoff, D. (2013). Spiritual and religious competencies for psychologists. *Psychology of Religion and Spirituality, 5*, 129–144.

Williams, M., & Penman, D. (2011). *Mindfulness: An eight-week plan for finding peace in a frantic world.* New York, NY: Rodale.

Wilson, K. G., & DuFrene, T. (2008). *Mindfulness for two: An acceptance and commitment therapy approach to mindfulness in psychotherapy.* Oakland, CA: New Harbinger.

Wilson, K. G., Sandoz, E., Flynn, M., Slater, R., & DuFrene, T. (2010). Understanding, assessing, and treating values processes in mindfulness- and acceptance-based therapies. In R. Baer (Ed.), *Assessing mindfulness and acceptance processes in clients* (pp. 77–106). Oakland, CA: New Harbinger.

Witte, J. (2005). *Religion and the American constitutional experiment* (2nd ed.). Boulder, CO: Westview Press.

Young, J., Cashwell, C., Wiggins-Frame, M., & Belaire, C. (2002). Spiritual and religious competencies: A national survey of CACREP-accredited programs. *Counseling and Values, 47*, 22–33.

Chapter 5
Ethics and Teaching Mindfulness to Physicians and Health Care Professionals

Michael Krasner and Patricia Lück

The Ethical Imperative of Attending to Burnout and Building Resilience in the Medical Profession

Michael Krasner

The Nature of Health Professional Suffering

> More than any other time in history, mankind faces a crossroads. One leads to despair and utter hopelessness. The other, to total extinction. Let us pray that we have the wisdom to choose correctly. (Allen, 1979)

This "Catch 22" is unfortunately the experience of all too many of today's medical practitioners. Physicians experience the same objectification and dehumanization frequently complained about by patients. Depersonalization is one of the cardinal features of "burnout" and evidence reported over more than a decade demonstrates that physicians experience burnout and related maladies such as depression, anxiety, and suicide at rates that exceed those in the general population (Shanafelt et al., 2003). Physician burnout is associated with poorer physical and mental health, and, not surprisingly, poorer quality of care, and patients of burned-out physicians experience poorer quality of caring (Crane, 1998; Haas et al., 2000). Affecting up to 60% of practicing physicians, evidence of burnout can be seen as early as third year of medical school (Dyrbye et al., 2006).

M. Krasner, MD (✉) • P. Lück, MD, MA
Olsan Medical Group, 2400 South Clinton Avenue H230, Rochester, NY 14618, USA
e-mail: Michael_Krasner@urmc.rochester.edu; patricialuck@me.com

© Springer International Publishing AG 2017 113
L.M. Monteiro et al. (eds.), *Practitioner's Guide to Ethics and Mindfulness-Based Interventions*, Mindfulness in Behavioral Health,
DOI 10.1007/978-3-319-64924-5_5

It is likely that burnout itself is a cultural phenomenon, reflecting the pace, complexity, and ongoing challenges found in the modern world. Holding much promise for the relief of suffering and already having brought under control many of the great scourges afflicting humankind, the world of medicine confronted only a handful of generations ago scarcities of water, food, and shelter. Commonplace infections no longer threaten one's survival or the survival of one's family. Despite these successes, stress-related medical conditions are epidemic and increasing and the future appears to only further this trend.

It is perhaps worth reviewing the history of modern, twenty-first century allopathic medicine, especially examining its foundations in the ancient world. Out of the Hippocratic tradition that took shape then, the ethical fundamentals that underpin the clinician–patient encounter can be viewed. Additionally, from the "mind-body" separation that took place in the centuries to follow, especially out of the enlightenment, some of the ethical challenges facing the modern medical practitioner can be better understood. This separation about the relationship between mind and matter, between subject and object, led to a dualism where mental phenomena are non-physical and the mind and body are separate and distinct. This Cartesian dualism, named for Rene Descartes, has influenced Western thought for centuries and has had a lasting impression on the study and practice of modern medicine. Some of its roots lie in classical Greek philosophy, from which also sprang forth many of our lasting ideas of modern science, in particular the art and science of medicine.

Roots of Twenty-First Century Medicine and Non-duality

The greatest mistake in the treatment of diseases is that there are physicians for the body and physicians for the soul, although the two cannot be separated.
    Plato (427–347 BCE)

If you lived on the Peloponnesian peninsula in the year 350 BCE and needed healing, you might first seek out a local healer in your community who practiced one of many forms of healing popular at the time. If you were not satisfied and still suffering, you might then journey, at great personal risk, to one of the prodigious healing temples of the ancient world such as Epidaurus, one of the better known Aesclepion temples. Asclepius was a hero and god of medicine in ancient Greek religion and mythology, and from the fifth century BCE many pilgrims flocked to the Aesclepion healing temples for cures of their ills. It is thought that Hippocrates began his career in Kos, the site of one of the most famous of these healing temples. On your way to such a temple you would meet travelers returning from their healing experiences. You might hear stories about their therapeutic experiences. This might have the effect of initiating the process of healing within yourself as anticipation built, stimulating your physiologic, neurologic, and immunologic systems, indeed the entire expectant forces of what is now known to include the powerful placebo effect (how many of us have patients who travel distance to our offices, telling us how much they feel better, just through the act of showing up in our clinics?).

Once arrived at Epidaurus, before even entering the temple, you may well participate in activities in the local community. You could take a swim at the local baths, shop at the marketplace, or go to the gymnasium. You might attend the theatre, and participate in the re-enactment of the mythological stories of the era as told through the words of the classical playwrights Euripides or Sophocles. The theatre of the time was an interactive one in which the audience was part of the action. It was a place where the collective mythos became personal, shared by both the players and the audience, where the great comedic and tragic stories would become personal and relevant, experienced by the one in need of healing, thus further initiating a transformation. It was a place where the nature of suffering was shared collectively, where illness and loss and grief were inseparable from the other experiences of life itself.

Finally, you would enter the healing temple. Once inside you would undergo purification rituals (think of the admitting process in a modern hospital, the donning of the hospital gown and the preparatory rituals for the modern surgery, rituals being about transformation). Within its walls, you would be attended to by physicians, healers, and priests who worked together. You would sleep and dream. Your dreams would be interpreted by a healer. Subsequently, a treatment plan would be devised which might include surgical procedures or a prescription from the pharmacopoeia of the time. Finally, you would be given instructions for care upon returning home. And then you would leave, returning home, hopefully healed, whole. And as you returned, you would share your experience of healing, and as a result be a source of inspiration, hope, and healing to others.

Case records exist from some of these encounters, inscribed in stone by the patients who experienced healing there. The detailed accounts of what occurred are obscure. Imagine pasting together the details of modern medical encounters, especially in the era of the electronic medical record where the narrative is created not through the syntax of human language but by the exigencies of templated phrases. However, what we read from these records are restoration narratives about a process that addressed suffering along many of its domains, and often required a transaction, a giving up something for a return to wholeness, not dissimilar to the modern insurance premium, co-pay, or lifestyle change prescribed within a modern medical encounter. Here is one example:

> Ambrosia of Athens became blind in one eye. She had laughed at being told of cures to the lame and the blind. But she dreamed that Asclepius was standing beside her, saying he would cure her if she would dedicate a silver pig as a memorial to her ignorance. He seemed to cut into her diseased eyeball and pour in medicine. When she woke in the morning she was cured. (OCR GCSE SHP Student Book chapter, n.d.)

At about the time of the pinnacle of this mythological-based health care system, an exciting and revolutionary new method, Hippocratic Medicine, was taking root. It is important to note that this new approach to medicine, with the empirical scientific paradigm that the Hippocratic corpus offered, radical in its implications, exciting in its promise, and transformative in its effects, was not accompanied by a rejection of the Aesclepion healing tradition of the time. It is felt that Hippocrates freed medicine from magic, superstition, and the supernatural, and used data collection and experimentation to demonstrate that disease was a natural process and the signs and symptoms of disease were the body's natural reaction to the disease process. However, rather than rejecting the earlier mythological worldview, it built upon and operated in concert with this ancient and culturally reflective approach. In fact, Aesclepion priests and healers regularly called upon Hippocratic practitioners to assist in the care of patients. The body–mind split that Plato lamented was perhaps somewhat mitigated by including these time-honored methods within the practice of Hippocratic Medicine. The value of traditional Aesclepion healing in this new approach to medicine is demonstrated in the opening line of the Hippocratic Oath which invokes the contemporary mythos:

I swear by Apollo Physician and Asclepius and Hygeia and Panacea and all the gods and goddesses, making them my witnesses, that I will fulfill according to my ability and judgment this oath... (National Library of Medicine, n.d.)

The Hippocratic Oath is one of the oldest binding documents in history and reflects the deepest intentions of the one taking it. Like the Bodhisattva vow described centuries later that commits one who takes the vow to an altruistic ideal for the sake of all beings, the Hippocratic Oath binds one to attend to the relief of another human being's suffering. Because disease and illness and their resultant suffering are inevitable parts of the human condition, the oath taken to practice the science and art of medicine is a daunting one. It is a statement of ethics, of professionalism, and of an ideal to uphold specific ethical standards. Among those standards are obligations to fellow human beings to treat and prevent illness, to respect privacy, and an understanding that these responsibilities include the patient and family's health and economic stability.

Although Hippocratic medicine was incorporated into the spiritual tradition extant in ancient Greece, the current structure and practice of Western allopathic medicine has been separated from cultural religious contexts. That split is in part a result of the historical role of organized religion, political trends, and modern science through the Early Modern (Renaissance), the Modern, and the Post-Modern eras. However, more recent trends related to broader movements within Medicine in developing patient-centered and relationship-centered approaches in medical care have brought into focus the need to examine the patient and the practitioners' relationships with the many domains of suffering, including the existential and the spiritual.

On a personal note, as a third-year medical student I was given a copy of an article without which I feel I would have been lost, with no compass directing me on the right path. Written by Eric Cassel and entitled *The Nature of Suffering and the Goals of Medicine*, I kept it close in my white coat side pocket and read it often (Cassell, 1982). Sometimes, I just touched it with my fingertips, especially at moments when I felt I was losing touch with the goals and vision that I held in becoming a physician. Through its words, I reminded myself that a patient's suffering results from a threat to biopsychosocial intactness. And that biopsychosocial intactness includes existential, spiritual, economic, relational, as well as physical domains. The article encouraged me to consider the cure of disease as not the only one of many ways to relieve suffering. More importantly perhaps, I learned that one could not assume to know the nature of the suffering experienced by patients without openly inquiring. And that inquiry, in some ways more intimate than the physical examination, touches on those personal and intimate areas of values, beliefs, cosmology, and spirituality.

With time and experience, I learned from patients the many territories of suffering at levels physical, emotional, spiritual, and existential. As I witnessed and participated in the rituals of medical education, I became initiated into the craft of medicine. As my nascent understanding grew through real relationships with real humans suffering from real diseases, this mission, the relief of suffering, illuminated for me that the Hippocratic Oath lives as more than an ideal but rather a flowing ever-present reminder of one's ethical responsibilities. I have little doubt that at the core of their motivations, this is true for my colleagues as well.

Relationship-Centered Care

> Nothing endures but change.
>   Heraclitus (535–475 BCE)

Relationship-centered care is an important framework for conceptualizing health care, recognizing that the nature and quality of relationships are central to health care and the broader health care delivery system (Beach and Inui, 2006). The existence of dynamic unending change as experienced at the micro and macro levels drives the illness experience, whereby no person alive is untouched. Near the time that Heraclitus lived, the historical Buddha gave a discourse named *Subjects for Contemplation* in which he presented the following regarding life's fragility: Each human is subject to aging, illness, and death; each will grow separate from all that is dear; and each is the owner and heir to all his or her actions (Bodhi, 2005). One can feel in these truths the multilayered dimensions of suffering described by Eric Cassell.

Amidst this awareness of one's mortality, human beings face the vital challenge of building a solid foundation upon which to live an inspired and rational life. Aaron Antonovsky's theory of health and illness, which he termed Salutogenesis, described several characteristics that help individuals develop resilience to stressors encountered in daily life, providing an individual with a *sense of coherence*, seeing life as a worthwhile challenge (Antonovsky, 1979). These include meaningfulness, manageability, and comprehensibility. Challenges are made more easily workable when they are understandable, when one has a sense of competency in addressing them, and when they can be understood in the context of one's personal cosmology.

Additionally, current understanding of human motivation posits three themes that drive human action and behavior even in the face of life's inevitable challenges.

They include: *Autonomy*—the universal urge to be causal agents of one's own life and act in harmony with one's integrated self; *Competence*—which refers to being effective in dealing with the environment in which a person finds oneself; and *Relatedness*—the universal desire to interact, be connected to, and experience caring for others (Ryan and Deci, 2002).

The importance of relationships in motivating the physician's work includes those with patients, patients' communities, and other health care practitioners. These relationships are central to quality of health care and are important in developing a paradigm of health care which integrates caring, healing, community, and the relationships involved including the patient, the practitioner, and the society. Consequently, health professional education should help developing practitioners to become reflective learners who understand the patient as a person, recognize and deal with multiple contributors to health and illness, and comprehend the role of relationship in health and healing.

In summary, movements in medicine toward relationship-centered care, also referred to as whole-person care, have evolved as a trend that asks all clinicians to turn toward the complex and multilayered ethical dimensions reflected in the Hippocratic Oath (Miller et al., 2010). These trends have resulted from a recognition that both the patient and clinicians' well-being are important. Individual and institutional approaches to personal health, population health, and effective health care delivery demand a deep understanding of the need to maintain a healthy clinical workforce for the sake of quality of care and quality of caring, but also as an ethical imperative for the relief of suffering. These trends include shared decision-making, greater patient autonomy, medical record transparency, greater disclosure of medical errors, and more detailed informed consent processes among others (Barry and Edgman-Levitan, 2012). The cultivation of mindfulness and the interventions that support it among health professionals can enhance the awareness of the connection between personal and professional well-being and the well-being of patients. In this way, it becomes an ethical act and a statement, to wake up, pay attention, notice the presence of judgment, and step into the present moment with patients.

The Ethical Challenges for Students and Medical Professionals

Patricia Lück

> To listen another soul into a condition of disclosure and discovery may be almost the greatest service that any human being ever performed for another.
>   Douglas Steere.

The fundamentals of medical ethics that serve as accepted medical practice and behavior include the generally accepted four principles of beneficence, non-maleficence, autonomy, and justice (Beauchamp and Childress, 2012). Beneficence means for the good of the patient; non-maleficence, to do no harm, is noted to go back to the time of Hippocrates as detailed earlier in this chapter; autonomy denotes respecting the capacity of the patient; and justice considers access to care within limited resources. Furthermore, the American Medical Association (AMA) lays out various responsibilities for the medical practitioner within the code of medical ethics that suggests a code of conduct with regard to the doctor–patient relationship, including: confidentiality; professional practice in best interest of the patient; support for access to care; and interprofessional relationships (AMA Code of Medical Ethics, June, 2001). While these certainly are taught in medical schools to a greater or lesser degree, the manner in which their multilayered complexity is enacted in practice is variable. Page, in a 2012 study attempting to measure the four principles and discover if they can predict ethical behavior, concluded that while medical ethics are valued they do not seem to directly influence the decision-making process, perhaps due the lack of a behavioral model that can describe or predict the use of these principles (Page, 2012). This variability shows up most vividly in that part of medical training referred to as the hidden curriculum. The hidden curriculum is that unconscious part of medical training, the behavioral modelling by senior colleagues, and the normative interactions of the training and treatment environment, that entrains students into the culturally and contextually common institutional approaches that they are being trained in. Lempp describes this as being that "set of influences that function at the level of organizational structure and culture. Including, for example, implicit rules to survive the institution such as customs, rituals, and taken for granted aspects" that can be categorized into six specific learning processes. These are identified as loss of idealism, adoption of a "ritualized" professional identity, emotional neutralization, change of ethical integrity, acceptance of hierarchy, and the learning of less formal aspects of "good doctoring" (Lempp and Seale, 2004). This transmission of these unwritten rules fosters greater distance rather than engaged intimacy with the patient. One of the identified processes involved in the hidden curriculum is that of change of ethical identity which may interfere consequently with the adequate development and fostering of the student's moral and ethical compass. This is especially active given the variety of experiences health care professionals and medical students encounter, which involve decision points of implicit and explicit ethics. Medical education policy makers have growing concerns about the erosion of ethical attitudes and behavior in medical students (Yavari, 2016). Yavari illustrates this when sharing their personal experience of witnessing patients being referred to in a derogatory manner by their senior colleagues and their shame at not speaking out against this behavior. Margie Shaw, of the division of medical humanities and bioethics at the University of Rochester Medical School, in conversation shared that she believes, given that the hidden curriculum by its very nature is not obvious, clinicians may benefit from more explicit training in medical ethics, especially in the practical aspects of applying medical ethics within the clinical setting. This highlights the perspective that not only is it important that medical ethics be taught while at medical school, but be taught in such a way that these principles are internalized and can readily be expressed and called upon in the medical decision-making process. How this internalization process may be effected is an area of interest when considering applications of mindfulness-based programs within the medical environment.

Derek Doyle, founding member of the International Association for Hospice and Palliative Care, offered this thought on receiving the Lifetime Achievement Award from the AAHPM in 2005: "I suggest to you that palliative medicine should be an exercise in befriending and sharing as much as an exercise in therapeutics or clinical pharmacology" (Doyle, 2005). With this, he affirmed that the doctor–patient relationship is grounded in the whole person, comprising skills that include the ability to turn toward the difficult conversations within the clinical encounter. Engaged communication promotes flexibility, warmth, and acceptance with an open-minded approach that is genuinely empathic, self-aware, respectful, and non-dominating in all interactions (Ekman and Krasner, 2017). This manner of communicating shows a level of connection that demonstrates awareness of possible communication barriers, personal bias, and expectations while still understanding and respecting the importance of resonance within the physician–patient encounter, as well as awareness of intra- and interpersonal perspectives. These skills can be cultivated through the practice of mindfulness-based programs (MBPs). Mindfulness-based programs challenge participants to a deep reflection of the ground that we inhabit. The contemplative practices at the heart of MBPs engage a quality of mind that can interrupt the automaticity of conditioned behaviors that may not promote ethical decision-making. Mindfulness training supports the development of attitudes that are grounded in self-awareness and deep listening with an awareness of different forms of communication and observational skills that embody attitudes which enable trust building within the professional, interprofessional, and interpersonal environment. This supports the ability to detach from one's own personal values, ideals, and beliefs while being intimately present for our patients (Krasner et al., 2009; Sibinga and Wu, 2010). Listening well and responding to the patient's own telling of their suffering could be the most important service we offer a patient in need, with awareness and communication skills sitting at the heart of cultivating ethical behavior and practice within the health care environment.

Relating to patients with a quality of intimacy, presence, wholehearted engagement, and turning toward rather than away from difficulties can be challenging for the physician to learn when medical education often encourages a deconstructed experience of personhood where one experiences bodies as cadavers, clinical cases, diseases, and patients with diagnoses first and foremost, before these bodies can be re-experienced and engaged with as whole persons (Good, 1994, p. 73). Medical education encourages an emotional neutralization and distancing which inculcates less intimacy into the clinical encounter, and persists, through the influence of the hidden curriculum, into the working lives of many physicians. This distancing impacts the lives of physicians through rejection of the intimate and personal parts in their engagement with patients, rendering these as something akin to a public performance, and not a real, lived and in-the-moment experience. This distancing not only impacts the therapeutic connection the physician may have with the patient but also risks the well-being of the patient through the risk of cognitive errors driven by the inattention this distancing can cause. The imperative to cultivate closer and more intimate, yet therapeutically safe relationships with patients therefore can be seen as not only for benefiting the well-being of the patient, but also to ensure greater emotional connection and balance for the physician.

Henry Marsh in his book *Do No Harm: Stories of Life, Death and Brain Surgery* illustrates how a physician, in this case a renowned and skilled neurosurgeon, risks errors of attention and judgment with his inability to contain the emotional discomforts that arise from within the patient encounter.

> Three days earlier the juniors had admitted an alcoholic man in his forties who had been found collapsed on the floor of his home, with the left side of his body paralysed. We had discussed his case at the morning meeting, in the slightly sardonic terms that surgeons often use when talking about alcoholics and drug addicts. This does not necessarily mean that we do not care for such patients, but because it is so easy to see them as being the agents of their own misfortune, we can escape the burden of feeling sympathy for them. (Marsh, 2014, p. 257)

With his description, Marsh clearly demonstrates the entrainment of junior doctors into certain behaviors of patient disdain that are characteristic of the hidden curriculum. This example, which threatens ethical considerations, includes showing a lack of empathy for, and bias against alcoholics and drug addicts through the "slightly sardonic terms that surgeons often use" as well as the perceived inherent dangers of the emotional burden, therefore relieving the physician of "the burden of feeling sympathy for them." Jodi Halpern, a well-known clinician and author on the role of empathy in the clinical relationship, asserts that the emotional receptivity of the physician helps the patient acknowledge their suffering by enabling words to be attached to the suffering, and that the emotionally engaged physician allows the patient to work through her own difficult emotions (Halpern, 2011, p. 145). This aspect can easily be neglected when clinicians are consistently exposed to the implicit teachings of the hidden curriculum, inhibiting their empathic development and extending into the ethical realm of practice.

The Importance of Empathy

The capacity for being ethically grounded shows up in the day-to-day lives of physicians through their interactions most vividly reflected in the physician–patient relationship. The capacity for awareness and the conscious ability to discern the impact of this relationship can be examined by looking at the decision-making process within the clinical encounter and the inherent risks embedded in it.

John Eisenberg, examining this decision-making process, asserts that patients desire physicians primarily to listen and be human, and outlines four areas that influence clinical decision-making: the characteristics of the patient; the characteristics of the clinician; the clinician's interaction with their profession and the medical system; and the clinician's relationship with the patient (Eisenberg, 1979). These four areas overlap within the clinical encounter and within each area the process of decision-making is vulnerable to uncertainty, to lapses of present-moment awareness, and as a consequence error is a constant possibility.

Eisenberg argues that: "The medical problem, together with the patients' characteristics … create the uncertainty inherent in the clinical encounter." Physicians
bring to clinical encounters their own reactions to clinical uncertainty, both cognitive and affective. While physicians may claim to practice "detached concern," professing to not be swayed by other considerations, this is "an ideal not necessarily
achieved." These overlapping areas, however, and the capacity of the physician to
remain intimate and close to the discomfort inherent within the medical encounter
significantly impact the clinical relationship.

Budd and Sharma found that many doctors are uncomfortable with the idea that
the relationships that they form with their patients can be crucial to the patient's
satisfaction or otherwise with their treatment, yet the importance of this relationship
is supported by the research (Budd and Sharma, 1994). Another example of the
importance of this relationship is evidence that demonstrates the decision to litigate
in medical errors is often associated with a perceived lack of caring and/or collaboration in the delivery of the health system, through its personification in the physician (Beckman et al., 1994). This relationship is influenced not just by what was
done during the medical encounter and the course of the treatment, but also the
manner in which it was done, contributing greatly to the success of the encounter
and the relationship.

Medical practice is filled with uncertainty. For the clinician, residing within the
personal moments and emotional aspects of meeting the patient, there are numerous
opportunities that can lead to improved decision-making that enhances patient care.
Danielle Ofri, in her book *What Doctors Feel*, demonstrates a clear understanding
of the four areas outlined by Eisenberg that influence the decision-making process
and emphasizes the affective dynamic of the clinical encounter (Ofri, 2013, p. 3).
She also concurs with Jerome Groopman in his book *How Doctors Think* when
illustrating this point: "Most [medical] errors are mistakes in thinking, and part of
what causes these cognitive errors is our inner feelings, feelings we do not readily
admit to and often don't even recognize" (Groopman, 2007). She notes that doctors
who are "angry, jealous, burned out, terrified, or ashamed can usually still treat
bronchitis or ankle sprains competently," but it is when "clinical situations are con-
voluted, unyielding, or overlaid with unexpected complications, medical errors, or
psychological components…[that]…factors other than clinical competency come
into play" (Ofri, 2013, pp. 2–3). These moments when medical care is at its most
uncertain and complex require the physician possess the capacity for awareness of
her own emotional discomfort, rather than a denial of and turning away from it. This
uncertainty and complexity requires that she be able to engage not only with the
private and personal aspects of the patient, but also with her own subjective experiences that affect the clinical decision-making process.

The quality of engagement during these challenging clinical moments impacts
multiple domains within clinical care: from the quality of care delivered including
errors and near-misses to the quality of caring experienced through the presence of
empathy and the compassion of the clinician; from the level of work-satisfaction
and perceived stress and its effects on clinician well-being to the toll of burnout and
the loss of self-efficacy or fear of personal inadequacy and failure; and from the

capacity for self-disclosure in the face of failure or errors to its impact on patient's trust. The perceived need for certainty and control over the clinical encounter by the physician stands in contrast to the enormous amount of uncertainty that is actually present. This uncertainty is inherent in the nature of the presenting patient's concerns, the need to gather and synthesize relevant information, and the ability to make appropriate decisions for diagnostic evaluations and effective treatment. Uncertainty in medicine is further influenced by the capacity to only partially master the vast amount of knowledge and skills needed, the uncertainty of the limitations and ambiguities of the knowledge and skills, and consequently the uncertainty of how these two relate (Gerrity et al., 1992). In medicine, it can be difficult to know how much one does or does not know in any given situation, and in which—an adequate or inadequate knowledge base—one is functioning at the present moment.

When patients present to the physician with a precipitously acute, or even a lingering chronic presentation, there may be a narrow window of opportunity which, when missed, creates a greater likelihood for error. The body, a complex system in itself, is not always well-appreciated or understood, especially at times by the person presenting with the complaint. The presentation of dis-comfort and dis-ease must be related by the patient to the clinician through the telling of a personal narrative, in a way that can be explored, interpreted, and investigated by the clinician that eventually leads to a plan of action. This all occurs within a dynamic that is open to misinterpretation, bias, stigma, and cultural misunderstandings. This complexity is compounded by the physician who may have been entrained into an approach of detached concern with limited curiosity about the individual details of the patient's life for fear of becoming too intimately involved. As a result, the likelihood of error in this scenario may further increase. Jodi Halpern found that curiosity about the patient's personal situation enhances medical effectiveness through the development of empathy and consequently intimacy in the patient–physician encounter (Halpern, 2011, p. 87).

The capacity to step into the emotional dynamic affecting the patient results in a connection and intimacy that allows the physician to listen to the patient embedded within the greater scope of needs and life itself, possibly preventing errors that could result from not listening carefully to the patient's needs, errors of attention and judgment. Sibinga and Wu point out that this element of "the performance of the individual clinician remains a crucial and largely unaddressed element of patient safety" (Sibinga and Wu, 2010). Furthermore, Sibinga connects mindfulness, as a debiasing strategy, to the clinician's capacity to counter their entrained cognitive dispositions unwittingly enhanced by the hidden curriculum.

When the professional ethic of to do no harm is unintentionally violated, many physicians find themselves deeply affected regardless of whether an error results in harm to the patient or not. Research with medical residents demonstrates that errors are associated with significant subsequent personal distress and impacts the levels of well-being, a decrease in empathy, lower quality of life, and increased levels of burnout and depression (West et al., 2006). Few resources go toward alleviating this distress. Most physicians have experienced the distressing realization that they have made an error, and the subsequent shame and exposure. Even though more emphasis is now being placed on disclosure of errors and training programs are developing within medical education to train for these eventualities, it is still with great emotional turmoil and distress that physicians face such occurrences. It is perhaps the loss of empathy in response to repeated exposure to emotional distress that is most pertinent here. Empathy is one of the capacities that allows the physician to stay closely connected to the relevant personal aspects of the patient experience, and empathic curiosity enhances the intimacy of the medical encounter and the physician–patient relationship. Therefore, the threat to empathy also threatens this important part of the patient–clinician relationship. In their yearlong resilience-building program of mid-career primary care physicians, Krasner and colleagues found significant improvements in empathy that strongly correlated with measures of mindfulness, supporting the value of mindfulness and contemplative training in improving empathy and psychosocial orientation within the practice of medicine (Krasner et al., 2009).

Intimacy—Why Does It Matter?

Faith Fitzgerald illustrates the power of intimacy and presence within the physician–patient relationship, describing the shift when the physician chooses to pause and listen deeply to the personal narrative of the patient without the immediate push to solve, but to instead remain present with the uncertainty and discomfort. (Fitzgerald, 1999) She, like Halpern, believes "it is curiosity that converts strangers […] into people we can empathize with." Curiosity is the spark that leads to empathy and connection, but resides in the intention held by intimacy and presence. A spark inhibited at times by aspects of medical education where anything less than purely biological medicine can be at times discouraged and discounted through the hidden curriculum. For Fitzgerald, there is a clear reward for both patient and physician in being curious:

> [T]o the patient it is the interest and physical propinquity of the physicians, which is therapeutic in and of itself. To the physician, curiosity leads not only to diagnoses but to great stories and memories, those irreplaceable "moments in medicine" that we all live for.

Historically, changes in medicine have mirrored societal movements toward greater individuality, from public to private within medical care, and from a more socially oriented approach to one more focused on the individual. This shift to the individual, however, requires the physician to correspondingly engage with the patient as an individual, and not as a system, something that has been a challenge in medical education, fixated as it has previously been on the approach of detached concern and valuing cognition over emotional attunement.

It is challenging for physicians to develop intimacy and clinical empathy with their patients rather than resort to detached concern even as this distance risks errors of attention and judgment, especially when the patient does not evoke natural affection in the physician. Research, however, into medical care and in particular with medical narratives informs us that for the patient, being listened to and heard, and feeling that one's personal story matters to the physician improves therapeutic connection and benefits the physician–patient relationship (Charon, 2006). This type of relationship when highlighted by curiosity about the patient's personal circumstance may decrease error formation caused by lapses of attention or judgment and ward against the tendency toward particular decisions that may be premature, incomplete, or inaccurate. Such a relationship may also increase patient compliance, and when mistakes do occur, decrease patient litigation (Beckman et al., 1994). The capacity for clinical relationship building, and furthermore the capacity to develop clinical empathy, attunes the physician to the other's experience and is cultivated through curiosity. In the words of Halpern, "Although a physician cannot directly will herself to empathize, by cultivating curiosity she can develop empathy" (Halpern, 2011, p. 130).

The subjective experiences that physicians have with their patients are not commonly explored in medical education, yet when physicians are asked to remember moments of intimacy and connection with their patients they do so through recalling specific patients they have cared for. For example, in a study of a group of Internal Medicine specialists asked about their most meaningful experiences in the practice of medicine, they recalled that relationships deepened through recognizing the common ground of each person's humanity and discovered and were deeply gratified by the intrinsic healing capacity of simply being present (Horowitz et al., 2003). In another investigation physicians enrolled in a yearlong training program focusing on mindfulness, self-awareness, and communication skills realized that patients notice when the physician can be present and listening, focusing on understanding and empathy, leading to greater effectiveness and sense of meaning in their work (Beckman et al., 2012). Rather than re-enforce a sense of alienation through detached concern, the physician's obligation is to mitigate this by cultivating a capacity for intimacy in the clinical encounter, a capacity that can be cultivated and supported by the practice of mindfulness.

The Personal

The following narrative illustrates previous points of ethics, empathy, and the hidden curriculum, and the subsequent mitigating effect of mindfulness. My own medical school experience impressed on me that medical education and care is neither ethically nor politically neutral. Having chosen to study at the University of Cape Town, I was a student during the turbulent final years of the apartheid regime in the 1980s. At medical school I was confronted with the realities of politically biased care with separation of patients, differentiated care, and inequitable resource allocation based on race and color. I witnessed the "colored" colleagues in my tutorial group being unable to examine any of the white patients. Distressed by much of this, I sought guidance from a renowned activist and mentor. Her sage and ethical advice was to continue to attend to the ethical standard of my own behavior as best I could within my day-to-day encounters with patients, colleagues, and staff. She advised me however within this day to day to keep an eye on the long view, especially the need for systemic change within health systems that impact patient care and patient caring. Underscoring this reality and wisdom of advice was my later understanding of Eisenberg's research that clinical decision-making process includes the four areas of influence of the patient, clinician, clinician–patient relationship, and importantly the clinician's interaction with their profession and the medical system. I developed an understanding that the expressed ethical dynamic of the medical system itself is influenced by the contextual reality of the political, social, and cultural milieu of its time.

Later, as an intern in an Australian clinical setting on surgical rotation I was challenged by the senior attending physician to keep a cancer diagnosis secret from a patient. This particular attending physician did not believe it was helpful to disclose distressing diagnoses and bad news to patients, especially to female patients, preferring to tell the husbands or families, and allowing them to make decisions regarding care as well as disclosure. This placed me in a difficult ethical dilemma when the patient herself asked me for my opinion and for disclosure to her of the diagnosis. Further discussion with the attending and appealing to him to reconsider his instructions on ethical grounds yielded no results. There was an additional threat to my career if I countermanded him.

I sought further assistance and advice, and after much thought concluded that my first duty was to my patient, who detecting a cover up was insistent that I be open with her. With the support of the nursing staff, I arranged a breaking bad news disclosure meeting, not simple for a young 24-year-old newly qualified physician. The outcome for my patient's mental and emotional well-being, and her capacity to make informed choices for her future care have left an indelible impact on the importance of trust and my ethical responsibility toward patients. I have learned a deeper understanding of disclosure imperatives, as well as gained insight into the hidden ethical pressures and impact of the hidden curriculum.

Needless to say, I was sidelined from further surgical assisting and received a less than complimentary end of rotation review. Fortunately, surgery was not my future specialty area. Had it been, I would be curious if my resolve in challenging my attending would have been as resolute in acting upon the ethical principles of beneficence and justice.

Ethical behavior in the workplace can differ substantially from that behavior in training situations (Soltes, 2017). It can be more difficult to adhere to ethical behavior when decisions at work are often quick, intuitive and set free of the slower reflective thinking of the training environment. These dynamics point to the importance of building awareness and attentional reflective training, training that mindfulness practice offers, to enhance the capacity for ethical behavior even in the reality of every day pressure-filled workplace environment.

Early in my palliative care career, I cared for a young man who impressed upon me the ethical imperatives of doing the least harm, of respecting individuality, autonomy, personal religious and cultural perspectives, as well as the value of presence and listening. He had terminal bone cancer and was experiencing severe and difficult to control pain. He was paralyzed and bedbound, requiring his medical visits to be made at home. As our visits progressed and trust between us grew we began to explore in greater depth his diagnosis and prognosis. Having experienced a brutally frank and traumatic diagnostic disclosure from his surgical specialist, he clung to the last vestiges of hope and the denial of his approaching death. As time progressed and he was met with open acceptance, patience, and empathic care from his caregiver team, he was moved to openly acknowledge his condition and begin to explore what that would mean for him.

He spoke at length about the initial diagnosis and various treatments he had been through. Like many young people, he had given little thought to being ill and especially the possibility of dying. Now, no longer taking things for granted, he was finding meaning in the small moments of spending time with his family, beginning to accept that the rapidly increasing growth of the tumors in his body meant this would eventually shorten his life. The moment that will always stay with me from this encounter was when he asked to discuss his growing cancer and what that may mean for him.

In anticipation of delivering difficult and perspective-changing news to him, I asked him how he wanted this news to be communicated. His only response was "gently." He wanted to be told gently, for me to communicate in a manner that treated him with respect, compassion, care, and dignity, with his personhood recognized as central to the clinical interaction. This was a plea to physician and patient alike to inhabit with full presence this moment of engagement, recognizing with awareness the ethical complexities inherent in every physician–patient relationship.

How do we inhabit moments like this ethically as a medical community? How do we gaze through that window into our mutually unfolding lives when faced with another's deep suffering, as we simultaneously stand on the other side of that window, with our lives gifted to us? An invitation to do so is beautiful echoed through the words of Mary Oliver in her poem *Wild Geese* where she reassures us that "you do not have to be good… you only have to let the soft animal of your body love what it loves." This is an invitation to show up for this moment just as we are, where in this moment we fully belong by virtue of being alive, with a realization that for now the "world offers itself to (y)our imagination" (Oliver, 1992, p. 110).

There is much that can draw us away from this moment of engagement. Not just the suffering of this moment, but also experiences from the past, as well as fear of pain or discomfort that is imagined to arise in the future. This fear of past, present, and future continues to push us toward a longed-for better-than-now future. A future more rosy than the one we fear, or the present we inhabit and turn away from. "Tell me about despair, yours, and I will tell you mine. Meanwhile the world goes on." Mary Oliver continues encouraging us to turn toward the suffering inherent in this moment, especially within the compassionate presence of another.

This process of hoping for a different future in the encounters with suffering is met most poignantly when facing death. Death, depending on your perspective, is perhaps the ultimate loss, or the ultimate goal of our lives. As the ultimate loss, it encompasses loss of life, self, all the relationships that tether us to this world.

Working through these anticipated losses is an important step in preparing for death. Central to this work is the presence of hope. Hope unattached to an outcome, but embodied in a capacity of trust and openness, becomes a sustaining supportive capacity. But when hope is attached to achieving a better and different outcome that may not be attainable, hope becomes an unending cycle of expectation, disappointment, and loss. In this way hope often coexists uneasily with the suffering experienced when facing difficulty and death. The nature of hope may change as the focus of life shifts for many in the final days from a "doing" mode to "being" mode, from achieving to experiencing, from giving to receiving, from controlling to accepting, from tomorrow to today, to right now this moment. Hope unattached to an outcome allows the present moment to unfold as it can, even in the face of difficult suffering.

Greenhut takes this perspective with her description of the kind of hope that keeps us from experiencing the present moment through its constant looking forward toward the future with imagined expectations that may not be realistic or even supported by the reality of the current situation (Greenhut, 1995). She argues that by overly imagining positive results in the future, we suffer the results of ignoring what is happening in the here and now. That despite the presence of pain and discomfort, the moments unfolding in the realm of now are the only ones we truly have. Within that now are the only moments in time we occupy that hold the possibility of choices to change our lives and of actually impacting the future. These moments of now, moments that we attune to within mindfulness practice, are not only inhabited by pain and fear, but frequently and simultaneously also contain moments of joy and delight that are so often missed by focusing on how things could be different. We can only live our lives fully when we let go of that part of hope that denies the present experience by seeking unrealistically to change the suffering we experience in this moment. Therefore, letting go of hope is not a giving up on dreams but a giving up on the fantasy that this moment can be any other way than it is. The process of turning toward what is here now and being with this reality as it unfolds is living *in hope* rather than *a hoping for* things to be different. This capacity for being with and turning the difficult is cultivated with a mindfulness practice.

One of my patients, close to death, fluctuated between the hope of recovering her sight and the fear of going blind, the hope of a cure and her fear of dying, the hope she would beat her cancer and the fear that she could not manage the dying process. When she was hopeful and looking to an anticipated positive future, she was upbeat, but with each subsequent loss she experienced—stopping chemotherapy, further growth of the tumor, increasing pain—she found herself to be more depressed and bereaved again. When she was able to interrupt this repeating loop of hope and fear, and express how she felt in all she was experiencing, she experienced a greater sense of calm and was more able to cope with her suffering and with the uncertainty of the journey she was on.

Living in the hope that one has the resources to manage the present moment, rather than hoping for a different outcome, fosters resilience and self-confidence in our journey. When we live "in hope" rather than "hoping for," we cultivate the belief and capacity in our own resourcefulness. When one can look at the future with equanimity, and be open to all outcomes, the present moment can be experienced as being okay despite the difficulties that may be present.

> Giving up hope does not take away our will to be alive. Rather, it gives us the strength to live in the present and to grow from our suffering. Releasing ourselves from hope allows us to accept life in the here and now regardless of its duration or the state of our health, and it helps us to gain as much from depression as we gain from joy. (Greenhut, 1995)

This meeting the moment with authenticity allows both the physician and the patient to be the person whose story has been lived authentically. In my experience as a palliative care physician who practices from a mindfulness perspective, I have found that being unattached to any particular outcome for my patients releases both of us from any need to show up other than how we already are. Being open rather than attached to outcomes may be the greatest gift that mindfulness and mindfulness-based programs have to offer when working within palliative care. Mindfulness lifts the need to have suffering present in any particular way; it meets suffering however it shows up with empathy, compassion, patience, acceptance, non-judging, curiosity, and beginner's mind, allowing paradoxically greater spaciousness for experiencing joy. A mindful palliative care approach also does not expect or strive for a particular death experience such as a so-called "good death." Rather, it allows the clinician to be present for whatever experience shows up, to cultivate the capacity for fierce embodied compassionate presence in the face of suffering. This capacity for presence cultivated through mindfulness training within medicine will be addressed in the following section on Mindful Practice in supporting the growth of a healthier community.

In an era of medical care driven by technology and in which patients decry the lack of the human connection within the clinical encounter, cultivating clinical intimacy and empathy, paying attention with curiosity and concern about how health professionals show up for ethical dilemmas, attending to the subjective and emotional dimensions of the clinical relationship, fostering curiosity, and listening closely to the personal and intimate concerns in the lives of patients may not only enhance the clinical experience of both the patient and the physician, but it may also decrease errors arising from lack of attention and poor judgment. I have found through my own medical practice in clinical palliative care and in my experiences teaching mindfulness, that an authentic embodied presence imbued with patience, non-judgment, kindness, and beginner's mind allows me to be less attached to outcomes that might be determined by my own needs, and allows me to deeply listen to the needs and suffering of my patients and class participants. Having less of a need for any particular outcome, whether it be in health, end-of-life care, or in teaching, but rather closely attending to what is actually present allows me to participate in the evolving outcome that is unfolding and revealing itself in the moment we live in with a deeper trust, greater compassion, and a greater quality of care and caring. I also believe this being unattached to outcome with patience, non-judgment, kindness, and beginner's mind strongly supports and encourages an ethical approach that is grounded in transparency, openness, integrity, autonomy, respect, mentorship, personal practice, self-awareness, and humility.

Mindful Practice: Supporting the Growth of a Healthier Medical Community

Michael Krasner

> Ars longa, vita brevis, occasion praeceps, experimentum periculosum, iudicium difficile.
> Art is long, life is short, opportunity fleeting, experiment dangerous, judgment difficult.
> Aphorismi, Hippocrates of Kos (460–370 BCE)

The first word of this aphorism, written not in Latin, but in Greek, is *tekhnê*, signifying that the art of medicine includes the technical. To paraphrase, medicine is a craft carried out with skill, acquired over a long period of study and practice, where the opportunities for learning are transient, yet require experiences of significant risk which challenge judgment. Patients, who at some point include every member of the human race—indeed all of us, suffer from illness. There has always been and will always exist a sense of urgency and need for those who skillfully practice the science and art of Medicine.

Mindful Practice

> The ultimate value of life depends upon awareness and the power of contemplation rather than mere survival.
> Aristotle (384–322 BCE)

Michael Kearney, palliative care physician, in his review of physician self-care, asserts that clinicians who adopt self-awareness-based approaches to self-care may be able to remain emotionally available in even the most stressful clinical situations (Kearney et al., 2009). These approaches paradoxically enhance the potential of the work itself to be regenerative and fulfilling for the physician.

He described the risks all clinicians have of compassion fatigue, and illustrates the possibility for *exquisite empathy*. This involves *highly present, sensitively attuned, well-boundaried, heartfelt empathic engagement* where practitioners are *invigorated rather than depleted by their intimate professional connections with traumatized clients*. It appears that this type of empathic connection protects clinicians against compassion fatigue and burnout.

But how does one cultivate a clinical presence that promotes *exquisite empathy* and assists healing in a bidirectional manner? One approach for the medical practitioner is through developing greater mindfulness—the quality of being fully present and attentive during everyday activities. Mindful practice can be described as the application of mindfulness in medical work, involving moment-to-moment purposeful attentiveness to one's own mental processes during daily work with the goal of practicing with clarity and compassion (Epstein, 1999). The development of greater mindfulness is enhanced through training in contemplative practices.

Research demonstrates that physicians who participated in a program on mindful communication experienced improvements in measures of well-being and demonstrated enhancement in personal characteristics associated with more patient-centered orientation to clinical care (Krasner et al., 2009). Additionally, burnout improved with decreased depersonalization and greater sense of personal accomplishment. This intervention included contemplative practices within which clinical narratives were shared among colleagues. Appreciative inquiry techniques focused discussion on capacities and strengths in sharing the narrative-based dialogues. The inclusion of self-reflective clinical storytelling highlighting positive aspects of challenging clinical experiences connected practitioners with regenerative and fulfilling aspects of their work.

Several themes emerged from these physicians' reflections on this program which was based on cultivating intrapersonal and interpersonal mindfulness (Beckman et al., 2012). These themes shed light on the ways in which the intervention enhanced physicians' ability to practice patient-centered care, improved their sense of well-being, and decreased burnout. They included (1) sharing personal experiences from medical practice with colleagues reduced professional isolation, (2) mindfulness skills improved the participants' ability to be attentive and listen deeply to patients' concerns, respond to patients more effectively, and develop adaptive reserve, and (3) developing greater self-awareness was positive and transformative, yet participants struggled to give themselves permission to attend to their own personal growth.

Additionally, participants reported that the program promoted self-awareness, presence, authenticity and greater effectiveness and meaning—at work and at home. It also helped to diminish their sense of isolation, helping them effectively and meaningfully share their experiences with peers in a facilitated, respectful, and supportive environment. Finally, participation in the Mindful Communication program enabled physicians to make time for self-development and to realize how lack of attention to oneself can erode the capacity to engage more effectively with peers, family, and patients. The following quote of one of the participants powerfully illustrates aspects of this:

> In general, I think that I am a pretty good listener. I will spend extra time with my patients if they need it, but I felt in some ways that it was kind of sucking me dry. I would be so empathetic, and then I would feel frustrated, like what else can I do?… I would think about patients at home, in the shower, thinking she can't get to her appointment, maybe I should pick her up and drive her…. I would empathize to the point of where I would be so in their shoes. I would start to feel the way that they felt and I mean, you know, take four of those in a row in a day, and I would be just wiped out … and, they don't really want to hear about me and my processes…. It's not that I don't empathize with them anymore, but [now] I feel OK just to listen and be present with them … and I think that in some ways that helps them more … and that is a wonderful thing that you can do for patients…. I just needed to learn that myself, I guess. (Beckman et al., 2012)

The health professional–patient relationship contains both technical and human aspects, and as discussed earlier one can refer to these as the *Hippocratic* and the *Aesclepian* aspects, respectively. The kinds of attention that are called for in the clinical encounter include both an observational stance and an intimately connected stance as reviewed by Dr. Lück. In the Flexner's Carnegie Foundation report of 1910 that has had substantial impact on the shape of medical education over the last century, not only was competency in the basic sciences emphasized, but equally was the importance of a liberal education (Flexner, 1910). Elements of medical education that include experiential and reflective processes, the use of personal narratives, integration of self and expertise, and candid discussion among learners are approaches suggested to meet the objectives of medical professional formation designed to integrate the art and science facets of quality medical care (Rabow et al., 2010).

Situated at the center of these elements, mindfulness can be considered a universal human capacity to foster clear thinking and openheartedness. It assists in developing a greater sense of emotional balance and well-being. The original purpose of mindfulness in Buddhism is to alleviate suffering and cultivate compassion. This suggests a role for mindfulness in medicine (Santorelli, 1998). Likewise, mindfulness facilitates the physician's compassionate engagement with the patient (Ludwig and Kabat-Zinn, 2008). It has also been suggested that mindfulness is a central competency for effective clinical decision-making (Epstein, 1999). This competency may be promoted through practicing attentiveness, curiosity, and presence as part of a medical educational approach for developing useful "habits of mind" (Epstein, 2003). Indeed, not only can mindfulness be seen as a core competency that can be cultivated, but it can also be looked at as a potential antidote to the depersonalizing effects of the current medical environment (Stange, 2003).

Mindful Practice was developed by physicians at the University of Rochester School of Medicine and Dentistry as an educational intervention, currently part of the required third-year medical student experience, designed to be used in medical student, graduate medical education (residency) and postgraduate continuing medical education for practicing physicians and other health professionals. It can be thought of as an adapted mindfulness-based program (Crane et al., 2016) specific to the medical community, within which are several "technologies" used to encourage practitioners to reflect and share clinical experiences that are challenging and meaningful. It is hoped that from these reflections, contemplative practices, and dialogues, a greater understanding of their own self as clinician/physician health professional, and of their relationship with their patients and with their work develop.

These "technologies" include the following:

1. The use of narratives, the actual stories of the clinician with their patients, influenced by the broad field of narrative medicine, which provides a way of understanding the personal connections between physicians and patients and the meaning of medical practice and experiences for individual physicians. It also reflects the physicians' values and beliefs, and how these become manifest in the physician–patient relationship, and how that connection relates to the society in which it develops. According to Charon, narrative medicine helps imbue the facts and objects of health and illness with their consequences and meanings for individual patients and physicians (Charon, 2001a, 2001b). Narrative medicine

in the Mindful Practice programs includes the sharing of stories that arise from the participants' clinical experiences and takes the form of reflection, dialogue and discussion in large and small groups, specific writing exercises, and journaling. Narratives are chosen by the participants about their own personal experiences of caring for patients. Thus, the narratives are grounded in the real lived experiences of the physicians, not in philosophical or rhetorical—what-ifs that impact on cognitive and emotional challenges.

2. Appreciative inquiry (AI) strives to foster growth and change by focusing participants' attention on their existing capacities and prior successes in relationship building and problem-solving (as opposed to an exclusive focus on problems and challenges). Much of medical training focuses on what is wrong rather than what is right. Patients are described in terms of problem lists, but there are no defined places to describe their strengths and resources. Morbidity and mortality rounds focus on analyzing bad outcomes, but there are few opportunities to explore effective teamwork and joint decision-making. The theory behind AI is that reinforcement and analysis of positive experiences with patients and families are more likely to change behavior in desired directions than the exclusive critique of negative experiences or failures (Cooperider and Whitney, 2005). Appreciative inquiry involves the art and practice of asking unconditionally positive questions that strengthen the capacities to apprehend, anticipate, and heighten positive potential. It is an inquiry tool that fosters imagination and innovation. The AI approach makes several assumptions: (1) for every person or group there is something that is working; (2) looking for what works well and doing more of it is more motivating than looking for what doesn't work well and doing less of it; (3) what we focus on becomes our reality and individuals and groups move toward what they focus on; (4) the language we use to describe reality helps to create that reality; (5) people have more confidence to journey to the future if they carry forward parts of the past; (6) we should carry forward the best parts of the past.

Traditionally, the steps of AI involve the following: (1) definition—what we wish to see or grow in ourselves and our groups; (2) discovery—what gives life; (3) dream—what might be; (4) design—what should be; and (5) delivery—what will be. AI's impact on fostering change includes a strengthening of the confidence and positive dialogue about the future, increased feelings of connection and participation, and an appreciative mind-set and culture.

In the Mindful Practice curriculum, the first two steps of AI definition and discovery are integrated into the structure of interpersonal dialogues in the sharing of participants' narratives. Participants are guided in using AI techniques when engaged in appreciative dialogues, discussion, and reflection. With the ongoing practice and support of skilled facilitation, this approach becomes second nature and is the predominant technique used for exploring the experiences that arise in the narratives, perceived through the quality of mindfulness.

The Mindful Practice program is facilitated in a modular manner, in which each module contains elements to cultivate greater mindfulness through contemplative practice and skills building. Additionally, each module includes a discussion of a challenging theme or dynamic in clinical work, and asks the participants to reflect on their own personal experiences related to theme. Participants then engage in dialogues sharing their experiences, and directing them to use the approach of appreciative inquiry to explore the inherent capacities they have for working with these challenges. Among the themes of Mindful Practice modules are burnout, meaningful experiences, errors, suffering, grief, attraction, self-care, and others (Krasner et al., 2009).

The Personal

My own journey toward the teaching of mindfulness approaches in my medical work began over 25 years ago when exploring a personal contemplative practice amidst the increasing pressures of building a practice of primary care internal medicine, experiencing the challenges of a growing family of three young children, and finding myself at the time emotionally exhausted as I entered what was still the early stages of my career. At about this time my father became ill with pancreatic cancer and almost immediately, influenced by the book *Full Catastrophe Living*, he also began a serious contemplative practice (Kabat-Zinn, 1990). We were both affected deeply by the personal effects of a mindfulness practice. For my father, he lived another 24 months, most of that in relatively good health and high function. For me, I began a deeper inquiry into the power of this approach for me personally as well as professionally.

Within a few years, I began mindfulness facilitation training, and then teaching MBSR, initially with patients, then a broader community of participants. Among these participants were physicians of all types, representing many specialties and from community as well as academic careers. Prompted by these colleagues I began to offer health professional-specific MBSR course with continuing medical education credit offered. From a facilitation standpoint, the experiences with these predominantly physician groups were qualitatively similar to other MBSR groups. However, I began to hear from these participants about the effects that the course experiences were having on the meaning they derived from their work and their enjoyment and commitment to medicine.

After a number of years, the opportunity arose to direct a project that, in part, led to the creation of the Mindful Practice program. This project, originally called *Mindful Communication*, included a collaboration with medical communication experts at the University of Rochester, and enrolled in the yearlong training project that was developed, 70 local primary care physicians. Simultaneously, our team also trained in another yearlong program faculty at the University of Rochester School of Medicine and Dentistry to facilitate Mindful Practice seminars as part of the required curriculum for all third-year medical students.

Since those "early years" in 2005–2007, and since the completion and report on the Mindful Communication project in 2009 (Krasner et al., 2009), the Mindful Practice program has continued to be a part of the medical school curriculum.

Additionally, new training approaches for practicing physicians and other health professionals has involved over 600 health professionals in intensive retreat-like trainings held locally and worldwide (see www.mindfulpractice.urmc.edu). I would like to briefly summarize some personal reflections on the experience of working with health professional colleagues, and how this relates to the ethics and teaching of mindfulness to physicians and health professionals.

It is difficult to encapsulate the experience in a few paragraphs, but perhaps it would be helpful for me to share my impressions from facilitating one of the Mindful Practice modules to physicians and other health professionals, so the reader can gain some insight into the power of mindful attention and awareness applied to challenges faced by clinicians. That module has to do with an exploration of errors. Errors is certainly one of the most challenging experiences for anyone to contemplate, especially the physician in which medical errors can have such grave consequences for the patients, and can be associated with fear, shame, humiliation, exposure, self-doubt, anger, and hosts of other emotional states for the clinician.

During this module, we explore together, through a dramatized video demonstration, the disclosure of a serious mistake in medical judgment by a physician to a patient's family member (the patient died as a result of this error). After this discussion, and supported by formal mindful practices including loving-kindness practice, the participants are then asked to share in pairs their own personal experiences, and to discover, through the process of appreciative inquiry, the capacities and successes that were present for them and are part of them through this difficult challenge, and can be carried forward into future challenges.

It would be an understatement to suggest that participation in this module is difficult. Many of the participants, however, are able to share their narratives of experiences they have had but have never spoken of, reflected on with a colleague, shared openly or even considered that there were any worthy qualities within themselves related to the experience. These often emotional, cathartic, and healing conversations allow the health professional to be able to rediscover the complexities and the possibility for different framing of experiences rather than a black-and-white dualistic understanding of an absolute orientation toward errors. Additionally, what arises out from these conversations is an almost universal recognition of the deep caring, compassion, concern, respect, and love by the clinician for the patient involved in the error. This, I think, helps reconnect the ethics of the professional—autonomy, beneficence, non-maleficence and justice—with not only the internal thoughts and feeling but also the actions of the clinician.

In 1925, Dr. Francis Peabody said to the graduating class at Harvard Medical School *One of the essential qualities of the clinician is interest in humanity, for the secret of the care of the patient is in caring for the patient* (Peabody, 1927). Mindful Practice helps connect health professionals with this caring dimension of the patient, and in doing so, becomes a process that supports the ethics of relationship of the health professional with the patient.

Conclusion

> A man who has been through bitter experiences and travelled far enjoys even his sufferings after a time.
> HOMER, The Odyssey

Jon Kabat-Zinn in his book *Full Catastrophe Living* presented the definition of mindfulness that guided the development of the Mindfulness-Based Stress Reduction Program (MBSR) as: moment to moment awareness (Kabat-Zinn, 1990, p. 2). Over time, this has become understood as the awareness that arises through paying attention on purpose in the present moment, nonjudgmentally. These definitions are accompanied by a number of attitudinal foundations that guided the cultivation of mindfulness: patience, non-judging, beginner's mind, letting go, trust, non-striving, and acceptance. At a recent symposium at John's Hopkins University in 2014 Kabat-Zinn offered an updated definition that included a more explicit ethical intention for the cultivation of mindfulness: *Mindfulness is the awareness arising from paying attention, on purpose in the present moment, non-judgmentally, in the service of self-understanding, wisdom, and compassion* (Kabat-Zinn, 2014).

This clarification of the definition of mindfulness for teaching within mindfulness-based programs reflects more explicitly the ethical intentions of self-understanding, wisdom, and compassion. It mirrors a growing recognition within the medical community for the need to be more explicit about the underlying professional ethics that not only support the provision of mindful health care, but also support the needs of the providers of health care. This emerging realization impacts the entire systemic professional ethics of health care itself. Promoting best practice in medicine includes paying attention to the patient as well as the physicians and other health professionals as people who, in order to deliver high quality and compassionate care, need to attend to the care of themselves as well.

For health professionals, the intentional turning toward the "full catastrophe" as a vocation and as an avocation on the surface may seem odd. For who would find not only a calling but also a deep enjoyment and satisfaction in attending to the aging, ill, and dying? Yet, as discussed earlier, the meaning found from simply being present to even the most difficult conditions and circumstances of their patients motivates the health professional (Horowitz et al., 2003).

We can begin to speculate why this might be. Might it be in the empathic resonance and recognition that supporting another human being's autonomy satisfies one's own desire for the same? Might it be in the beneficent actions by health professionals that one experiences the power of giving and receiving? Might it be in the efforts to do no harm, that non-malfeasance also helps the health professional to avoid harm herself? Might it be in the simple act of caring, utilizing one's knowledge and skills regardless of who the patient is or where she comes from or what her values are, that the health professional experiences the power of justice enacted within a moment of contact, and can see the reflection of that justice as the moral imperative flowing bidirectionally?

For physicians, physicians-in-training, and other health professionals, turning toward the most difficult and challenging aspects of the human condition with exquisite empathy may actually prevent burnout and the associated diminution in quality of care and quality of caring. Mindful awareness and communication skills sit at the heart of cultivating ethical behavior within the health care environment. Mindfulness itself creates the "ethical space from which to see, think, speak, act, and work in ways that are not conditioned by reactivity" (Batchelor, n.d.).

While working with practicing physicians and medical students in coursework designed to develop mindfulness, the sharing of their reflections about clinical narratives they are part of provides a rich source of meaning and relationship-centered connection. At the conclusion of these courses, students or practitioners are often asked to write their own Hippocratic Oath. From these words, we can all gain faith in those who practice the art and science of Medicine, and who will care for us as we age, become ill, and die.

> I promise to always put the patient at the center of my practice. I will treat the human being and try to consider the world in which he lives…I will try to stay aware of my own feelings, beliefs and biases as I treat my patients…I will remember that I am only one link in a long chain of caregivers…I will try to remember that neglecting my own health and well being may negatively affect my patients. Really caring about myself and my patients should be at the center of what I try to do. (Medical Student)

References

Allen, W. (1979, August 10). My speech to the graduates. *New York Times*, 25.

AMA Code of Medical Ethics. (2001). Retrieved March 26, 2017, from https://www.ama-assn.org/sites/default/files/media-browser/principles-of-medical-ethics.pdf

Antonovsky, A. (1979). *Health, stress and coping.* San Francisco, CA: Jossey-Bass Publishers.

Barry, M. J., & Edgman-Levitan, S. (2012). Shared decision making-the pinnacle of patient care. *The New England Journal of Medicine, 366*, 780–781.

Batchelor, S. (n.d.). A Buddhist Brexit: A secular reimagining of the dharma may help us face political calamity. *Tricycle Magazine, 26*(Spring).

Beach, M. C., & Inui, T. (2006). Relationship-centered care: A constructive reframing. *Journal of General Internal Medicine, 21*(Suppl 1), S3–S8.

Beauchamp, T., & Childress, J. (2012). *Principles of biomedical ethics* (7th ed.). Oxford: Oxford University Press.

Beckman, H. B., Markakis, K. M., Suchman, A. L., & Frankel, R. M. (1994). The doctor-patient relationship and malpractice: Lessons from plaintiff depositions. *Archives of Internal Medicine, 154*(12), 1365–1370.

Beckman, H., Wendland, M., Mooney, C., Krasner, M. S., Quill, T. E., Suchman, A. L., & Epstein, R. M. (2012). The impact of a program in mindful communication on primary care physicians. *Academic Medicine, 87*(6), 1–5.

Bodhi, B. (2005). *In the Buddha's words: An anthology of discourses from the Pali canon.* Boston, MA: Wisdom Publishers.

Budd, S., & Sharma, U. (1994). *The Healing bond: The patient-practitioner relationship and therapeutic responsibility.* London: Routledge.

Cassell, E. (1982). The nature of suffering and the goals of medicine. *New England Journal of Medicine, 306*(11), 639–645.

Charon, R. (2001a). Narrative medicine: Form, function and ethics. *Annals of Internal Medicine, 134,* 83–87.

Charon, R. (2001b). The patient-physician relationship. Narrative medicine: A model for empathy. *Journal of the American Medical Association, 286,* 1897–1902.

Charon, R. (2006). *Narrative medicine: Honoring the stories of illness.* Oxford: Oxford University Press.

Cooperider, D. L., & Whitney, D. (2005). *Appreciative inquiry: A positive revolution in change.* San Francisco, CA: Berrett-Koehler.

Crane, M. (1998). Why burned-out doctors get sued more often. Medical Economics, 75(10), 210–212., 215–218.

Crane, R. S., Brewer, J. A., Feldman, C., Kabat-Zinn, J., Santorelli, S. F., Williams, J. M. G., & Kuyken, W. (2016, December 29). What defines mindfulness-based programs? The warp and the weft. *Psychological Medicine,* 1–10.

Doyle, D. (2005). Dr. Doyle receives Lifetime Achievement Award from American Academy of Hospice and Palliative Medicine. *International Association for Hospice and Palliative Care Newsletter, 6*(2).

Dyrbye, L. N., Thomas, M. R., Huschka, M. M., Lawson, K. L., Novotny, P. J., Sloan, J. A., & Shanafelt, T. D. (2006). A multicenter study of burnout, depression, and quality of life in minority and nonminority US medical students. *Mayo Clinic Proceedings, 81*(11), 1435–1442.

Eisenberg, J. (1979). Sociologic influences on decision-making by clinicians. *Annals of Internal Medicine, 90*(6), 957–964.

Ekman, E., & Krasner, M. (2017). Empathy in medicine: Neuroscience, education and challenges. *Medical Teacher, 39*(2), 164–173.

Epstein, R. (1999). Mindful practice. *Journal of the American Medical Association, 282*(9), 833–839.

Epstein, R. (2003). Mindful practice in action (II): Cultivating habits of mind. *Families, Systems & Health, 21,* 11–17.

Fitzgerald, F. (1999). Curiosity. *Annals of Internal Medicine, 130*(1), 70–72.

Flexner, A. (1910). *Medical education in the United States and Canada: A report to the Carnegie Foundation for the Advancement of Teaching.* Boston: Updyke.

Gerrity, M. S., Earp, J. A. L., DeVellis, R., & Light, D. (1992). Uncertainty and professional work: Perceptions of physicians in clinical pratice. *American Journal of Sociology, 97*(4), 1022–1051.

Good, B. (1994). *Medicine, rationality, and experience: An antropological perspective. Lewis Henry Morgan Lectures.* Cambridge: Cambridge University Press.

Greenhut, J. (1995). Living without hope. *Second Opinion, 21*(1), 27.

Groopman, J. (2007). *How doctors think.* Boston, MA: Houghton Mifflin Harcourt.

Haas, J. S., Cleary, P. D., Puopolo, A. L., Burstin, H. R., Cook, E. F., & Brennan, T. A. (2000). Is the porfessional satisfaction of general internists associated with patient satisfaction? *Journal of General Internal Medicine, 15*(2), 122–128.

Halpern, J. (2011). *From detached concern to empathy: Humanizing medical practice.* Oxford: Oxford University Press.

Horowitz, C. R., Suchman, A., Branch, W. T., & Frankel, R. M. (2003). What do doctors find meaningful about their work? *Annals of Internal Medicine, 138*(9), 772–776.

Kabat-Zinn, J. (1990). *Full catastrophe living: Using the wisdom of your body and mind to face stress, pain and illness.* New York, NY: Bantam Dell.

Kabat-Zinn, J. (2014). *Mindfulness and learning: An interdisciplinary symposium.* Baltimore: Johns Hopkins University.

Kearney, M. K., Weininger, R. B., Vachon, M. L., Harrison, R. L., & Mount, B. M. (2009). Self-care of physicians caring for patients at the end of life "Being connected … a key to my survival". *Journal of the American Medicial Association, 301*(11), 1155–1164.

Krasner, M. S., Epstein, R. M., Beckman, H., Suchman, A. L., Chapman, B., Mooney, C. J., & Quill, T. E. (2009). Association of an educational program in mindful communication with burnout, empathy and attitudes among primary care physicians. *Journal of the American Medical Association, 302*(12), 1284–1293.

Lempp, H., & Seale, C. (2004). The hidden curriculum in undergraduate medical education: Qualitative study of medical students' perceptions of teaching. *British Medical Journal*, *329*(7469), 770–773.

Lück, M. (2015, September). *Intimacy in the clinical encounter: It's not what you think*. MSc Medical Humanities Dissertation, Kings College, London.

Ludwig, D., & Kabat-Zinn, J. (2008). Mindfulness in medicine. *Journal of the American Medical Association*, *300*, 1350–1352.

Marsh, H. (2014). *Do no harm: Stories of life, death and brain surgery*. London: Weidenfeld and Nicholson.

Miller, W. L., Crabtree, B. F., Nutting, P. A., Stange, K. C., & Jaén, C. R. (2010). Primary care practice development: A relationship-centered approach. *Annals of Family Medicine*, *8*(Supplement 1), S68–S79.

National Library of Medicine. (n.d.). Retrieved February 12, 2017, from National Library of Medicine Website: https://www.nlm.nih.gov/hmd/greek/greek_oath.html

OCR GCSE SHP Student Book chapter. (n.d.). Retrieved February 12, 2017, from OCR GCSE History A: Medicine through time: https://www.pearsonschoolsandfecolleges.co.uk/AssetsLibrary/SECTORS/Secondary/SUBJECT/HistoryandSocialScience/HistoryChapters/OCRGCSESHPStudentBookchapter.pdf

Ofri, D. (2013). *What doctors feel: How emotions affect the practice of medicine*. Boston, MA: Beacon Press.

Oliver, M. (1992). *New and selected poems*. Boston, MA: Beacon Press.

Page, K. (2012). The four principles: Can they be measured and do they predict ethical decision making? *BioMed Central Medical Ethics*, *13*(10), 1–8.

Peabody, F. (1927). The care of the patient. *Journal of the American Medical Association*, *88*, 877–882.

Rabow, M., Remen, R., Parmelee, D. X., & Inui, T. S. (2010). Professional formation: Extending medicine's lineage of service into the next century. *Academic Medicine*, *85*, 310–317.

Ryan, R. M., & Deci, E. L. (2002). Self-determination theory and the facilitation of intrinsic motivation, social development, and well-being. *American Psychologist*, *55*, 68–78.

Santorelli, S. (1998). *Heal thyself: Lessons on mindfulness in medicine*. New York, NY: Bell Town.

Shanafelt, T. D., Sloan, J., & Habermann, T. M. (2003). The well-being of physicians. *American Journal of Medicine*, *114*(6), 513–519.

Sibinga, E. M. S., & Wu, A. W. (2010). Clinician mindfulness and patient safety. *Journal of the American Medical Association*, *304*(22), 2532–2533.

Soltes, E. (2017, January 11). Why it's so hard to train someone to make an ethical decision. *Harvard Business Review*.

Stange, K.C., Peigorsh, K.M., Miller, W.L. (2003) *Families, Systems and Health, 21*, 24–27.

West, C. P., Huschka, M. M., Novotny, P. J., Sloan, J. A., Kolars, J. C., Habermann, T. M., & Shanafelt, T. D. (2006). Association of perceived medical errors with resident distress and empathy: A prospective longitutdinal study. *Journal of the American Medical Association*, *296*(9), 1071–1078.

Yavari, N. (2016). Does medical education erode medical trainees' ethical attitude and behavior? *Journal of Medical Ethics and History of Medicine*, *9*, 16.

Part II
Ethics in Mindfulness-based Interventions and Programs

Chapter 6
The Moral Arc of Mindfulness: Cultivating Concentration, Wisdom, and Compassion

Lynette M. Monteiro

Introduction

The use of mindfulness-based interventions (MBIs) has grown significantly in the last decade, influenced the philosophy of psychology, and has become a highly investigated clinical intervention. Its use in the treatment of depression, anxiety, pain, trauma, and several other psychological disorders has been reasonably supported by research outcome studies (Khoury et al., 2013). However, the practice of mindfulness is also a personal one that extends into my professional life, not just as a select set of tactics I think may benefit my clients. In 2003, when (Segal, Williams, & Teasdale, 2012) published their influential book on mindfulness-based cognitive therapy (MBCT), I felt confident that the concepts I valued in Buddhism could be translated into a therapeutic program with sensitivity and care. Training in Jon Kabat-Zinn's program of mindfulness-based stress reduction (MBSR; Kabat-Zinn, 2013; Segal et al., 2012) at the Center for Mindfulness, University of Massachusetts, however, revealed the challenges of attaining competency in this modality, holding the integrity of the program and our professional ethics, and exercising discernment in how the skills developed in a mindfulness-based program are put to use.

Since then I've trained in several types of mindfulness programs and have experienced the main challenge as an evolving exploration of ethics and mindfulness. Although this topic has been addressed frequently, it has been presented in a manner that inclines us towards an understanding of ethics in mindfulness as inseparable from the spiritual path, holy on one hand and a risky process to include in psychotherapy on the other. Although one would be tempted on first glance to say the Buddhist scholars are in the former category and the Western secular mindfulness

L.M. Monteiro, PhD (✉)
Ottawa Mindfulness Clinic, 595 Montreal Road, Suite 301, Ottawa, ON, Canada K1K 4L2
e-mail: lynette.monteiro@gmail.com

© Springer International Publishing AG 2017
L.M. Monteiro et al. (eds.), *Practitioner's Guide to Ethics and Mindfulness-Based Interventions*, Mindfulness in Behavioral Health,
DOI 10.1007/978-3-319-64924-5_6

143

practitioners are in the latter, the truth is that the issues of ethics and mindfulness are and have been close to the heart of early adopters of secular mindfulness-based interventions and who then developed what are now called Second-Generation mindfulness programs (Van Gordon, Shonin, & Griffiths, 2015; Singh et al., 2014).

The divisiveness in the various stances towards the issue of ethics and mindfulness has not prevented a quiet revolution of programs designed and developed with sensitivity to the spiritual and secular protocols and processes. The chapters in this section are exemplars of how this complex route from and between spiritual practice to secular application has been navigated. It gratified and astonished me, in reading these chapters, to see that we had each approached the issue of creating and refining our programs by drawing from our professional training that was coextensive with our Buddhist practice.

In this essay, I offer an exploration of some overarching themes in the development of these programs that strive to hold the integrity of mindfulness as it was intended to be transmitted. Of necessity, some aspects of design and development have been left out in the chapters so that a deeper understanding of the rigor and discipline required for each program could be the central focus. Among these are two essential topics that also have received glancing coverage in the extant literature: teacher training and scope of application of mindfulness programs. My exploration of these and other topics in this essay is not intended to offer any resolution for the dilemmas arising from training teachers of mindfulness programs in embodied ethics in short time frames or the ethics of teaching mindfulness to populations like the military, greedy capitalists, or others who are suspected of using mindfulness to do unconscionable harm. I hope to simply raise the net so that the threads and the spaces they define are slightly more visible and available for ongoing conversations about responsible caring.

Ethics and Mindfulness

To explore the ethics of responsible caring, I am drawing from both my own process of growing as a teacher and trainer in the field of MBIs and the challenges of developing our mindfulness program (Mindfulness-Based Symptom Management; MBSM). As an eternal teacher-in-training in various mindfulness interventions, ethical issues related to competency, skillfulness, and my understanding of the therapeutic relationship are crucially important. Developing a mindfulness program curriculum that held its Buddhist roots with transparency while honoring the need for a secular translation presented a specific challenge. Issues we needed to address included informed consent, evidence-based practice and practice-based evidence, and respect for the diverse religious and spiritual affiliations of participants were central to program delivery. And finally, as a Buddhist who has taken up a vow to act in ways that prevent social and individual violence, the call to provide mindfulness teachings to organizations whose functional intention is antithetical to the principles of not doing harm required a deep examination of how mindfulness practices might be misused or misappropriated. (This topic is explored further in the next section.)

Let me begin with an overview of the issues of mindfulness and ethics as they are informed by Buddhist and psychological models.

Concepts of Mindfulness and Ethics

Mindfulness and ethics are interdependent in that neither can exist in any form without the other. In the Buddhist concept of dependent arising, neither has a separate identity or existence. The activities or practices of mindfulness cultivate concentration and insight; the intention of practice is clarity, both of perception and of choices in thoughts, words, and deeds. And it is in the interstitial space between perception and choice that the complex issues of ethics, values, and virtues arise.

Using a weaving metaphor, Crane et al. (2016) describe MBSR and MBCT (first-generation mindfulness programs) as the warp of the fabric of mindfulness programs while the weft reflects the individualization of the curriculum and context of the program. While the metaphor is compelling, it places MBSR and MBCT in a privileged position and limits the different threads that also can form the warp of the fabric. It is possible, as the second-generation programs push at the edge of those limits, that the warp is something other than, deeper than the philosophies or perspectives of first-generation programs.

The overarching theme in the chapters of this section arises from theories and concepts of responsible caring thereby introducing warp threads with an ethical texture. Each chapter represents the application of mindfulness in a lay, secular context with a specific intention of addressing twenty-first century individual and collective ills, find their ground. Bruno Cayoun, describing and supporting mindfulness-integrated cognitive behavioral therapy (MiCBT), offers a careful and syncretic approach to treating psychological distress. Patricia Jennings and Anthony DeMauro ground the CARE program in the ethic of responsible care. Frank Musten and I detail the development and application of mindfulness-based symptom management (MBSM) as the convergence of Thich Nhat Hanh's teaching of ethics and the ethics of care in the work of Carol Gilligan and Joan Tronto (Gilligan, 1993, 2011, 2014; Tronto, 1993). Pittman McGehee, Christopher Germer, and Kristin Neff explore the necessity of self-compassion in the cultivation of core values and the virtues of loving-kindness, compassion, equanimity, and joy support those values.

James Kirby and colleagues and David Addiss extend the concept of responsible caring to the ultimate intention of cultivating mindfulness. If, from the Buddhist perspective, the arc of mindfulness practice is a moral one, then its landing zone is in the field of compassion. In fact, it is hard to imagine compassion as anything less than the highest ethic, the cause for which we all devote our time and energy, independent of our disagreement over the number of ethical angels dancing on the meditation cushion.

The programs presented in this section are carefully designed to uphold the inseparability of mindfulness and ethics, and stand up well against the criticisms of secular mindfulness as bereft of ethics as contained in the Buddhist teachings of mindfulness. At the same time, I have found it important to challenge the prevailing view that any perceived absence of specifically Buddhist ethics is the same as a total absence of ethics. Western psychology offers two very prominent models and lines of inquiry into moral development and cultivation of virtues. Ruth Baer's chapter in this book addresses the latter and therefore the topic will not be included here; however, the field of moral development does play a significant role in helping us understand the human capacity to care and be compassionate as well as the failure to do so. Further, Narvaez's work on neurobiology and human morality (Narvaez, 2014; Rest & Narvaez, 1994; Rest, Narvaez, Bebeau, & Thoma, 1999) and Bandura's work on moral disengagement (Bandura, 2016) serve the field of mindfulness well in extending our understanding of the complexities of cultivating moral judgment and action. In psychotherapy itself, ethics are a central issue in its training and practice. The complexity of ethics, values, and virtues is addressed by Tjeltveit (1999), Pope and Vasquez (2016), Pettifor, Sinclair, and Gauthier (2011), and the various professional association guidelines for psychologists, physicians, psychotherapists, and counsellors. Thus, not only are mindfulness and ethics inseparable, ethics and any psychologically focused intervention—be it a general program or treatment—are equally inseparable.

The question, however, remains: what are we pointing to when we speak of ethics and mindfulness? In this regard, McCown's body of work (McCown, 2013, 2014, 2016; McCown, Reibel, & Micozzi, 2010) is central to the exploration of ethics and mindfulness as a relational construct. Recent commentaries to Monteiro, Musten, and Compson (2015) are rich in their examination of the issue of implicit and explicit ethics in mindfulness with the most striking comment being that the subtle influences of a Judeo-Christian cultural frame must be included in any exegesis of the topic (Amaro, 2015). In effect, Amaro is pointing to the relational frame of culture and our often-unexamined presumption of its privilege. Still I believe the topic remains confounded both by language and a view of the topic as monolithic. In my growing understanding, there are two aspects to this topic and it may serve the discussion well to differentiate between them: ethics *of* mindfulness and ethics *in* mindfulness.

Where the first section of this book, led by Compson, Gunther-Brown, and Baer's chapters, has touched on the ethics *of* mindfulness, this second section (and the subsequent one) offers the ways in which ethics can be and are contained *in* mindfulness. The former, ethics *of* mindfulness, may be seen to examine the virtues and pitfalls of translating a spiritual practice into a secular frame; it can also include examinations of the appropriateness and intentions of training certain populations (military, corporate moguls, etc.). The latter, ethics *in* mindfulness, opens the discussion to the thoughtful development of mindfulness programs such that they hold the integrity of mindfulness: the cultivation of concentration, wisdom, and compassion.

It may be necessary then to look at the Buddhist and Western conceptualizations of ethics and mindfulness not as two colliding cultures, but as a convergence of thoughts and philosophies that had their origins two and a half centuries ago. A common theme in both conceptualizations is the concept of mindfulness as a moral arc, and I explore the implications of that view with an eye on its relevance to program development and training of those who aspire to teach these programs.

The Moral Arc in Buddhist Practice

Buddhist ethics are a practice of developing the Noble Person, one who is aware of both the truth of suffering and its corollaries of impermanence, fluid self, and inherent unsatisfactoriness (Harvey, 2000, 2013). The core teachings of Buddhism are that life is challenging because of our reactivity to the inevitable pain of being human by becoming resistant, clinging, or confused about the direct experience itself. The solution, the Buddha taught, is to become aware and awake to the myriad ways we avoid reality and to engage in a rigorous practice of clarifying and concentrating the mind. It begins with ethics, which is cultivated from an aspiration to be virtuous in thought, word, and action and from that base to cultivate wisdom and compassion in how we live our lives (Gombrich, 2009/2013).

Harvey (2000) describes the process of cultivating ethics in the Buddhist Path as a series of stages which begin with the cultivation of virtues. He goes further to suggest that this cultivation occurs through influence and inspiration by "good examples" and the motivation arises from a "preliminary wisdom." Following from this establishment of a virtuous base, the cultivation of concentration through meditation can lead to clarity and wisdom. Gombrich (2009/2013) points out that the strength of the Buddha's teachings lay in turning brahminical or caste-bound practices of his time into ethical commitments thereby transforming ritual as externalized doing (offering sacrifices) into an act of purifying one's mental state. In other words, by placing intention and moral action in the same frame and in the hands of the practitioner, the teachings emphasize individual autonomy and responsibility for one's own experiential process.

At the same time, ethics in the Buddhist framework are not solely about personal improvement or personal salvation. The ultimate trajectory of practice is the cultivation of compassion, and we might say that in Buddhism compassion is the highest ethic. Compassion is one of four interconnected noble states of being called the *brahmaviharas* or a way of love; the others are loving-kindness, resonant joy, and equanimity (Monteiro & Musten, 2013). As we clarify our mental states and develop a discerning wisdom in our thoughts, words, and actions, these states become a natural inclination of mind. They interact with each other, supporting and amplifying our capacity to be kind-hearted, understand and appreciate the joy of others, be matter-of-fact with the vagaries of life, and to fully know the suffering that others feel and to wish better for them.

However, the ability to engage with the world through the lens of this state of being requires steadiness in the face distress (ours and that of others), clarity of knowing what is required in our relationship to our own experience and that of others, and the willingness to act in a way that minimizes harm. In other words, the foundation of love is mindfulness, and the practice of mindfulness is the intention to love. Holding this map of practice in mind, let us now look at the ways Western psychology has addressed the issue of ethics and the development of a virtuous person.

The Moral Arc in Western Psychological Practice

Western psychology is no stranger to the topics of moral development and applied ethics. Baer (2015) cogently outlines the ways in which psychological models and research can contribute and have contributed to the cultivation of virtues and values in secular mindfulness. One of those models began with the work of Lawrence Kohlberg on moral development (Kohlberg, 1976; Rest & Narvaez, 1994) and placed the understanding of moral actions in the individual's determination of right and wrong rather than a process of forced socialization to cultural norms. This latter view had been a means of promoting a sense of positive adjustment by diminishing any incongruence between personal moral reasoning and one imposed by cultural norms.

Rest and Narvaez (1994) argue that the field of moral development does not present a uniform set of concepts and the research was confounded by approaches based on a large range of psychological—and often competing—theories. They propose a Four Component Model comprising moral sensitivity, moral judgment, moral motivation, and moral character, which offers a broader process-oriented framework. The model also addresses the issue of moral failure, that is when moral action could/should, but fails to occur. This closely parallels Buddhist practices that include unskillful actions to be "put down" and skillful ones to be taken up (Aitken, 1984). The model is not cast as a logical progression; however, it seems intuitive that moral sensitivity is required as a foundation, an awareness of how our actions affect others. Moral judgment plays a role in determining a course of action; however, it presumes a clarity of vision with respect to the relational aspects of any situation. That is, a simplistic determination of right or wrong may be as harmful as not making a decision. Moral motivation brings to light the clarity and intentionality required in moral decision-making; understanding the impact of competing values and their sequelae plays a role in knowing the higher-level ethic required in each situation as well as making the choice that is best practice for the situation. Moral character is defined as the strength or fortitude to make difficult moral decisions and is likely the source of moral failure even if the previous three components are present and developed.

The Four Component Model offers two subtle perspectives relevant to mindfulness practice. First, there is an implicit principle of cultivating the capacity of the individual through awareness of moments of moral failure that can then be used as opportunity for maturity; that is, the capacity to see and experience an incongruence between the action required and the action taken can lead to wisdom in future experiences. I choose the term "incongruence" deliberately because when we become aware of how we have behaved and the way it is inconsistent with our intentions and therefore our values, we tend to refer to those instances as somehow being "not me." Incongruence also infers a pre-existing condition of intention or a ground of values from which we operate. In this latter sense, it parallels the Buddhist idea of intention in action.

The groundswell of mindfulness programs and practices reflects, through psychological diagnostic terminology, the results of a lack of awareness or disconnect between ideal and actual, "should have" and "did," "should be," and "is." Research into burnout (M.P. Leiter, Frank, & Matheson, 2009; M.P. Leiter, Jackson, & Shaughnessy, 2009; Maslach & Leiter, 1997) and its causes suggests burnout results in part from an incongruence between trying to adhere to stated organizational values and the actual lived or expected behaviors. For example, an organization may have stated values to provide quality and compassionate health care for all persons, but fiscal demands and personnel shortfalls may result in operating principles that do not reflect the stated values. The pressure to provide health care under such circumstances can result in the factors of burnout, including helplessness to take ethical stands against an employer. The cultivation of mindfulness as a practice of awareness and clarity might foster better decision-making and relationship-building in such circumstances.

In their chapter, Jennings and DeMauro address the ways mindfulness training assists teachers in meeting the demands of a stressful workplace, their commitment to their students, and their need to attend to personal well-being. The prosocial classroom theoretical model Jennings and DeMauro propose addresses the social and emotional competencies that play a significant role in self-care and eventual well-being. The feedback received from the teachers who participated in the CARE training suggests a shift in important aspects of the teacher–student relationships towards greater empathy and compassion.

The second perspective offered by the Four Component Model is the vision of moral development as a moral arc of practice rather than a process of dealing with complex decision-making through algorithms or rule-bound actions. As with Buddhist practices of mindfulness, the model begins with the cultivation of an aspiration to learn from and cultivate relationships that serve self and others well. The practice of developing awareness gives rise to sensitivity to the impact of our actions on ourselves, others, and the world around us. In the context of mindfulness programs, participants come with a range of awareness of their own suffering and it would not be an exaggeration to say much time in practice is spent resisting the reality that suffering is present. The arc of practice then is one of developing clarity and steadiness in the face of suffering and learning how to be patient with the inconsistencies and incongruences of thought, word, and action we all experience.

The post-Kohlbergian direction was towards an elucidation of ethics of care by Carol Gilligan (1993, 2011, 2014) and her colleagues (Fisher & Tronto, 1990; Gilligan & Attanucci, 1988; Tronto, 1993; van Nistelrooij, Schaafsma, & Tronto, 2014). As we (Monteiro and Musten) explore in our chapter and McGehee and his colleagues proposed in their chapter on Mindful Self-Compassion, the concept of care for self and others is a moral stance incorporating the elements of responsibility in the context of relationships. These relationships are viewed not only as interpersonal ones, but also our internal relationship with our ideals. By inviting an explicit exploration of the ethics of (self) care and caring through the Five Skillful Habits, a core practice in the MBSM curriculum, the intent is to open awareness to the incongruence between ideal values and actual or lived ones.

This approach to the cultivation and clarification of personal ethics is consistent with Buddhist practices that promote not just the renunciation of what leads to harm, but also the cultivation of what results in good (Aitken, 1984). Thich Nhat Hanh's formulation of the Five and Fourteen Mindfulness Trainings (Hanh, 2005, 2007) opens with the words, "Aware of the suffering caused by" and establishes both an acknowledgment of the impact of our actions and a commitment to transforming those that are unskillful or cause harm. This attitude of what to put down and what to take up becomes relevant in the following discussion of the domains of secular mindfulness in which ethics play a significant role.

In his chapter, Bruno Cayoun describes the development of MiCBT as a "theoretically congruent and technically complementary" convergence of cognitive behavioral therapy and Buddhist teachings (see also Cayoun, 2011). The arc of MiCBT is the cultivation of compassion which Cayoun views as central to healing and preventing relapse. Creatively, to integrate a conscious intentionality to cultivate ethics in their practice, he invites participants in MiCBT to take up "five ethical challenges" each week. He also points out that intentional harmful actions are likely attempts to reduce unpleasant sensations and increase pleasant ones. And, consistent with the issue of becoming aware of incongruence in our actions, he points out that without becoming aware of the potential ethical "breaches" in our actions, the practice of mindfulness may not be able to foster a generalizability of ethical actions.

Three Domains of Secular Mindfulness

In mindfulness-based programs (MBPs), the issue of ethics emerges in three domains:

- The training we receive and offer to effectively use mindfulness approaches.
- The sensitivity with which we translate what are Buddhist (or the very least Buddhist-informed) concepts and implement these practices with populations that may not be comfortable or resonate with them.
- Our awareness of the impact of mindfulness practices on individuals and groups who may misappropriate their use.

In writing about ethics in mindfulness, I've organized these domains as training the teacher of mindfulness, developing the teachings (or content) of mindfulness programs to reflect and honor their origins, and sensitivity to those who are taught mindfulness (Monteiro et al., 2015).

Training the Teacher

The subtext to the three chapters in this section is the training of qualified teachers so that these programs can be delivered with consistency and program integrity. Although training as a mindfulness practitioner/teacher is available globally, and the programs that offer training have strict criteria, these tend to focus on attaining deliverable skills and are measured by competencies in various domains (Crane, Kuyken, Hastings, Rothwell, & Williams, 2010; Evans et al., 2014). What is not given opportunity in the high demand for qualified teachers is necessary time for the cultivation of the individual so that the ethical frame is eventually embodied.

One argument made for the exclusion of explicit ethics in mindfulness programs is that teachers of mindfulness have their professional ethical codes that protect participants (Kabat-Zinn, 2003, 2011; Williams & Kabat-Zinn, 2013). This argument ignores the reality that mindfulness programs are not always conducted by regulated health care professionals and, while we do not dismiss the commitment of nonregulated professionals to safeguard their clients, there is a higher ethic of providing protection and allowing for recourse and redress in cases of harm, especially when dealing with vulnerable populations. Given the incidence of mental health issues in a general population (in Canada, 20% of the population at any time is at risk for experiencing a mental health challenge), the probability of a significant percentage of participants having mental health challenges in any program is high. Thus, appealing to professional ethical codes is necessary, but it is an insufficient factor in ensuring the safe and effective delivery of mindfulness programs.

Even with a professional Code of Conduct to support us (CPA, 2015), it is not a simple solution to safeguard our participants. As health care practitioners we hold in delicate balance our respect for individual differences, the potential of our subtle influences, our own ethical convictions, and are called upon to reflect on and make ethical decisions that are putatively objective (Monteiro, 2016). This clarity of self requires the cultivation of our capacity for self-awareness, emotional regulation, and compassion. They are directly connected to *Principle II: Responsible Caring* (CPA, 2015) and its corollaries of competence and self-knowledge in ways not limited to knowing the evidence-based research. However, the "rub" of training lies in the length of time it takes to become a skilled mindfulness teacher or therapist. And the challenge for me was not to become so reliant on the practices as strategies and techniques at the cost of cultivating an embodiment of what those practices intend— the cultivation of the whole person. Key developmental questions here include the way in which we may allow such practices to shape our personal worldview and how to trust the trajectory of our training so that we can proceed with confidence.

The common factor in all mindfulness programs is the emphasis on the inherent wisdom of the participant and the therapist as the co-facilitator of the process of healing. McCown (2013) describes this as a co-created fluid interaction that is primarily relational. In this regard, the paradigm shift of mindfulness approaches is from a hierarchical relationship to one that is interactive, from one of the therapist as the subject-matter expert to being a co-explorer of a complex landscape. However, as he points out, in establishing its *bona fides* as an evidence-based treatment, the philosophy of mindfulness paradoxically has highlighted the individual, inner experience without a corresponding emphasis on the cultivation of the co-facilitator, the therapist.

Supporting the need for the cultivation of the facilitator/therapist, there is evidence that therapists who have engaged in mindfulness training experience shifts in their capacity to be present and hold the relational space. In a qualitative study, (Lee, Paré, & Monteiro, in press) investigated the impact of mindfulness on the way therapists interacted with their patients. The subject therapists reported changes in their ability to be present in session, to honor the client's position, and to listen actively. Aggs and Bambling (2010) reported increased well-being in therapists (from a wide range of health care sectors) after an 8-week mindfulness training course and greater attitude of equanimity within the work of therapy.

In the context of the *Principle II: Integrity of the Relationship & Section III.10* (CPA, 2015), mindfulness offers the therapist an opportunity to cultivate a way of being with self and other that is aware, connected, and respectful. By developing an approach that is curious and compassionately investigative, the process of evaluating "how their personal experiences, attitudes, values, social context, individual differences, stresses, and specific training influence their activities and thinking" (CPA, 2015) becomes less threatening and more likely to aid in the development of a skillful psychologist.

While attention and open awareness are important aspects of practicing mindfulness, compassion is the core intent of the path of mindfulness and can be considered the highest ethic of practice. Self-compassion, in turn and as McGehee and colleagues note in their chapter, is noted to be an initiator in the cultivation of compassion for others (Neff, 2011; Solhaug, Eriksen, & de Vibe, 2016). Patsiopoulos and Buchanan (2011) report that training in self-compassion enhanced self-care, reduced job-related stress, and increased effectiveness with clients. Participants also reported compassion as an emergent quality of practicing self-compassion. The authors suggest that inclusion of self-compassion as part of therapist training could be important in preventing therapists' burnout and healing relationships in the workplace. This is important in the light of research that suggests a core feature of burnout is cynicism towards the populations being served (Leiter, 2008; Maslach & Jackson, 1984; Maslach & Leiter, 2008). While Mol, Kompanje, Benoit, Bakker, and Nijkamp (2015) suggest burnout factors can negatively impact the quality of patient care and, through job attrition, an eventual loss of skilled professionals, Fernando, Skinner, and Considine (2017) demonstrated that a brief mindfulness intervention impacted tendencies to help or like patients among medical student, but this was also moderated by levels of self-compassion.

Training the Mindful, Compassionate Psychologist-Ethicist It is evident that our ability to hold the ethical space in our professional role relies on clarity of mind and compassion for self and others. However, mindfulness and compassion training, while considered valuable in the cultivation of a therapist, invite mixed opinions of when to introduce these practices. Segal (quoted in Boyce, 2016) stated that introducing mindfulness practices in postgraduate training as clinical skills invites a reliance on mindfulness as a tool rather than an enhancement of a matured, insightful therapeutic practice. The research indicates differently for both well-being and therapist's skills. Danilewitz, Bradwein, and Koszycki (2016) reported positive impact of a mindfulness program on medical students with respect to their well-being and clinical effectiveness. Halland et al. (2015), in a study of mindfulness for psychology students, reported increases in problem-focused coping with those scoring higher on emotional reactivity benefiting from reduced avoidance-focused coping by seeking social support. Felton, Coates, and Christopher (2013) noted increases in self-compassion and confidence in preventing burnout in the future among master's-level health care counselling students. The students also indicated there was reduced emotional reactivity and increased empathy for their clients. Thus, despite the concerns expressed by Segal (in Boyce, 2016), training in mindfulness and self-compassion appears to have a positive impact in the cultivation of therapists-in-training with a suggestion of confidence in dealing with future challenges of being a health care professional.

Cultivating mindfulness and compassion are important for both the mindfulness teacher-in-training as well as the seasoned practitioner. In their chapter, Kirby, Steindl, and Doty connect the cultivation of compassion to the motivation to help others, a manifestation of an ethical stance to suffering. They also suggest that this motivation has evolved from the mammalian caring motivational system and through the vagal system allows for prosocial behaviors. In turn, both prosocial affiliation and the ability to connect with the suffering of others can lead to a globally compassionate approach. In his chapter, Addiss takes the necessity for cultivating compassion and its impact on ethical discernment onto the global stage. Global health, he proposes, needs mindfulness, but the process is complex and requires deep sensitivities to language, culture, economies, power differentials, and an awareness of our biases. He states flatly that "good intentions are not enough," but rather a place to start. In fact, by tying together compassion and justice, Addiss brings us full circle into the ethic of care: the work of Gilligan and her colleagues that informed and inspired the chapters in this section.

How the ethic of care has been explored here is key for developing mindfulness in health care professionals who connect with vulnerable populations. The cultivation of emotion regulation, changes in perspective of the self, and compassion (Hölzel et al., 2011; Monteiro, 2015) are thus not only primary areas relevant to mindfulness and training programs, but are also crucial in fostering our capacity to care well for those who seek our skills.

Developing the Teachings

Mindfulness and ethics are inseparable. Each supports the other through the cultivation of intention, attention, and awareness of the quality of mind we bring to our experience (Shapiro & Schwartz, 2000). However, whether ethics should be part of a mindfulness curriculum is a tinderbox discussion with lines drawn between Buddhist traditionalists and secular modernists. There are arguments that insist it is implicit in the deportment of the teacher and that making it explicit inappropriately imposes values (Kabat-Zinn, 2011), and other perspectives that insist explicit ethics is honest and respectful of the origins and purpose of mindfulness (Amaro, 2015; see also Gunther Brown in this book). I have struggled with this aspect ethics and mindfulness more than any other aspect of program development. I know that we cannot rely solely on vicarious learning (deriving values from those we observe) and I am aware that therapeutic relationships are not "values-neutral" (Monteiro, 2016). These two issues were central in the choices we made to include value-driven goals in developing an ethics-based mindfulness program (Monteiro, Nuttall, & Musten, 2010). I am also deeply aware that informed consent means being fully transparent about the origins and purpose of mindfulness. However, the complexity of holding all these frames is daunting and sometimes introduced unintended consequences in their implementation. For example, potential participants tended to become frustrated and even anxious with our initial information sessions where we strove overly much to be clear about the origins of the program and the need for "fully informed consent."

Nevertheless, those moments of embarrassment and discomfort gave rise to important questions and opportunity for discernment. Because mindfulness is a relational process, it requires cultivating an "ethical space" (McCown, 2013). So, these are the critical questions I ask: How do we include ethics in a way that is transparent because wise discernment of our choices is the intent of mindfulness? How can we offer values-motivated goals as practices yet remain respectful of cultural and individual diversity? How do we develop awareness of the subtle influences of our values, be they Judeo-Christian, Buddhist, or secular? Jane Compson addresses some of these issues in her chapter in the context of the issues raised in the previous section.

These questions are challenging not only because they impose a cognitive load on an already complex process of explaining mindfulness to potential participants, but because they do not lend themselves to definitive answers. And perhaps, as I am slowly beginning to suspect, we also are not asking better questions. When we frame the question as something to be done, something to be included or excluded in a manualized format, I believe we are missing the deeper issue of the relationality of a mindfulness program. To extend McCown's terms (McCown, 2014, 2016), we are trying to fill the space with things we need to be doing rather than simply waiting for the potentiality of a relationship to emerge.

McCown and colleagues (2010, 2013) have defined and illustrated a complex and elegant model of the way in which mindfulness becomes the container, an ethical space, from which growth arises, including the growth of any curriculum we purport to be teaching from. It resonates with verse 11 of the Tao Te Ching (Red Pine, 2009):

Thirty spokes converge on a hub
but it's the emptiness
that makes a wheel work.
pots are fashioned from clay
but it's the hollow
that makes a pot work
windows and doors are carved for a house
but it's the spaces
that make a house work
existence makes a thing useful
but nonexistence makes it work.

Nevertheless, it is important to hold both the ephemeral process of letting the program teach itself and having a map of the landscape in which the practices can mature in some logical progression to the benefit of the participants (which includes the teacher). What threads these two seemingly contradictory factors together is in the interaction between teacher and participant, the Inquiry.

Inquiry as Love As with all relationships, the seeds of connection blossom through attention. In a mindfulness program, the inquiry is the direct meeting of two individuals in a way that transcends their roles as teacher/therapist and participant/client. There are very few explorations of this aspect of a mindfulness program and it is a challenge to train as a skill. The primary injunction—if one can have injunctions in an ephemeral process—is that the inquiry process is not an opportunity to give advice, ask leading questions, assert expertise, or otherwise engage in a desire for a specific outcome. We come close to its intention if we can view inquiry as a process of nourishing a fragile and tentative step into a deep realization that may be either painful or joyous or both. Leitch (personal communication) describes it as being a half-step behind the participant and being motivated by curiosity as their journey unfolds.

Crane (2009) describes the inquiry process as a set of concentric circles that the dialogue moves among. It begins with the exploration of the experiential awareness of the direct experience, proceeds to a recognition of the relational aspect of the experience to personal patterns and tendencies, and lastly moves to the outward-most circle of how this learning informs a new way of meeting the experience. Crane (2015) writes that its aim is:

> to reveal and bring into conscious awareness automated and unrecognized habits and patterns of thinking and feeling and to make known some of the properties of thoughts and feelings. The manner of attending to the experience, the teacher, and the relational process are all thus aiming to offer an embodiment of the attitudinal qualities of mindfulness. (p. 1105)

The interchange is designed and practiced as an exploratory, open-ended dialogue grounded in the moment (and often requiring a reminder to return to this moment). It requires the teacher be fully present, embodying that presence with no agenda to direct or shape the exchange. In that stance, the teacher models equanimity as a full and fearless willingness to be present to whatever is arising. In the MBSM program, we approach inquiry through the same framework as the overall program with Shapiro and Schwartz's (2000) model of mindfulness as *intention-attention-attitude (stance)* guiding the interconnected circles of dialogue.

The inquiry takes place between two people, one who has offered a narrative and the other who offers their presence in the unfolding of the narrative. The purpose of the inquiry is to clarify what is being reflected, to explore obstructions that keep the narrative from being heard in its totality (going into past or future, distraction, asking for advice, etc.). The overarching intention of the inquiry is to allow the teacher and participant to meet in the time and space of the direct experience.

Often the participant offers a narrative that is tangled with past and future. The initial question posed in the present is the trigger for various stances that can be judgments of the participant's performance in the present, anxieties about their future, or avoidance of the arising internal emotional states. The inquiry is an effort to embody the three elements of mindfulness: Intention, Attention, and Attitude/ Stance, and we begin by bringing attention to the immediate experience, exploring the stance, and finally cultivating an intention to observe more closely. Even though the structure seems formulaic, the frame of IAA is held lightly and the dialogue is often a dynamic movement among the three factors. Overlaid on this is the teacher's own attention to themes of pushing away, holding onto, or being confused about aspects of the experience. This awareness is not offered to the participant as received wisdom; rather it serves to shape invitational questions about the immediate experience. Table 6.1 illustrates the inquiry process in a dialogue between teacher and participant.

One could hypothesize that the inquiry has healing or reparative qualities because it is a nonjudgmental and unconditional acceptance of the participant's experience. In the teacher's willingness to be fully present to distressing emotions or uncertainty, the inquiry process is a co-creation of the four mental states of loving-kindness, equanimity, appreciative or resonant joy, and compassion. As such, it can also be an opportunity for the participant to turn towards their own suffering with the same mental qualities. And finally, if we view resistance, clinging, and confusion as harmful and contributing to unskillful choices, their reduction can be an opportunity to cultivate antidotes of wisdom, generosity, and acceptance/clarity as virtues that result in better outcomes.

Who Is Taught

At one level this domain is related to ethics *in* mindfulness by posing the question, "How does the curriculum need to meet the needs, especially ethically, of the population being taught?" At another it is more deeply a question of the ethics *of* mindfulness where the question is "Should we teach mindfulness to populations that can misappropriate the skills?" Perhaps the most contentious issue in the debate of

Table 6.1 Inquiry dialogue incorporating intention, attention, and attitude or stance to experience

Note: While in theory intention-attention-attitude (stance) can seem a logical progression, in practice we explore it as an iterative, organic process. In this example, the dialogue is entered at the attentional level.

ATTENTION: This level of inquiry is intended to open the speaker to the sense dimensions of the experience.
Inquiry after the practice: *What did you notice?*
Speaker: I couldn't do it. It was hard to stay focused.

Inquiry: *What else did you notice?*
Speaker: I was everywhere, all over the place. It hurt.

Inquiry: *So, as you're describing this, I'm noticing some judgment of yourself, your performance. You also said it hurt. What sensations did you notice that told you it was hurting?*
Speaker: My knees hurt. I must not be doing it right.

Inquiry: *Your knees hurt. Is there a sensation that describes the hurt?* (Narrowing the focus to the sensations and letting the judgment go.)
Speaker: Pain. It throbbed, ached.

Inquiry: *And then what happened?*
Speaker: I moved it and it got less painful. But I didn't know if that was the right thing to do.

Inquiry: *So you noticed it was painful, ached. Then you moved into it and made a change which changed the sensations.*
(Tying together attention and sensations; awareness of impermanence of sensations.)

ATTITUDE/STANCE: The second level of inquiry is intended to explore the speaker's stance (aversion, clinging, confusion) to the experience.
Inquiry: *If I can go back to the sensation of pain you felt, how did you meet that? What was your attitude to it?*
Speaker: I was angry that it was happening. I got irritated that the session was going on for so long.

Inquiry: *You were pushing back against the length of the session. What else did you notice?*
Speaker: I just kept getting angry. It wouldn't stop.

Inquiry: *What sensations signaled for you that it was anger?*
Speaker: Tight, tense, feeling in my gut.

Inquiry: *And what was your stance to the anger? How did you meet that?*
Speaker: I don't know. I didn't like it. It was all frustrating.

Inquiry: *And as you're speaking about it now, what are you noticing?*
Speaker: I'm tense, tight. Frustrated because I sound stupid.

Inquiry: *And right now, how are you meeting that tension, tightness?*
Speaker: I don't like it.

Inquiry: *So there's a lot of pushing back going on. In the past and in this moment.*
(There can also be clinging to a past experience—a good meditation/body scan for example. Or there can be confusion about an experience—this is where the need to know arises, the "why" questions. This particular example touches on the identification with the experience—i.e., a sense of fixed self.)

INTENTION: The third level of inquiry explores one possible way of creating intention in the practice.
Inquiry: *Would it be ok if we take a moment and bring attention to that tension, wherever it is in your body* (might even localize it before)? (Speaker agrees to try) *Let's breathe into it as you did with the body scan. Create the intention in your mind to pay a gentle attention to it right here, now. Only being curious about it.* (Invites the whole class to engage in this.)
(After about a minute): *What are you noticing now?*
Speaker: It's less.

Inquiry: *Can you say more about what you're noticing that tells you it's less?*
Speaker: It's not as tense, there's a relaxation in my gut, it feels better.

Inquiry: *So, when we bring our attention to the discomfort, approach it rather than push it away, something changes. In this case, it became less. In other cases, it may change in a different way. In all cases, we're practicing a different stance to the experience.* (Letting go of assumptions of how the experience should be.)

mindfulness between Buddhists traditionalists and secular practitioners arises when mindfulness is taught in organizations that do not uphold the absolute interpretations of "do no harm." These would include military, police, and businesses viewed as oppressing vulnerable populations (see chapters in the next section). In a subtle way, traditionalists (Buddhist or otherwise who view secular mindfulness as bereft of ethical content) might also include anyone who wants to learn mindfulness for "symptom relief." The assumption is that any approach whose goal is symptomatic relief would only provide superficial and short-sighted skills, and this would be both at the cost of a deeper transformation and the potential of misusing the skills. I have watched this hardline stance soften recently as both sides attempt to see that "symptom relief" is a necessary beginning to deeper transformation, especially in cases of police and military members with PTSD. Of course, as a health care professional, my professional ethics also caution against being the one who dictates where, how, and how far our clients wish to go in their journey with us. As noted in Compson and Monteiro (2015), mindfulness training is akin to physical training for health; some may use the training to maintain good health while others may use it to run marathons. Mindfulness training offers opportunities; given the opportunity, the decision of which direction to travel with it is individual.

Nevertheless, as someone who works with police and military organizations and teaches these populations, I find myself on the knife's edge of ensuring the intention of the organization to teach their members mindfulness remains congruent with the intention of their employees to cultivate wise discernment and that they have the freedom to do so. Yet, how can this balance be held and can we ever know the final application of our work? The chapters in this section and subsequent sections describe programs that can be and are applied to a range of presentations. Frank Musten, in his chapter leading the next section, addresses the complex issues embedded in the decision to offer mindfulness to certain populations that are perceived to be problematic in how the training may be used.

In the following chapters, CARE (Jennings and DeMauro), MiCBT (Cayoun), and MBSM (Monteiro and Musten) are employed with populations presenting with psychological distress. MBSM has been developed not only for stress and pain management, but is also offered to military, police, paramedics, and civilian members of these organizations who have been diagnosed with PTSD and Operational Stress Injuries (OSI), which includes moral injuries. It is also a contributor to a program on building resiliency for active duty soldiers in the Canadian Armed Forces. The dark reality of our current economic and cultural climes is that these programs are also a means of maintaining and returning participants to the very nature of work that can be or has been the source of their distress. The concerns raised by Buddhist practitioners (Purser, 2015; Purser & Loy, 2013; Titmuss, 2013) that mindfulness applied blindly or superficially as symptom relief can result in suppression of emotions and oppression of the individual need to be acknowledged. However, there is also a need for contextual understanding that the degree of psychological distress first and foremost calls for us to address the existing suffering. Whether this results in the production of automatons who return to the frontlines to kill or maim with impunity remains to be demonstrated. In the absence of this latter evidence, it does seem that the ethics of care requires us to address the suffering of the individual without judging them for a life decision they made.

And finally, the concerns that mindfulness can or might be weaponized by persons with poorly developed ethics, especially if taught without the ground of ethics, are equally applicable to anyone participating in a program. Every group has the potential of hosting individuals with a range of personality styles and perspectives that allows for the misuse of mindfulness skills. While all the need for caution discussed earlier may be appropriate in how one constructs, models, and instructs mindfulness, there is something important missed in the discussion of ethics *of* mindfulness. That is, neither the participant nor teacher arrives *tabula rasa*; their ethics and values are already present in the room. In other words, in the debate about ethics *of* mindfulness, a far more complicated picture emerges when content, teacher, and client are taken as a threefold interaction of *already existing* values and ethics.

Conclusion

The design and development of a mindfulness program is complicated and complex. The effort put into a system of thought that holds its integrity of theory and concepts in application is considerable. In our own experience with the development of MBSM, it took almost a decade of tinkering, training, and receiving teachings from a wide range of warm, generous, brilliant teachers who challenged our assumptions and forced revisions when the practices did not reflect the intention of every component. It was and continues to be a humbling process.

Even more humbling is to see the commonalities among the chapters in this section as we each drew from familiar and disparate grounds. Cognitive behavioral therapy, moral development and ethics of care, Buddhist psychology, and the common infrastructure of secular mindfulness design have come together to produce very different programs in this section and the next. The arc of our practice is a moral one with the intention to land in a field of compassion. And even if the programs seem differently designed, the intention is the same: to relieve the suffering of the world so that wisdom and compassion can benefit all beings in our circles of care. May the merits of our efforts benefit all beings.

References

Aggs, C., & Bambling, M. (2010). Teaching mindfulness to psychotherapists in clinical practice: The Mindful Therapy Programme. *Counselling and Psychotherapy Research, 10*(4), 278–286.

Aitken, R. (1984). *The mind of clover: Essays in Zen Buddhist ethics*. New York: North Point Press.

Amaro, A. (2015). A holistic mindfulness. *Mindfulness, 6*(1), 63–73. https://doi.org/10.1007/s12671-014-0382-3

Baer, R. (2015). Ethics, values, virtues, and character strengths in mindfulness-based interventions: A psychological science perspective. *Mindfulness, 6*(4), 956–969. https://doi.org/10.1007/s12671-015-0419-2

Bandura, A. (2016). *Moral disengagement: How people do harm and live with themselves.* New York: Worth Publishers.

Boyce, B. (2016, August). Is mindfulness the future of therapy? *Mindful, 48–56.*

Cayoun, B. A. (2011). *Mindfulness-integrated CBT: Principles and practice.* Chicester: Wiley-Blackwell.

Compson, J., & Monteiro, L. (2015). Still exploring the middle path: A response to commentaries. *Mindfulness, 7*(2), 548–564. https://doi.org/10.1007/s12671-015-0447-y

CPA, C. P. A. (2015). *Code of ethics for psychologists.* Retrieved from http://www.cpa.ca/aboutcpa/committees/ethics/codeofethics

Crane, R. S. (2009). *Mindfulness-based cognitive therapy: Distinctive features.* New York: Routledge.

Crane, R. S., Brewer, J., Feldman, C., Kabat-Zinn, J., Santorelli, S., Williams, J. M., & Kuyken, W. (2016). What defines mindfulness-based programs? The warp and the weft. *Psychological Medicine.* https://doi.org/10.1017/S0033291716003317

Crane, R. S., Kuyken, W., Hastings, R. P., Rothwell, N., & Williams, J. M. G. (2010). Training teachers to deliver mindfulness-based interventions: Learning from the UK experience. *Mindfulness, 1*(2), 74–86. https://doi.org/10.1007/s12671-010-0010-9

Danilewitz, M., Bradwein, J., & Koszycki, D. (2016). A pilot feasibility study of a peer-led mindfulness program for medical students. *Canadian Medical Education Journal, 7*(1), e31–e37.

Evans, A., Crane, R. S., Cooper, L., Mardula, J., Wilks, J., Surawy, C., … Kuyken, W. (2014). A framework for supervision for mindfulness-based teachers: A space for embodied mutual inquiry. *Mindfulness, 6*(3), 572–581. https://doi.org/10.1007/s12671-014-0292-4

Felton, T. M., Coates, L., & Christopher, J. C. (2013). Impact of mindfulness training on counseling students' perception of stress. *Mindfulness.* https://doi.org/10.1007/s12671-013-0240-8

Fernando, A. T., Skinner, K., & Consedine, N. S. (2017). Increasing compassion in medical decision-making: Can a brief mindfulness intervention help? *Mindfulness, 8*(2), 276–285.

Fisher, B., & Tronto, J. C. (1990). Toward a feminist theory of caring. In E. Abel & M. Nelson (Eds.), *Circles of care.* Albany, NY: SUNY Press.

Gilligan, C. (1993). *In a different voice: Psychological theory and women's development* (revised ed.). Cambridge, MA: Harvard University Press.

Gilligan, C. (2011). *Joining the resistance.* Cambridge: Polity Press.

Gilligan, C. (2014). Moral injury and the ethic of care: Reframing the conversation about differences. *Journal of Social Philosophy, 45*(1), 89–106.

Gilligan, C., & Attanucci, J. (1988). Two moral orientations. In C. Gilligan, J. V. Ward, & J. Taylor (Eds.), *Mapping the moral domain.* Cambridge, MA: Harvard University Press.

Gombrich, R. (2009/2013). *What the Buddha thought.* Bristol, CT: Equinox Publishers.

Halland, E., de Vibe, M., Solhaug, I., Friborg, O., Rosenvinge, J. H., Tyssen, R., … Bjørndal, A. (2015). Mindfulness training iproves problem-focused coping in psychology and medical students: Results from a randonized controlled trial. *College Student Journal, 49*(3), 387–398.

Hanh, T. N. (2005). *Interbeing: Fourteen guidelines for engaged Buddhism.* Berkeley, CA: Parallax Press.

Hanh, T. N. (2007). *For a future to be possible: Buddhist ethics for everyday life.* Berkeley, CA: Parallax Press.

Harvey, P. (2000). *An introduction to Buddhist ethics.* Cambridge: Cambridge University Press.

Harvey, P. (2013). *An introduction to Buddhism: Teachings, history and practices* (2nd ed.). Cambridge: Cambridge University Press.

Hölzel, B. K., Lazar, S. W., Gard, T., Schuman-Olivier, Z., Vago, D. R., & Ott, U. (2011). How does mindfulness meditation work? Proposing mechanisms of action from a conceptual and neural perspective. *Perspectives on Psychological Science, 6*(6), 537–559.

Kabat-Zinn, J. (2003). Mindfulness-based interventions in context: Past, present and future. *Clinical Psychology: Science and Practice, 10,* 144–156.

Kabat-Zinn, J. (2011). Some reflections on the origins of MBSR, skillful means, and the trouble with maps. *Contemporary Buddhism*, *12*(1), 281–306.

Kabat-Zinn, J. (2013). *Full catastrophe living: Using the wisdom of your body and mind to face stress, pain, and illness*. New York: Bantam.

Khoury, B., Lecomte, T., Fortin, G., Masse, M., Therien, P., Bouchard, V., … Hofmann, S. G. (2013). Mindfulness-based therapy: A comprehensive meta-analysis. *Clinical Psychology Review*, *33*, 763–771.

Kohlberg, L. (Ed.). (1976). *Moral stages and moralization: The cognitive developmental approach*. New York: Holt, Rinehart, & Winston.

Lee, T., Paré, D., & Monteiro, L. M. (in press). Exploring the experiences of therapists after participating in an intensive mindfulness program. *Journal of Counseling and Spirituality*.

Leiter, M. P. (2008). A two process model of burnout and work engagement: Distinct implications of demands and values. *Supplemento A, Psicologia*, *30*(1), A52–A58.

Leiter, M. P., Frank, E., & Matheson, T. (2009). *Values, demands, and burnout: Perspectives from national survey of Canadian physicians*. Paper presented at the American Psychological Association.

Leiter, M. P., Jackson, N. J., & Shaughnessy, K. (2009). Contrasting burnout, turnover intention, control, value congruence and knowledge sharing between Baby Boomers and Generation X. *Journal of Nursing Management*, *17*(1), 100–109. https://doi.org/10.1111/j.1365-2834.2008.00884.x

Maslach, C., & Jackson, S. (Eds.). (1984). *Burnout in organizations* (Vol. 5). Beverly HIlls, CA: Sage.

Maslach, C., & Leiter, M. P. (1997). *The truth about burnout: How organizations cause personal stress and what to do about it*. San Francisco, CA: Jossey-Bass.

Maslach, C., & Leiter, M. P. (2008). Early predictors of job burnout and engagement. *Journal of Applied Psychology*, *93*(3), 498–512.

McCown, D. (2013). *The ethical space of mindfulness in clinical practice: An exploratory essay*. Philadelphia, PA: Jessica Kingsley Publishers.

McCown, D. (2014). *Mindfulness: Fulfilling the promise at last, with a relational view*. Paper presented at the Beyond the Therapeutic State: Collaborative Practices for Individual and Social Change, Drammen, Norway.

McCown, D. (2016). Being is relational: Considerations for using mindfulness in clinician-patient settings. In E. Shonin, W. van Gordon, & M. D. Griffiths (Eds.), *Mindfulness and Buddhist-derived approaches in mental health and addiction* (pp. 29–60). Switzerland: Springer.

McCown, D., Reibel, D., & Micozzi, M. S. (2010). *Teaching Mindfulness: A practical guide for clinicians and educators*. New York: Springer.

Mol, M. M. C. v., Kompanje, E. J. O., Benoit, D. D., Bakker, J., & Nijkamp, M. D. (2015). The prevalence of compassion fatigue and burnout among healthcare professionals in intensive care units: A systematic review. *PloS One*, *10*(8), e0136955. https://doi.org/10.1371/journal.pone.0136955

Monteiro, L. (2015). Dharma and Distress: Buddhist teachings that support psychological principles in a mindfulness program. In E. Shonin, W. Van Gordon, & N. N. Singh (Eds.), *Buddhist foundations of mindfulness* (pp. 181–215). New York: Springer.

Monteiro, L. (2016). Implicit ethics and mindfulness: Subtle assumptions that MBIs are values-neutral. *International Journal of Psychotherapy*, 210–224.

Monteiro, L., & Musten, R. F. (2013). *Mindfulness starts here: An 8-week guide to skillful living*. Victoria, BC: Friesen Press.

Monteiro, L., Musten, R. F., & Compson, J. (2015). Traditional and contemporary mindfulness: Finding the middle path in the tangle of concerns. *Mindfulness*, *6*(1), 1–13.

Monteiro, L., Nuttall, S., & Musten, R. F. (2010). Five skillful habits: An ethics-based mindfulness intervention. *Counselling and Spirituality*, *29*(1), 91–103.

Narvaez, D. (2014). *Neurobiology and the development of human morality*. New York: W.W. Norton.

Neff, K. D. (2011). *Self-compassion: Stop beating yourself up and leave insecurity behind*. New York: William Morrow.

Patsiopoulos, A. T., & Buchanan, M. J. (2011). The practice of self-compassion in counseling: A narrative inquiry. *Professional Psychology: Research and Practice, 42*(4), 301–307.

Pettifor, J., Sinclair, C., & Gauthier, J. (2011). The 25th Anniversary of the Canadian Code of Ethics for psychologists. *Canadian Psychology, 52*(3), 149–235.

Pope, K., & Vasquez, M. (2016). *Ethics in psychotherapy and counseling: A practical guide* (5th ed.). Hoboken, NJ: Wiley.

Purser, R. (2015). Clearing the muddles path of traditional and contemporary mindfulness: A response to Monteiro, Musten, and Compson. *Mindfulness, 6*(1), 23–45.

Purser, R., & Loy, D. (2013). Beyond McMindfulness. *Huffington Post*. Retrieved from http://www.huffingtonpost.com/ron-purser/beyond-mcmindfulness_b_3519289.html website: http://www.huffingtonpost.com/

Rest, J., & Narvaez, D. (Eds.). (1994). *Moral development in the professions: Psychology and applied ethics*. Hillsdale, NJ: Lawrence Erlbaum Associates.

Rest, J., Narvaez, D., Bebeau, M. J., & Thoma, S. J. (1999). *Postconventional moral thinking: A neo-Kohlbergian approach*. New York: Psychology Press.

Segal, Z. V., Williams, J. M., & Teasdale, J. D. (2012). *Mindfulness based cognitive therapy for the prevention of depression relapse* (2nd ed.). New York: Guilford Press.

Shapiro, S. L., & Schwartz, G. E. (2000). The role of intention in self-regulation: Toward intentional systemic mindfulness. In M. Boekaerts, P. R. Pintrich, & M. Zeidner (Eds.), *Handbook of self-regulation* (pp. 253–273). San Diego, CA: Academic Press.

Singh, N., Lancioni, G., Winton, A., Karazsia, B., Myers, R., Latham, L., & Singh, J. (2014). Mindfulness-Based Positive Behavior Support (MBPBS) for mothers of adolescents with autism spectrum disorder: Effects on adolescents' behavior and parental stress. *Mindfulness, 5*(6), 646–657.

Solhaug, I., Eriksen, T. E., & de Vibe, M. e. a. (2016). Medical and psychology student's experiences in learning mindfulness: Benefits, paradoxes, and pitfalls. *Mindfulness, 7*(4), 838–850.

Titmuss, C. (2013). The Buddha of mindfulness. The politics of mindfulness. http://christophertitmuss.org/blog/?p=1454. Retrieved from http://www.christophertitmuss.org/

Tjeltveit, A. C. (1999). *Ethics and values in psychotherapy*. London: Routledge.

Tronto, J. C. (1993). *Moral Boundaries: A political argument for an ethic of care*. New York: Routledge.

Van Gordon, W., Shonin, E., & Griffiths, M. (2015). Towards a second generation of mindfulness-based interventions. *Australian & New Zealand Joyrnal of Psychiatry, 49*(7), 591–592. https://doi.org/10.1177/0004867415577437

van Nistelrooij, I., Schaafsma, P., & Tronto, J. C. (2014). Ricoeur and the ethics of care. *Medical Health Care and Philosophy, 17*, 485–491.

Williams, J. M., & Kabat-Zinn, J. (2013). *Mindfulness: Diverse perspectives on its meaning, origins and applications*. New York: Routledge.

Chapter 7
The Purpose, Mechanisms, and Benefits of Cultivating Ethics in Mindfulness-Integrated Cognitive Behavior Therapy

Bruno A. Cayoun

Asserting that an unethical life leads to and maintains suffering is not a statement that requires empirical evidence from the scientific literature. It is evident in daily life. We just need to reflect on our own life and that of those we love. No matter what values we uphold, we are unlikely to wish or enjoy being harmed in any way. The personal experience of being lied to or spoken to in a harmful way is not acceptable to anyone. Similarly, no one wishes to be robbed or killed. We implicitly shun performing these actions, and doing this is not simply based on a sectarian or value-ridden set of rules. This also applies to inappropriate sexual conduct and intoxication. Moreover, harmful behavior such as stealing, killing, harmful speech, and sexual inappropriateness is more likely to be enacted under the influence of drugs or alcohol-induced intoxication. Those who engage in these actions are also suffering, as will be discussed later in this chapter. Accordingly, a patient who learns to refrain from such basic harmful actions is likely to benefit, along with those with whom they live. Clinicians know too well how failing to do so jeopardizes therapy outcomes and promotes relapse. This chapter discusses the roles and benefits of ethics in Mindfulness-integrated Cognitive Behavior Therapy (MiCBT). Since the rationale for applying ethics in MiCBT originates from Buddhist psychology, a brief overview of the roles of ethics in Buddhism may be helpful. The original terminology in Pali language is italicized.

B.A. Cayoun, DPsych (✉)
Mindfulness-integrated Cognitive Behavior Therapy Institute, Hobart, Tasmania, Australia
e-mail: bruno.cayoun@mindfulness.net.au

© Springer International Publishing AG 2017   163
L.M. Monteiro et al. (eds.), *Practitioner's Guide to Ethics and Mindfulness-Based Interventions*, Mindfulness in Behavioral Health,
DOI 10.1007/978-3-319-64924-5_7

Ethics in Buddhism

Ethical values and guidelines existed in ancient civilizations, including that of Egypt, Greece, and India, well before Buddhism emerged just over 2500 years ago. In Buddhist psychology, ethics serve several purposes, all of which have at the same goal: to decrease suffering. As such, ethics for a wholesome life are not based on a dogmatic belief system—although many Buddhists prevent unethical behavior by fear of "bad karma" and perform "good actions" out of hope for a good rebirth. However, one of the appealing aspects of Buddhist education is its emphasis on ethics as a means of protecting oneself and others from being harmed, because we are likely to feel safe in the presence of someone dedicated to doing no harm. Deliberate effort toward ethics is an act of compassion and insight, which we will discuss later in this chapter.

An important aspect of Buddhist education is that it explicitly prohibits evangelistic behavior, such as teaching someone who does not ask for it, or trying to convert someone to Buddhism. Accordingly, it would not be appropriate for a therapist aligned with Buddhist values to push their views and values, including ethics, on anyone. Nonetheless, ethics are at the forefront of the Buddhist psychological system, as expounded in the Eightfold Path (Bodhi, 2000), where the path of wisdom begins with commitment to ethical behavior. Such commitment protects the student from harmful behavior and is a corequisite for psychological maturation. In fact, it would be inconceivable to teach mindfulness for the sake of developing mindfulness skills alone, as a self-serving technique. Doing so would result in attention training that may not translate to appropriate action. The relationship between attention and action is discussed in more detail below, along with the traditional teaching that mindfulness is best used as an inner vehicle to navigate decision-making and behavior in the least harmful way and lead to insight and compassion. Ethics in Buddhist psychology plays several roles, each serving a greater system of education (See Jayasaro, 2011, for discussion). Some of these are summarized below.

Ethics as Protective Factors

Several levels of commitment to ethical conduct are encased within sets of guidelines, which rely heavily on one's ability to be mindful. A monk or nun observes 227 rules, clustered into four categories of ethics. The "five precepts" are the most commonly used for laypeople:

1. Refraining from using harmful speech. This includes language that is harsh, voluntarily inaccurate and misleading, critical of others (e.g., backbiting), untimely (wasteful of people's time), and useless (e.g., just speaking to get others' attention). Thus, mindfulness is indispensable in our effort to use speech that is *true, timely, kind, respectful,* and *useful.*

2. Refraining from taking lives. This includes the life of all sentient beings. It also conveys the importance of respecting the environment since damaging it will damage the habitat of animals who depend on it. In terms of livelihood, following this precept would include refraining from performing actions that can kill or harm oneself and others physically, such as fabricating or selling weapons, and driving recklessly.

3. Refraining from taking what is not given. The translated term "not taking the non-given" is the accurate traditional descriptor, which could be easily summarized as "not stealing." However, we may inadvertently take what is not actually given on a daily basis while not associating it with "stealing," because the notion of stealing tends to be associated with a salient crime that is directly reprehensible. Taking the non-given includes, but is not restricted to, typical acts of theft. It involves taking financial advantage to someone else's detriment—whether this is a contextually acceptable behavior or not—using the work phone or other facilities for personal use without permission, borrowing goods or money which we are not sure to return, plagiarism, taking away a person's rights, or taking credit for someone else's work. Engaging in this last action can sometimes be subtle. For example, in an academic context, taking the non-given may involve reading or hearing about someone else's unpublished concept, idea, or methodology and publishing an article based on it without acknowledging the original source just because the original source has not yet been published and the author is not well known. However, since this self-oriented behavior can harm, it is considered unethical and this precept can provide guidance to protect both parties from such harm.

4. Refraining from inappropriate sexual conduct. This includes all harmful actions related to or involving sex. Besides obvious sexual abuse, it also includes putting pressure on a partner for sex, using manipulative approaches to gain sexual favors, nonconsensual extramarital sex. In our Western, secular understanding of mindfulness and ethics, it is sometimes difficult to perceive the boundaries of what constitutes the potential for harm. For example, in the case of abstaining from flirtatious behavior, especially between two people who do not seem to be committed to someone else, this sounds prohibitive and difficult to see how this relates to mindfulness and ethics. As with other precepts, this is a contextually flexible precaution to prevent harm that has nothing to do with a dogmatic "right" and "wrong" action. For example, the Australian Psychological Association (APS) Code of Ethics for psychologists stipulates that the psychologist should not have a sexual relationship with a patient for a minimum of 2 years following discharge, even though both individuals may be single. Although this sounds reasonable, the unfortunate harm to patients reported over the years has led the APS to also include the need to first explore with a senior psychologist the possibility that the former patient may be vulnerable and at risk of exploitation, and encourage the former patient to seek independent counselling on the matter. Interestingly, the APS suggests developing an "ethical antenna." This is another way of saying "be mindful of potential harm," rather than merely prohibiting some actions.

5. Refraining from taking intoxicants. This is mostly understood as involving the use of alcohol and what are typically considered illicit drugs. Indeed, alcohol and cannabis were used in the days of the Buddha. There are two main reasons for this precept. One is to maintain our health and respect for human life. The other is to preserve our ability to use mindfulness to maintain the four previous precepts. When intoxicated, it is easier to speak inappropriately, kill, steal, and break healthy sexual boundaries because of the decrease in response control and increased impulsivity that accompany intoxication. Some monastics (e.g., Jayasaro, 2011) have also proposed that intoxication is not limited to a consequence of using a substance, and extends to all new types of addiction, including the dysfunctional use of social media and the Internet, as well as the devices used to access them.

"Right Mindfulness"

Theravada Buddhism teaches us that our ability to increase awareness of ethical behavior largely depends on the effort to remain mindful and to keep our mental and emotional states in check (Jayasaro, 2011). This is because in Buddhist psychology, as summarized in the Eightfold Path (Bodhi, 2000), mindfulness is a tool, not a goal. It is a means of exploration that develops to enable a sincere examination of our own nature, desires, and habits, just as a pathologist uses a microscope as an investigative tool to understand pathogenic phenomena. It is not a cure in itself, but rather a means to an end. Since mindfulness is not always understood in this way in the West, it may be useful to differentiate focused and sustained attention training (*samadhi*) from mindfulness (*sati*), as originally taught by the Buddha in "The Great Discourse on the Foundations of Mindfulness" (*Mahāsatipatthāna Sutta*) (Walshe, 2012). Before exploring Right Mindfulness, it is important to explore how the secularization and modernization of mindfulness has resulted in some linguistic and conceptual inaccuracy, an issue that has been acknowledged by others (e.g., Dreyfus, 2011). The resulting potential for misinterpretation is explored first, so that the concept of Right Mindfulness is better understood and applied to the issue of ethics.

Most readers of mindfulness-related publications would have come across the notion that mindfulness involves a purposeful and sustained attention that excludes complex cognitive elaboration ("judgment") (e.g., Kabat-Zinn, 1994). Although useful and elegant in its economy, this type of definition can lead to erroneous interpretations and practice methods that distance the meditator from the original teaching. If it were simply to pay attention "on purpose, in the present moment, and non-judgmentally" (Kabat-Zinn, 1994, p. 4), then a cat sitting attentively in front of a mousehole, ready to jump on his prey, would be a mindful cat. A sniper paying purposeful attention in the present moment, ready to kill, following orders and not making any judgments, would also be a mindful sniper. Certainly, these kinds of activities require great attentional capacity and inhibitory control over intrusive stimuli that can be transferred to other contexts, but can we shoot someone mindfully? As described below, Buddhist psychology asserts that the "mindful" aspect of the attentional effort includes a higher order cognitive process able to differentiate right from wrong (benign from harmful) action. A mindful mode of information processing incorporates focused attention, but does not content itself with accepting the present moment. It *must* be free from the mental attitudes of craving and aversion, and free from identification with the experience. It is not enough to be attentive and accept whatever arises in the present without means of extinguishing learned responses, especially since what arises can be harmful. Other authors are beginning to express this point more explicitly (Desbordes et al., 2015).

Other misunderstandings can also occur because of clichés or poorly expressed concepts and their related instructions. For example, when an MBI therapist tells patients that mindfulness requires "being" and not "doing" without clear explanations, confusion can arise in various domains. First, what does "being" really mean? In appearance, sitting with eyes closed and peacefully noticing what arises in the present moment appears to fit the suggestion of "being," but the devil is in the detail, as they say. Practicing mindfulness accurately is far more about doing (and undoing) than being. Focusing and keeping attention on the breath at the entrance of the nostrils while inhibiting cognitive and interoceptive stimuli emerging in conscious awareness and systematically shifting attention back to the breath is unarguably a very busy task, tapping three executive functions simultaneously (signal detection while attending, inhibition of the learned response, and attention shifting) (Bishop et al., 2004; Cayoun, 2011). There is now established neurological evidence that mindfulness practice is a busy mental task. Imaging studies have repeatedly shown that increased activation in the default mode network (DMN; day dreaming and self-referential processing) occurs systematically when the brain is at rest, and deactivates significantly during attention-demanding tasks ("doing"), especially during mindfulness practice (Farb et al., 2007; Gard et al., 2011). This provides neurological evidence that mindfulness is a "doing" mental action. Although some teachers and clinicians may hold an accurate understanding of the practice itself, cliché terms such as these can derail the student's attention from the correct method. Moreover, even when the brain is not subjected to performing a task, the systematic activation of the DMN produces spontaneous autobiographical memories, expectations of future self-related events (Buckner, Andrews-Hanna, & Schacter, 2008; Fox et al., 2005), or even ruminative brooding that co-emerge with body sensations (Lackner & Fresco, 2016). This means that "just being" occurs neither during meditation, nor during rest. Since being awake involves a deliberate or involuntary mental activity, Buddhist teachings train students to "do" wholesome actions and prevent unwholesome ones.

In his teaching of the Eightfold Path, and in detail in his discourses on the establishment of mindfulness (*Mahāsatipatthāna Sutta;* Walshe, 2012), the Buddha's explicit explanation of "Right Mindfulness" (*sama sati*) is difficult to ignore—note that the term "Right Mindfulness" is translated from the Pali *sama sati*, which is meant to be understood as "correct," "comprehensive," "full," or "profound," which allows a continuum of practice accuracy, rather than a rigid assumption of a fully right or fully wrong practice. It also allows the context to mediate the correctness of the practice. The Buddha's description of Right Mindfulness advances that mindfulness is practiced accurately and is wholesome only if "clear comprehension" (*sampajanna*) accompanies attention (*sati*). Clear comprehension is expressed as a fourfold process, as translated here by Venerable Bhikkhu Lokopalo (Lokopalo, 2010):

1. Clear comprehension of what is useful, purposeful (*satthaka sampajano*)
2. Clear comprehension of what is beneficial, wholesome (*sappaya sampajano*)
3. Clear comprehension of the context of awareness (*gocara sampajano*)
4. Clear comprehension of reality as a process of impermanence (*asammoha sampajano*)

Practicing mindfulness accurately (with *sampajanna*), rather than attention control training alone, inevitably leads to the progressive realization of three universal phenomena: (1) everything is continually changing (*anicca*), (2) therefore there is no permanent or substantial self (*anatta*), and (3) ignoring this and maintaining attachment to a false sense of intrinsic self leads to various forms of suffering (*dukkha*). To the extent that the mindfulness practitioner realizes these phenomena, the will and ability to disidentify from one's sense of self can occur, along with the "letting go" of attachment to the related habits of craving and aversion (Hart, 1987). This is not to say that training in sustained and focused attention is not beneficial. Indeed, the benefits of attention training are reflected in helpful neuroplasticity occurring in numerous domains of therapy, from stroke rehabilitation (Dimyan & Cohen, 2011) to attention-bias modification treatments for anxiety (Hakamata et al., 2010). However, calling attention training "mindfulness" is a misrepresentation of what it is and unhelpful because practitioners may miss important aspects of mindfulness and their resulting benefits, including the cultivation of ethics. In contrast, the Buddha's original instructions in the *Mahāsatipatthāna Sutta* (Goenka, 1998; Walshe, 2012) about establishing mindfulness specify that mindfulness needs to be cultivated with clear comprehension at four interactive levels of experience (*in the Buddha's words*): the body (*kaye kayanupassi viharati atapi sampajano satima …*), body sensations/interoception (*Vedanasu vedananupassi viharati atapi sampajano satima …*), mind/mental states (*Citte cittanupassi viharati atapi sampajano satima …*) and mental objects/thoughts, images, etc. (*Dhammesu dhammanupassi viharati atapi sampajano satima …*).

Being mindful, in the Buddhist sense, means noticing the arising of, and interactions between, these phenomena while remaining aware of their transient and impersonal nature. Suffering is understood to be the consequence of our inability to let go of that with which we identify. Thus, suffering is a function of one's attachment to an illusory self ("I") and its associated agents ("my"). If practiced as originally taught, mindfulness acts as the unbiased monitoring of phenomena spontaneously emerging in conscious awareness. Clear comprehension is often synonymous with wisdom in the *suttas*; for instance, in the *Digha Nikaya Tika* (Walshe, 2012, DN 2. 376): "*Samantato pakarehi pakattham va savisesam janati ti sampajano*": "One who understands the totality clearly with wisdom from all angles (of whatever is manifesting) or who knows distinctly has *sampajanna*" (trans. Lokopalo, 2010).

Ethics as a Condition for the Cultivation of Right Mindfulness

From the above description of mindfulness, a decrease in suffering depends on our ability to be aware and less reactive when things change, based on the understanding that *change is the norm*. In contrast, performing an unethical (harmful) action necessitates a craving or aversive reaction. The voluntary acts of injuring or killing someone, and speaking harshly or backbiting are expressions of aversion. Similarly, voluntary acts of taking the non-given and sexual misconduct are expressions of craving. Intoxication may be maintained by positive or negative reinforcement, or both, and can be accompanied by either craving or aversion accordingly. In line with Buddhist teachings, Jon Kabat-Zinn is also of the view that ethical behavior is a necessary basis for mindfulness practice:

> The foundation of mindfulness practice, for all meditative enquiry and exploration, lies in ethics and morality, and above all, the motivation of non-harming. Why? Because you cannot possibly hope to know stillness and calmness within your own mind and body […] if your actions are continually clouding, agitating, and destabilizing the very instrument through which you are looking, namely, your own mind (Kabat-Zinn, 2005, p. 102).

This is one of the reasons for which attending a traditionally taught Buddhist meditation retreat requires registrants to commit to observing strict ethical conduct during the retreat; at least the five ethical precepts cited earlier, often adding a commitment to complete celibacy for the duration of the retreat. In traditional Buddhist teaching, taking mindfulness training without initially committing to ethical conduct is simply inconceivable, theoretically unsound and technically unsuccessful. When we are mindful, we know that we are about to act, or that we have acted, in discord with our ethics and can feel the constrictive somatic experience of anxiety without having to avoid it. The clear understanding that body sensations arise and pass away, while not associating them with our sense of self, will prevent the reinforcement of reactions. Keeping in mind a clear comprehension of phenomena allows the willingness and greater capacity to be patient and equanimous (*Upekkha*; Cayoun, 2011; Desbordes et al., 2015). The same applies to feeling other emotions and to some health conditions, such as chronic pain (Cayoun, Simmons, & Shires, 2017).

Thus, traditionally taught mindfulness is understood as an *informed* exploration of the present moment and a corresponding means of *holding in mind* what is beneficial from what is harmful (*kusala* from *akusala*), with clear discernment, from moment to moment, whether one is meditating or not. It has been proposed that this notion of embodied ethics fuses cognitive dimensions and ethical qualities (Grossman, 2015). It is not surprising that the translation of the Pali *sati* as "mindfulness" remains ambiguous among authors, some of whom describe it in terms of "remembering" (Gethin, 1998; Sharf, 2014). As traditionally practiced, mindfulness is used to remain aware of the potential harmful mental, verbal, or physical actions, as well as the intention that may precede them (Jayasaro, 2011). It requires maintaining an awareness of speech, actions, and intentions without identifying with them, remaining honest and humbled by the reality of our current mental state. In turn, this truthfulness assists in accepting others' ethical flaws and contributes to a compassionate attitude.

Thus, Buddhist psychology teaches that ethical living and mindfulness are inter-dependent and inseparable (Jayasaro, 2011). When one is absent, the other suffers. When we lack mindfulness, emotional reactivity stimulates and facilitates harmful intentions and actions. When we lack ethics, the agitation produced by harmful intention and action hinders the practice of mindfulness and its benefits. Since the interdependence of ethics and mindfulness is relevant in the context of MBIs, we now turn to the cultivation of ethics in Mindfulness-integrated Cognitive Behavior Therapy (MiCBT).

Cultivating Ethics in MiCBT

Unless a sound theoretical rationale for introducing ethics in therapy exists, adher-ence to therapy and therapy outcome can be hindered by both therapists and patients' mental representations of ethics, as will be discussed later (see also Baer, 2015, for discussion). Since clinicians using MiCBT are trained to use a scientist-practitioner approach, they provide a clear and ecologically valid rationale for integrating both mindfulness training and ethical behavior in CBT. The rationale is encased within the co-emergence model of reinforcement (Cayoun, 2011), which describes in a verifiable way how operant conditioning can be deepened to better understand how behavior is subconsciously reinforced. Accordingly, this section briefly describes the model to provide a useful mechanistic behavioral framework and related ratio-nale for the inclusion of ethics in MiCBT.

The Co-emergence Model of Reinforcement

The co-emergence model of reinforcement (CMR) is a neurophenomenological approach to operant conditioning, grounded in the Buddhist psychological princi-ples of "dependent origination" and "the five aggregates" of personal experience (Narada, 1968). One of the central teachings of the Buddha is the teaching on ego-lessness (*Anattalakkhana Sutta*) found in the connected discourses (*Samyutta Nikaya*; Bodhi, 2000). In this teaching, he described what constitutes the very essence of what we erroneously perceive as a "self," in terms of five most basic physical and mental processes that allow experiences to occur. These have been translated as the "five aggregates" (*pancakkhandha*). These are (1) matter (*rupa*), (2) consciousness (*Vinnana*; pronounced "vinyana"), (3) sensation (*vedana*), (4) per-ception (*sania*), and (5) mental formation or volition (*sankara*), which is the propen-sity to react. He explained that none of these factors constitute a permanent "self," and identification with them perpetuates suffering. Although a detailed description of these mechanisms is beyond the scope of this chapter, they become increasingly obvious as one practices "Right Mindfulness" and are central to acquiring a deeper understanding of Buddhist psychology, from which the CMR is partly derived.

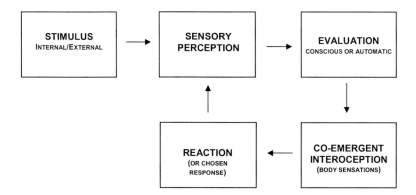

Fig. 7.1 Components of the co-emergence model of reinforcement during equilibrium in information processing (Adapted from Cayoun, 2011)

The basic components of the CMR are pictorially represented in Fig. 7.1 and can be briefly described as follows (See Cayoun, 2011 and 2015 for a comprehensive account). First, Sensory Perception arises, whether triggered by internal stimuli (body sensations, thoughts, and images from imagination or memory) or external stimuli (e.g., five senses stimulated by the environmental cues). Note that even new stimuli may be perceived as known by association. Second, sensory information is filtered by the evaluation system to make sense of the information. Evaluation can occur without conscious cognitive processing when categorization of the stimulus has been reinforced over time; that is, when it is "automatic." Evaluative processes can be observed on a dimension of personal importance, where stimuli are perceived as being more or less related to one's sense of self (values, needs, personality, beliefs, autobiographical memories, expectations). As mentioned earlier, self-referential processing is associated with the activation of brain pathways forming the "default mode network" (DMN), with activation of the medial prefrontal cortex (mPFC), posterior cingulate cortex, and lateral parietal cortex (Buckner et al., 2008; Fox et al., 2005). The more one takes things personally, the greater the activation in this network, leading to the elevated activation of the third component, Interoception.

Whether the evaluation is conscious and slow, or subconscious and fast, self-referential processing stimulates body sensations, as reflected neurologically in patients with chronic pain (Gard et al., 2011; Grant, Courtemanche, & Rainville, 2011; Mansour, Farmer, Baliki, & Apkarian, 2014) and depression (Farb et al., 2007, 2010). Note that *non*-co-emergent body sensations also occur directly via sensory perception due to common experiences (e.g., kinesthetic feedback during movements, digestion, and pain) and are not the consequence of evaluation. However, the automatic evaluation of such body sensations may lead to additional ("co-emergent") body sensations, which are activated through different neurological pathways (Farb, Segal, & Anderson, 2013; Zang et al., 2014; Zeidan & Vago, 2016). The model of co-emergence posits that evaluation co-emerges spontaneously with interoception in two ways. Firstly, the more the evaluation of the stimulus is self-referential (associated with "I," "me," and "mine"), the more intense the co-emerging body sensations. Secondly, the more the evaluation is associated with information that is deemed agreeable, the more pleasant the co-emerging body sensations. Similarly, disagreeableness leads to unpleasant sensations. Imaging studies and reviews on how motivation shapes interoceptive inference support this basic everyday reality (see Farb et al., 2015, for a review). The insular cortex is central to the detection of emotions and the mapping of physiological responses to emotions, and passes the information to other brain regions (Lutz, Brefczynski-Lewis, Johnstone, & Davidson, 2008). The insula is anatomically positioned to serve as an interface between afferent processing mechanisms and cognitively oriented modulatory systems, and has been associated with the experience of both emotions and physical pain (Farb et al., 2007; Starr et al., 2009).

Fourth, the reaction system is triggered, depending on the intensity and type (hedonic tone) of body sensation. Unless one is trained to practice equanimity, the probability of a reaction is a function of interoceptive intensity. More intense body sensations trigger stronger reactions. Moreover, the type of reaction is a function of hedonic tone. Unless specifically trained to alter innate brain wiring, sufficiently intense pleasant sensations lead to craving reactions, such as repeated behavior, and sufficiently intense unpleasant sensations lead to aversive reactions, such as avoidant behavior. Accordingly, the model advances that people neither react to the stimulus nor to its evaluation. They react because of body sensations: the *consequence* of evaluation. It follows that the reaction is reinforced if the craving or aversive reaction produces the desired outcome—craving producing more pleasant sensations or aversion producing less unpleasant ones.

A stress response causes a disequilibrium state in the information system, whereby attention is depleted from sensory systems (Sensory Perception and co-emergent Interoception) and reallocated to the Evaluation and Reaction systems (See Fig. 7.2). From a survival perspective, this allows the rapid evaluation of potential threats and defensive reaction. For example, when a stimulus is ambiguous, rapid retrieval of mental representations of the stimulus replaces the actual perception of the stimulus. In other words, "what it is" is replaced by "what it is like," and often "what it is like *for me*." The evaluation produces a spontaneously co-emerging sensation in the body to which we barely pay attention, and to which we react immediately assuming that the internal experience is an accurate measure of what the stimulus represents. When this attentional bias is sustained for long periods, the associated neural activation in frontolimbic networks (including mPFC, insula, and amygdala) strengthens, leading us to be over-judgmental (inflated Evaluation) and overreactive (inflated Reaction). This has been observed repeatedly in patients with chronic pain (Apkarian, 2008; Baliki, Geha, Apkarian, & Chialvo, 2008; Baliki et al., 2012; Gard et al., 2011; Mansour et al., 2014) and in patients with chronic depression (Farb et al. 2010; Siegle et al., 2007). Both genetic and environmental conditions can lead to brain reorganization which maintains a disequilibrium state among these four components (as per Fig. 7.2), manifesting in behavioral expressions that clinicians often assign to neurosis or problematic personality trait.

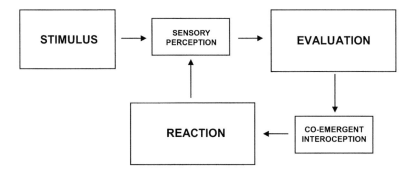

Fig. 7.2 The co-emergence model of reinforcement during disequilibrium in information processing (Adapted from Cayoun, 2011)

This neurophenomenological account integrates the essence of operant conditioning and extends its scope by proposing that *all* conditioning principles rely on operant learning and the locus of reinforcement is interoception (body sensations), subserved by the insular cortex. This also means that harmful behavior is conditioned and its perpetuation can be minimized through training. According to the co-emergence model, doing harm through reactive behavior starts with a strong body sensation, whether pleasant or unpleasant. Since behavior is prescribed by interoceptive salience interacting with hedonic tone, learning to become increasingly aware of how we think (Evaluation) and equanimous with how it spontaneously makes us feel (Interoception) decreases the need to react with craving and aversion (Hölzel et al., 2010). The learned response is increasingly extinguished (Hölzel et al., 2016) and ethical decisions and actions become more accessible. Furthermore, prolonged practice of mindfulness has been shown behaviorally and neurologically to decrease the emphasis on Evaluation and Reaction and increase the emphasis on Sensory Perception and Interoception, making us less judgmental and reactive, and more objective with what we experience in the present moment (Brewer et al., 2011; Farb et al., 2010; Ingram, Atchley & Segal, 2011; Lackner & Fresco, 2016; Taylor et al., 2011; Zeidan & Vago, 2016). This understanding of how mindfulness training deconditions our reactive habits and recreates an equilibrium state among the four components is the guiding theoretical principle for the four stages of MiCBT, which are briefly described below.

The MiCBT Model

Mindfulness-integrated Cognitive Behavior Therapy (MiCBT; Cayoun, 2011) may be defined as a theoretically congruent and technically complementary integration of traditional mindfulness training (as taught in the lineage of Ledi Sayadaw, Saya Tetgyi, Sayagyi U Ba Khin, and later S. N. Goenka) and traditional CBT that

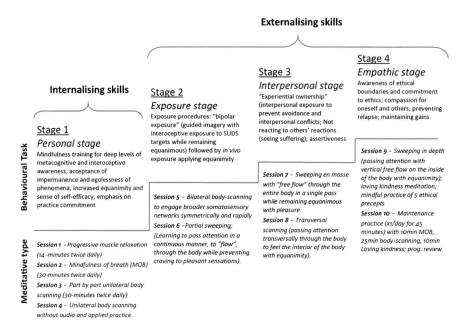

Fig. 7.3 The 4-stage model of Mindfulness-integrated Cognitive Behavior Therapy (adapted from Cayoun, 2011)

provides a transdiagnostic approach to help patients address emotional distress rapidly across a wide range of disorders. MiCBT is an evidence-based approach that can be delivered individually or in group. It has been shown to effectively reduce anxiety and depression in a range of conditions (e.g., Bahrani, Zargar, Yousefipour, & Akbari, 2017; Farzinrad & Kamal, 2013; Kumar, Sharma, Narayanaswamy, Kandavel, & Reddy, 2016; Roubos, 2011; Scott-Hamilton & Schutte, 2016; Scott-Hamilton, Schutte, & Brown, 2016; Senderey, 2017; Yazdanimehr, Omidi, Sadat, & Akbari, 2016). MiCBT typically lasts eight to 12 sessions, but it is flexible enough to be extended for longer periods with more severe and complex conditions. The four stages of MiCBT are summarized in Fig. 7.3 (see Cayoun, 2011, 2015; Cayoun, Francis & Shires, 2017, for a comprehensive implementation protocol).

Following standard clinical assessment, "Stage 1" (the "Personal Stage") begins with an intrapersonal focus. The first set of skills involves paying attention to our inner experiences to manage attention and emotions through four modes of experience: bodily activities, body sensations, mental states, and mental contents (such as thoughts and images). Stage 1 teaches important skills, such as metacognitive and interoceptive awareness, and equanimity. Once these valuable skills have been developed, usually over 4 weeks for most people, patients are less distracted, their attention is more focused in the present, they are less likely to nurture unhelpful thoughts, sleep is generally improved, and they are markedly less emotionally reactive. They can then invest these intrapersonal skills into the second part of the program, Stage 2.

In Stage 2 (the "Exposure Stage"), patients learn to overcome the anxiety that leads them to establish unhelpful avoidance of distressing situations and actions, such as socializing, driving in the city center, meeting colleagues for coffee at work, speaking to family members, or looking for a job. Pronounced avoidant behavior found in such conditions as specific phobia or post-traumatic stress disorder is also addressed. The act of overcoming avoidant habits instills in patients a great amount of self-confidence and self-efficacy. By the end of Stage 2, patients have acquired sufficient skills to begin "Stage 3," where they apply mindful exposure skills to address challenging interpersonal situations.

In Stage 3 (the "Interpersonal Stage"), patients learn that people's reactivity is only a reflection of their suffering, rather than an expression of a fundamental maliciousness. Patients learn not to react to others' reactivity, as they have understood through Stage 1 that people react based on what they feel (as per the co-emergence model), not because of the triggering situation they are facing. Just as they have learned not to take their own suffering personally, they learn to extend this to others. They do so by remaining mindful that people's reactivity is a normal and expected consequence of their unawareness of how reinforcement takes place when they allow craving and aversion. At the same time, patients also keep in mind that people lack insight into the processes of change. They remain aware that most are not trained in mindfulness and equanimity and would most probably react less or differently if they were; this paves the way for compassion. As in other models, (e.g., Kramer, 2007), learning these skills enhances interpersonal insight, genuineness, and friendliness in their relationships. They also learn proficient communication skills that increase their sense of efficacy during difficult interactions.

Finally, in "Stage 4" (the "Empathic Stage"), patients externalize attention further outward toward others and learn to remain tolerant and more objective about the deeper nature of their reactivity and suffering. They develop compassion instead of reacting to their own and others' reactivity, through a training in empathy and harm-prevention. At this juncture, patients tend to discern their most wholesome values and see what is truly important to them. Insight and kindness are sufficiently developed to make them feel connected within themselves and to others. Accordingly, their choice of action is increasingly mindful of what constitutes potential harm, which they learn to prevent out of compassion.

We now turn to a rationale for which being kind to ourselves and others is central to Stage 4. There are three principal reasons for which MiCBT dedicates this whole therapeutic stage to the development of empathy, grounded in loving-kindness meditation, and ethical living. These are the cultivation of compassion, relapse-prevention, and the cultivation of joy and well-being.

The Cultivation of Compassion

Since low sense of self-worth is also a major maintaining factor and cause of relapse in depression, there is a good rationale for cultivating kindness and compassion for oneself and others. There is also evidence that empathic and compassionate mental states can be enhanced through the practice of loving-kindness meditation (Jazaieri et al., 2012). Two main brain areas are particularly relevant to the ability to produce compassion; the insula (central for interoceptive awareness) and the junction between the right temporal and right parietal lobes, which is central for perceiving the mental and emotional states of others (Lutz et al., 2008). These two regions provide an important neural substrate for the ability to maintain fulfilling relationships and a sense of connectedness with others and are markedly more developed in experienced meditators than in novices (Lutz et al.).

Through the stages of MiCBT, the gradual awareness of the processes of suffering in oneself and others prepares patients for a compassionate attitude. Understanding the co-emergence model of reinforcement, they are already primed to be attentive to a context of legitimate and universal suffering. During Stage 4, patients learn that they are the first recipients of the emotions they generate and they train to choose carefully what emotion to promote and what emotion to let go. As part of the rationale (based on the co-emergence model) for Stage 4 presented to patients, we typically ask them, using the Socratic dialogue, "When you create anger toward someone, who is feeling it first?" Because of the markedly increased interoceptive awareness developed through mindfulness meditation, they typically answer "me." We continue, "And what do you think the person with whom you are angry is feeling? Is he or she also feeling this heat and agitation in their body just because you are angry with them?"…"Ok, and when you are kind with someone and you feel a genuine connection, friendliness, and compassion for someone, what is it that you are feeling?" Their typical answer is, "Warm," "light," or "tingling." We continue, "If this is the case, even if someone seems to have done you wrong, what kind of feelings do you think would benefit you most in the long run?"…"How likely are you to relapse if you are not as affected by people's reactivity, if you understand their suffering and if you feel more compassionate on a daily basis?" Since it becomes evident to patients that "self-compassion helps to engender and is engendered by mindfulness" (Neff, 2004, p. 29), a rationale for compassion training based on cognitive-reappraisal is usually sufficient. While this framework draws from Buddhist concepts, it is also supported by Western psychological approaches to compassion and altruism. Should the patient be interested, both lineages can be shared and sensitivity is extended to questions of whether the patient feels that Buddhist values are being imposed.

In the first week of Stage 4, patients are taught loving-kindness meditation, which has consistently been taught as part of mindfulness training in Buddhist teachings (Hart, 1987; Salzberg, 1995). As taught in MiCBT, loving-kindness meditation is only taught in Stage 4, usually from the eighth or ninth therapy session. Practitioners focus on benign and often pleasant sensations at the center of the chest and other body parts that co-emerge with positive affirmations, in the form of kind thoughts and well-wishing for ourselves and others (e.g., "May I be kind to myself" and "May I share my equanimity with all beings"), based on traditional methods. It also includes thoughts of acceptance while pairing pleasant body sensations with memories of people with whom patients may have been in conflict or with whom they expect to be in conflict in the future, in a way that acts as a counterconditioning method and helps prevent relapse. It lasts approximately 10 min and is practiced at the end of each daily mindfulness meditation practice. Evidence suggests that just a few minutes of loving-kindness meditation can increase one's sense of social connectedness on both explicit and implicit levels, which may help decrease social isolation (Hutcherson, Seppala & Gross, 2008). In turn, the probability of relapse triggered or maintained by social isolation decreases.

A clear differentiation between empathy and compassion is useful, as empathy and goodwill toward others during meditation alone is not necessarily grounded in daily action. In contrast, *compassion is the will to extend oneself for the purpose of minimizing one's own or another's suffering*. Compassion may remain a genuine intention and propensity for action, or become a fully fledged action if the intention is sufficiently intense. Nonetheless, acts of compassion are often reserved for best friends, colleagues, family members, the old lady crossing the road, or the puppy dog lost in the street. Unless they are prescribed by an organized spiritual or religious system, daily acts of compassion are hard to come by, especially when a person's mental health is jeopardized and a state of disequilibrium overfocuses attention on self-related concerns. For a compassion training anchored in daily behavior-regulation, the most congruent type of action is ethical action. While helping someone may be motivated by various personal needs, including validation and social desirability, intentional ethical acts are not necessarily overt and are likely to emanate from a sense of connectedness and compassion.

Acting ethically also eliminates the cognitive dissonance that one faces when swatting a mosquito or squashing an ant after practicing loving-kindness meditation. Wishing all beings to be well is inconsistent with killing willingly. Similarly, reacting so strongly while experiencing unpleasant body sensations triggered by the resentment of the insect is inconsistent with the correct practice of mindfulness, which necessitates a state of equanimity, "an even-minded mental state or dispositional tendency toward all experiences or objects, regardless of their affective valence (pleasant, unpleasant or neutral) or source" (Desbordes et al., 2015, p. 357). Indeed, unethical behavior is incongruous with both compassion and mindfulness. We cannot be mindful and kind, and intentionally harmful at the same time. In line with traditional Buddhist teachings, it seems that the first condition for a reliable acquisition of mindfulness skills is to prevent harmful actions. Provided it is motivated by care and kindness, rather than duty, fear, or guilt, I propose that ethical living is the most grounded, productive, and transformative act of compassion toward oneself and others.

In Stage 4 of MiCBT, patients also learn to ground empathy through the practice of the five precepts described earlier. These five ethical principles fall within the Western understanding of "doing no harm" and are usually endorsed by both patients and therapists for that very purpose. Patients are asked to undertake "five ethical challenges" for 1 week, as behavioral experiments. They are asked to pay continuous attention to their speech, to whether they are taking something that is not offered freely, to behavior that threatens or takes the lives of others, to the way they perform sexual acts, and to their potential craving for intoxicating substances such as alcohol or illicit/non-prescribed drugs. They are asked to notice the type of body sensation that co-emerges with a harmful intention, to prevent the response to the sensation, and to prevent the harmful behavior by the same token. They are also asked to "collect the data" in a dedicated ethical challenges diary and bring it to the therapist at their next session. It is made clear to patients that committing to these ethical challenges for a week must be an act of compassion and has nothing to do with adherence to a dogmatic morality. This promotes a sense of agency over their choices, rather than a restriction. After this short period, patients may choose to adopt whichever ethical principles they have found beneficial during that short trial period, and make future attempts at integrating others that are more challenging for them.

This process often clarifies the patient's value system. We often note the frequent life-changing decisions that patients make during and following this practice. Among the many cases, I recall someone who decided to divorce because he finally accepted that he and his partner had not been interested in staying with each other for many years, which he then saw as a lie. Both are now remarried and they remain good friends. Another person realized that he never acknowledged that he was (mildly) addicted to gambling. He then began to perceive it as a form of "intoxication" and decided to end his habit after that week. Some commonly choose to commit to a casual partner and start a family, others choose to travel or change job. Patients' most important values seem to be brought to the fore.

As mindfulness skills develop sufficiently, it becomes evident that genuine compassion unambiguously leads to ethical behavior. Moreover, for ethics to produce compassion, there must be an intention to prevent harm, and this is a compassionate mental state. We never think, "he really prevented this person to be harmed because he lacks compassion." Equally, we don't think, "she really doesn't care about his well-being because she is very compassionate." This would not make sense at all. We may also think, "I wonder what was his true motivation for remaining polite at the meeting today, because he usually doesn't hesitate to humiliate his staff." When wholesome behavior is not coupled with compassion, it is not credible or personally beneficial. It may benefit others, but also reflect fear, guilt, conceit, or unwholesome hidden interests.

Of course, this seems rather remote from the treatment of a patient referred for spider phobia. Nonetheless, the simple act of monitoring body sensations while in the presence of a spider before killing it or running out of the room helps create some distance between the feeling and the reaction. Applying equanimity while experiencing the viscerosomatic sensations of anxiety allows access to executive functions (Kirk, Downar, & Montague, 2011) and some degree of acceptance that the spider is also a sentient being, that it has the right to live and a role in our ecological system. Attention is no longer biased toward "self-preservation." Not harming the spider is not only an ethical behavior, it is primarily an act of compassion. Compassion leads indubitably to ethical conduct, and ethical conduct is a prerequisite for compassion. Importantly, since compassion training produces neuroplasticity (Lutz et al., 2008), the continued effort to prevent harm through compassion is more important than the object of compassion toward which it is directed. Whether the effort is related to the person nearest to our heart or a spider in the bush, it wires the brain in the same way. It makes us more compassionate and less prone to dissatisfaction and reactivity. This also means less prone to relapse, as is discussed below.

The Prevention of Relapse in Common Mental Health Disorders

Cultivating compassion through kindness and ethical boundaries facilitates self-regulation skills. In contrast, feeling self-hatred or disconnected from others is a major cause of relapse into depression and a lack of happiness in general. From the CMR perspective, an overactive self-referential system of evaluation leads to over-reactivity and the consequent disequilibrium state. In turn, this increases the probability of relapse. One way to maintain an equilibrium state is to ensure that patients' attitude toward themselves is kind, and that their ability to be aware extends to others and is not limited to their experience. This decreases the emphasis on self-referential processing and reactivity when exposed to common stressors (Neff, Kirkpatrick, & Rude, 2007). Patients are also more able to acknowledge their role in adverse situations without feeling overwhelmed with emotions and can reduce their reactions "in ways that are distinct from and, in some cases, more beneficial than self-esteem" (Leary et al., 2007, p. 887).

One of the causes for relapse is undoubtedly the inability or unwillingness to maintain helpful ethical boundaries. For instance, poor anger management tends to promote impulsivity and harmful reactions, such as hurtful speech, cascading into relationship conflict and emotional distress. Lying, stealing, or using divisive speech at work may lead to endless workplace conflicts that trigger further episodes of anxiety. Inappropriate sexual behavior may break a circle of friends, leading to isolation and a rejection schema, and relapse into depression. The likelihood of unethical behavior and relapse increases with intoxication. Using drugs and alcohol can also precipitate depressive, anxious, delusional, or psychotic states, especially if the patient experienced them prior to treatment. Unlike harming people by means of speech or physical action, using alcohol is an accepted societal value. An expensive bottle of wine brought to a party will even attract praise and gratitude—two strong social reinforcers. Accordingly, avoiding alcohol is more complex and less appealing than preventing non-rewarded behavior.

Once intoxicated by a substance, it becomes difficult to detect common sensory input (Oscar-Berman & Marinkovic, 2007). Cognitive control, often called "executive functions" (working memory, attentional and inhibitory control, cognitive flexibility, reasoning, problem-solving, and planning), is also jeopardized (Jääskeläinen, Schröger, & Näätänen, 1999). "Refraining" from unethical actions requires behavioral output mechanisms that involve a specific executive function called "response inhibition." Inhibitory functions can be trained, even in children with ADHD (Cayoun, 2010). However, they are impaired under intoxicated states and controlling our action becomes either too demanding or impossible (Abroms, Fillmore, & Marczinski, 2003; Marinkovic, Rickenbacher, & Azma, 2012). For example, practicing mindfulness of breath (*anapanasati*) after a glass of wine or using marijuana is futile because we are trying to inhibit the learned response to emerging thoughts before returning our attention to the breath (an executive function known as attention shifting or cognitive flexibility) while THC and alcohol have a disinhibitory effect on our response (Koelega, 1995; Marczinski & Fillmore, 2003; McDonald, Schleifer, Richards, & de Wit, 2003). The consequence is poor concentration. In the context of effort toward ethics, the brain's capacity to inhibit an unwanted, or wanted but inappropriate, action is reduced to the extent that one is intoxicated. It becomes difficult to prevent harm even though we may be inclined and able to do so when not intoxicated.

Case-conceptualizing unethical behavior through the CMR reveals that an intentional harmful action is always an attempt to reduce and curtail unpleasant body sensations, or amplify and prolong pleasant ones. Negative and positive reinforcement (respectively) of harmful behavior takes place when this goal is achieved. Whereas mindfulness-derived ethical behavior requires interoceptive awareness and inhibition of craving and aversion (equanimity), harmful actions are best understood as learned responses originating from past causes and current conditions. That is, the lack of ethics reinforces craving and aversion. The assumption that a person harms another because they are "abnormal" or "evil" is not helpful, as there is little hope or clear direction for improvement. Habitual harmful actions are to be *unlearned* to promote well-being, rather than suppressed based on the right and wrong derived from cultural or religious values. A person benefits most from performing ethical actions when they emerge from compassion.

Accordingly, ethics are presented to patients as a *protection*, not a restriction or punishment. Patients learn to respect them and enjoy practicing them as they also nourish their sense of self-worth, as will be discussed below. They are told that their challenge will be to monitor their actions in daily life and prevent the five types of harmful action from taking place *to the best of their ability*. Patients do not perceive this as a rigid and daunting task because it is presented to them as a set of experiments from which to learn. They are encouraged to make it interesting by positioning themselves as a beginner, a student, rather than someone who "*should* know better." This is consistent with Buddhist education and practice while remaining culturally neutral. They learn to remain equanimous and be compassionate with themselves when they don't succeed. They learn that not positioning themselves as special (especially good or especially capable) can make the perception of failure more acceptable if things don't go to plan. It is usually humbling and relieving for them to be in the beginner's seat.

With practice, patients become more aware that healthy remorse for harmful actions directs attention to others, whereas guilt directs attention to their sense of self. Since guilt overemphasizes self-referential processing, patients are asked to prevent its proliferation. They are encouraged to be attentive to the consequences of their behavior on themselves and others, while still being kind to themselves and to strengthen their commitment to prevent future harm. With more refined mindfulness skills, they also notice and prevent harmful speech directed to themselves (e.g., self-loathing). MiCBT trains patients to prevent relapse into symptoms of depression or anxiety by (1) being mindful of early interoceptive distress cues while remaining equanimous, (2) remaining kind, tolerant, and compassionate with themselves and others, and (3) applying non-harming behavior across contexts. These three interactive and interdependent skill-sets help patients establish a genuine sense of connectedness and belonging that acts as protective factor against relapse.

Although a good rationale delivery goes a long way, some patients can be occasionally reluctant to engage with the experiment. We have identified two main fears to embrace ethics. One relates to their potential history associated with ethics, such as childhood experiences of religious constraints. The other is a fear of abandoning habits and things to which they are attached and with which they identify. Given that we identify with sensory pleasures and habitual behavior (e.g., gambling, intoxication, inappropriate sex, aggressiveness, gossiping, reckless driving, misappropriation, pursuing a cult of popularity, and chasing fame), abstaining from these ultimately leads to a fear of abandoning who we are. Since unethical behavior is reinforced by craving and aversion, and mindfulness training reduces both, it is possible to let go of our fear of embracing ethics by practicing mindfulness accurately, as discussed earlier.

The Cultivation of Joy and Well-being

Living a meaningful life contributes to a sense of well-being, but life cannot be meaningful for a person who does not believe he or she is interesting, likeable, and worthy in the eyes of others. The fundamental problem underlying a low sense of self-worth is that we perceive who we are as a real, substantial and permanent self. Even though there are no differences in intrinsic value between humans, we attribute an intrinsic difference by perceiving ourselves as unique, uniquely good or bad, uniquely beautiful or ugly, uniquely intelligent or unintelligent. This imagined self-image is reinforced over time through the updating pathways of the brain's DMN, sometimes called the "Me network" (Schwartz & Gladding, 2011). Unfortunately, an emphasis on the sense of self accentuates our sense of being different and separated from others. In turn, isolation creates anxiogenic and depressogenic cognitive vulnerabilities (Ingram et al., 2011). Patients with a low sense of self-worth tend to compare themselves with others and nurture their sense of inadequacy and defectiveness. In addition, when parents are unable to make a child feel unconditionally worthy, the child grows with an over-externalized locus of self-worth. The parents may inadvertently reserve their praise, or their attention altogether, for good performance at school or doing the chores at home. This feeds the probability of future performance anxiety in adulthood. The difficulty to internalize the sense that he or she is a worthy human being in the eyes of others makes the adult over-reliant on external feedback to reinforce their sense of worth. The same applies to self-care. If our sense of self-worth is poor, there is little reason for taking care of our body and mind. In sum, having "too much self" in mind creates unhappiness.

Fortunately, an over-externalized locus of self-worth can be internalized through a compassion training that integrates a respect for ethical boundaries. Learning to be kind and not making harmful decisions can make us feel worthy. Patients regularly report how proud they are for having saved a few ants from the usual careless stroke of their sponge while cleaning, or how strong they feel for not having had alcohol in the past few weeks. Their joy and increased hope arise from a deep sense of self-efficacy. Hence, a greater sense of self-worth helps internalize the locus of self-care, which in turn increases self-efficacy. Indeed, patients at Stage 4 of MiCBT rely less on the therapist to adopt health-related behavior. They take more responsibility for their health and activities by acting on values that are wholesome. This is often reflected in their tendency to make important decisions that can change existing relationships, initiate new ones, or start a new kind of life effortlessly. This includes the choice of a less harmful livelihood, born from a value of ethical living. We witness people's need for personal growth, and their liberating realization that their unhappiness was maintained by a lack of maturation, rather than flaws in their personality. Accordingly, the effort to outgrow what causes a lack of joy and well-being seems to be a better fit than "curing a mental illness." From a developmental perspective, maturing requires a growing awareness of the consequences of one's actions and those of others. Awareness of ethics is integral to the maturation of consciousness; it is integral to wisdom.

When patients, and people in general, decrease their focus on the self, they are more able to see others as they are. An ant on the kitchen bench is no longer a dirty or threatening pest to be wiped away with crumbs. It is a living animal that works very hard most of the day to feed the collective of its nest. It is vulnerable yet repeatedly taking risks of being killed while in search of food or water in the proximity of humans. Out of compassion, patients will keep their kitchen clean and the sink dry, so that ants are less likely to gather there and be harmed. Even if a patient has nothing else to feel proud about, going to sleep while processing the memory of their day's wholesome actions and interactions can produce a sense of meaning and joy. They recall that they saved lives, returned someone else's lost item, or held back on using intoxicants out of their own compassion and effort, an effort that is based on virtues which no one can take from them. If sufficiently repeated, they feel that they *become* virtuous because their effort to prevent harm arises from within. It is not a consequence of boundaries imposed by other people. Both ethical living and sense of self-worth are being internalized, rather than being reliant on external achievements and validation from others. Moreover, well-being is enhanced by a sense of connectedness with others, including animals and plants. Patients derive a sense of affiliation and life meaning by having *others* in mind, caring about them, and preventing harm to them. Feeling that we matter to others makes our life meaningful.

Nonetheless, adherence to ethical values can emerge from lifelong schematic models (systems of beliefs), some of which are unhelpful or even destructive. I recall one of my patients who was tremendously committed to his religious faith and became extremely depressed and anxious after he admitted to his wife that he was addicted to child pornography. They both agreed that she would stay in the marriage if he immediately abstained from visiting pornography websites and let go of his addiction. He sought professional help once he realized that he could not disentangle himself from his addiction. His approach was to pray to God to give him "the strength to banish the evil and become a good person." I also recall a depressed patient who had learned early in life that reducing people's suffering should be a daily duty which requires smiling to them. Her mother also told her that people who do not smile to others are not worthy in the eyes of God. She would become anxious when unable to smile to people on her low days. Both clients had initially mistaken Stage 4 of MiCBT for a religion-related exercise, one that rendered their sense of self-worth conditional upon external agents.

Hence, the therapist carefully observes the patient's motivation for applying ethics. Using a dedicated ethics diary, the therapist asks what the benefits in remaining mindful and equanimous were while attempting to prevent harm in the recorded situations. If the patient did not pay attention to their intentions and co-emerging body sensations (see Figs. 7.1 and 7.2), his or her motivation may depart from the task and the direction of attention may have been toward the self. If necessary, the therapist gently clarifies that the task is to study the emerging sensations and prevent the response so that harm to themselves or others does not occur. They are told that the goal is not to "become a good person," because they are neither good nor bad, they just have to note what intention and behavior produce suffering or happiness and learn from them. Eventually, most patients can grasp the idea that ethical living is to decrease suffering, rather than inflating one's sense of self ("the ego"). If ethics-related guilt and conceit are prevented, awareness of ethical boundaries and commitment to them increase their sense of self-worth and the potential for joy and well-being.

Implications for MBI Programs

Ethics in Behavioral Science and the Traps of Cognitive Dissonance

Most of us, most of the time, in most situations, know what is harmful and what is not. It is not that we are uneducated about ethics or not aware of what to prevent. It is usually a lack of awareness and inhibitory control under certain conditions, such as high arousal or intoxication. Mindfulness of behavior that differentiates benign from harmful consequences to explicitly prevent harm is a valuable behavior-regulation method. It is an ideal way of grounding empathy into a daily effort to think and act compassionately, and is by no means a form of dogma or enforced values.

Clinicians are required to take the problem of harming behavior seriously into account and act on it to minimize the risk of harm. For instance, the code of ethics for psychologists and psychiatrists in most countries requires the clinician to tell patients at the outset that he or she is mandated to breach confidentiality if the patient shows a genuine risk of self-harming or harming others. The clinicians' and researchers' adherence to a strict code of ethics is also mandatory and taught to interns at universities as an important part of their course curriculum. This adherence is universally endorsed and does not seem to provoke any confusion or disagreement with regard to psychological science, on the basis that a code of ethics is a protective aspect of our work, not a dogmatic restriction. Moreover, adhering to good practice standards and ethical codes of conduct for teachers and trainers of Mindfulness-Based Stress Reduction (MBSR) and Mindfulness-Based Cognitive Therapy (MBCT) has been expressed as an important priority (Crane, 2016).

Given that ethical guidelines are so strictly imposed on clinicians and researchers while concurrently perceived as beneficial, could basic ethics help our patients too? Could what is beneficial to a clinician be also beneficial to others? What if a patient raised in an abusive family, who also verbally abuses his own partner and children, could learn to use non-harmful speech? What if a patient who has been frequently unfaithful, and whose partner is deeply hurt and depressed, could learn how to prevent promiscuity and restore a harmonious marriage? Since much of people's suffering presented to clinicians involves ethical issues, could therapy be an ideal context for carefully introducing ethics education?

According to Monteiro (2016, p. 213), "explicit ethics refer to the overt and specific inclusion of an ethics or values-based framework in the MBI curriculum. Implicit ethics refers to the assumptions that awareness in and of itself suffices for ethical thought, speech, and action to emerge as well as be congruent with the individual's self and world view." Ethics are sometimes thought to be implicitly acquired through the development of mindfulness. Indeed, the more we are aware of our intentions and actions, the less we are likely to act in an impulsive and harmful way. When mindfulness is taught accurately, along with equanimity (Cayoun, 2011; Hart, 1987; Holzel et al., 2016), it enables the prevention of mildly arousing and low-impact harmful action. However, rapid and strongly arousing impulses will simply not allow metacognitive and interoceptive awareness, and response inhibition may be too slow to prevent harm. As highlighted by Kabat-Zinn (2005, p. 103), "If we are continuously creating agitation in our lives, and causing harm to others and to ourselves, it is that agitation and harm that we will encounter in our meditation practice, because that is what we are feeding." Unless our attention is primed to detect potential breaches of ethics through remaining mindful of our intention to prevent harm, the maturation and generalizability of ethical behavior is questionable.

As explained earlier in this chapter, this matter has nothing to do with religious values or religious education. Nor is it about changing patients into "good people." It is about not doing harm, which is part and parcel of healthy psychological maturation and emancipation. Since both therapy and ethical living share the purpose of alleviating suffering, it seems to make perfect sense to include ethics education carefully into therapy and teach our patients what we clinicians have learned and adhere to in daily life. This is not a "Buddhist thing." It is common sense. Yet, this difference is not always clear in the community of colleagues who implement MBIs and there is a concern among some therapists and teachers that explicitly including ethics in therapy may be an imposition on some patients' values (See Baer, 2015;

Crane, 2016; Monteiro, 2016; Monteiro, Musten & Compson, 2014; Shonin, van Gordon, & Griffiths, 2015, for discussions).

This is perhaps a consequence of insufficiently recognizing important pitfalls. For instance, there is a case where teaching ethics in therapy could trigger guilt and destructive shame. Take the example of a patient with borderline personality disorder (BPD) who self-harms to decrease the severity of dissociative states or anger-based arousal states. Since shame is highly likely to be an established habit in BPD (Peters, Geiver, Smart, & Baer, 2014), proposing that self-harm is unethical without placing this proposition in the context of a compassion training could lead to more guilt, shame, and self-harm to decrease the arousal that shame causes. Although this occurrence would be unlikely when ethics are implemented within a compassionate MBI, the implications of teaching explicit ethics are important to consider. Another pitfall relates to conceit. For example, being ethical for the purpose of "being spiritual" directs our attention to the self. If it makes us "special" or "good," it makes others ordinary or bad. Wise observation reveals that people's actions are sometimes skillful and wholesome and at other times not. Whereas performing good deeds and orienting our lives toward "the greater good" is wholesome in Buddhist psychology, the desire to "be good" reinforces the unfounded assumption of a self, an "ego." Accordingly, performing wholesome actions with the self in mind is neither in line with the original Buddhist teaching of egolessness (*anatta*), nor a good rationale for ethics education in the context of the Western scientist-practitioner approach.

However, the question of whether to include ethics explicitly or not in MBIs also seems to be related to the issue of identity and the preservation of who we are, both for the MBI clinician and their patients. Understandably, since ethical conduct is a major feature of most theistic systems, the implicit association between ethics and religion may mislead some MBI teachers and clinicians into thinking that educating our patients to act ethically, in a non-harmful way, imposes spiritual or religious values on them and falls outside the context of secular Western therapy. It has been argued that this view is partly caused by a misunderstanding of the reason for which traditional Buddhist psychology promotes ethical living (Grossman, 2015).

Thus, on the one hand, we may hold ethics in high esteem for the management of our own lives and career as therapists, while at the same time holding back on sharing this highly beneficial system of harm-prevention with our patients. I propose that this cognitive dissonance is unhelpful and divisive in our attempts to assist the MBI community to grow, and would be best acknowledged. Poor philosophy, or "unwholesome skepticism," permits the refutation of a belief based on another belief, one's own or one's in-group. Given its ramification in clinical practice, psychological science cannot afford a competition of views and must refocus attention on evidence. Despite the increasingly loud debate on this topic, we are still without any evidence whatsoever that teaching ethics in MBIs is perceived negatively by patients, or that MBIs are less efficacious when ethics education is included in the intervention. The reverse is also true. We are yet to see controlled studies examining the differential outcomes of implicit and explicit ethics in MBIs. Such studies are now needed. For example, randomized controlled trials examining MBSR or MBCT with and without explicit ethics would be invaluable. This would also be very poignant with Mindfulness-Based Relapse Prevention (MBRP), which is used to prevent relapse into substance abuse. Exploring the possible differential effects of including ethics in MBIs would be especially informative across contexts and patient populations. For instance, we would expect that additional benefits produced by the inclusion of ethics in inmate populations would reduce the rate of recidivism and reincarceration (e.g., Bowen et al., 2006).

Integrating Ethics in MBIs

An effect of cultivating mindfulness is an improved perception of the consequences of our daily intentions and actions. The processes of cause and effect become clearer. Actions that are harmful to oneself or to others tend to reinforce or maintain an existing psychological condition and are counterproductive during therapy. This is partly because humans are social beings and much of our difficulties either arise from interpersonal experiences or are strongly affected by them. Therefore, it would seem valuable to gently introduce an exercise in ethics into MBIs where the explicit training of ethics is not yet part of the curriculum. References to Buddhist values would not be necessary since ethical behavior is a universal act of maturity and a necessity for healthy survival. This has already been done successfully with Mindfulness-Based Symptom Management training (e.g., Monteiro & Musten, 2013; Monteiro, Nuttall, & Musten, 2010).

For example, as in MiCBT, this could consist of extending one's informal practice of mindfulness to monitor how body sensations arise when we intend to, or are about to, perform a potentially harmful action. By feeling in detail the nature of the body sensation, staying with it equanimously until it subsides and knowing that it will pass, patients become able to prevent the harmful action or, at the very least, take more responsibility for performing it. This exposure method is presented as using ethics "as a hook for mindfulness" or "using mindfulness to prevent harm." Although people may be given more directions, this attenuated introduction does not specify what type of harmful action to prevent and bypasses the potential association with a moralistic value system. Given Kabat-Zinn's dedicated chapter on ethics in MBSR (Kabat-Zinn, 2005), this approach is likely to be congruent with the practice and delivery of MBSR and its directly related models, such as MBCT (Segal, Williams, & Teasdale, 2002) and MBRP (Bowen, Chawla, & Marlatt, 2010).

There are three conditions for successful training with all types of new skill-acquisition, including mindfulness training and ethical behavior: *frequency*, *duration*, and *accuracy* of training (Cayoun, 2015, Scott-Hamilton & Schutte, 2016). Accuracy of training is the most important aspect—hence the aforementioned description of "Right Mindfulness"—because we can inadvertently waste a lot of time and energy if the practice targets brain pathways that are unrelated to the skills we seek to develop. Moreover, inaccurate practice can harm, especially if we practice it often and for long periods. The desired skills emerge to the extent that the practice is accurate. However, only occasionally reminding ourselves to refrain from causing harm is not likely to become a habit and will remain a top-down effort. Similarly, paying attention to our intentions and actions for a few seconds daily is not likely to make the task easier over time. There is evidence that the less we practice mindfulness in formal meditation, the less skilled our brain is in coping with ruminative brooding (Hawley et al., 2014). This is because habit-building relies on neuroplasticity, which depends on the amount and frequency of brain stimulation (Cramer et al., 2011).

Does one size fit all with ethics training? It is not likely, but the need for ethics is universally beneficial and necessary for preventing relapse. Ethics are only wholesome when they are context-sensitive. They must be "alive" and cannot be applied out of blind faith in "dead scriptures." When they are adaptive, they reach their optimum efficacy. In Buddhist teachings, this is referred to as "the Middle Way," which Ajahn Jayasaro broadly defines as the optimum maximum means of moving away from the unwholesome (craving, aversion, and ignorance of impermanence) and increasing the wholesome (Jayasaro, 2013). Consequently, if a seemingly ethical action, such as telling the truth, is about to cause more suffering than withholding it, then telling the truth becomes unwholesome. For example, if armed burglars attack you in your house and ask if you are alone, it is not a good idea to tell them that your child is hiding in the basement. By adopting a middle way, patients perform the least harmful action in the given circumstances. This is adaptive and prevents the risk of becoming dogmatic and rigid in the approach to ethical living.

Therapists are in a privileged position to promote compassion and interconnectedness in the community. Having witnessed well over a thousand patients undertakes the MiCBT program in the past 16 years, I do not have a single doubt that teaching ethics in the community enriches it. We often speak of "the greater good" or being kind, but what does this mean in terms of attitude? Unless these notions are materialized into concrete actions, it is just good philosophy. Having a small but clear set of guiding principles, such as the five precepts, and making an effort to be mindful of them can assist in preventing harm. Then, through wholesome behavior and intention, it becomes possible to integrate kindness, compassion, and the notion of greater good.

Summary and Concluding Remarks

In this chapter, I explained how compassion is developed through integrating daily training in empathy (loving-kindness meditation) with five basic ethical attitudes and boundaries in daily life. We discussed how and why compassion training requires actual actions to minimize harm and promote well-being for oneself and others. I explained why it is not possible to develop wisdom without compassion and that compassion cannot be authentically established across contexts without ethics. We also examined how, in MiCBT and in traditional Buddhist teachings, ethics are practiced out of compassion, rather than duty, guilt, or conceit.

I discussed the idea that we often relapse into psychological conditions because we have not let go of harmful attitudes; we can't resolve problems with the means that created them. I proposed that the reason for including such ethical attitudes (born from compassion) is to prevent relapse by valuing one's own and others' well-being. Doing so makes us connect with ourselves and others, including animals and plants, in a compassionate way, a way that is diametrically opposite to the way we feel when we are anxious or depressed, thereby acting as a buffer against relapse.

Moreover, I described the mechanisms of reaching a sense of self-worth in ethical and unethical mental states, with an emphasis on the fact that we cannot develop genuine happiness (which we are all seeking) with means that bring suffering, such as harmful actions. I clarified how a true and reliable sense of self-worth and well-being can only emerge from one's mind (as does one's sense of suffering) and how cultivating a mindfulness-based effort to prevent harm for oneself and others increases one's sense of self-worth. Without a profound appreciation of, and respect for, ethical boundaries, our well-being and that of others doesn't seem to matter.

Finally, I discussed some of the implications of the above in MBIs. Perceptual bias and cognitive dissonance were identified: practicing ethics appears essential to the clinician for good practice and healthy relationships between colleagues and with patients, while at the same time perceiving the explicit teaching of the same ethics to patients as an imposition of religious values to be avoided. I have then proposed ideas for future research, and a way of including a simple exposure-based approach derived from MiCBT to gently introduce ethics education in other MBIs.

I hope that this chapter has provided you with novel and reassuring ideas that encourage you to train yourselves and your patients with the full potential of mindfulness, combined with universally acceptable ethics and compassion. It is said that when an old lady came to pay respect to the Buddha lying on his death bed, she asked him to teach her how to ease her suffering. Despite being told that the revered 80-year-old teacher was too tired to teach, she insisted that she would not accept anyone else to teach her in case they alter his original teaching. At these words, the Buddha rose out of compassion and offered her these few words as a summary of the teaching: "Abstain from performing harmful actions, perform skillful actions, and keep on purifying [deconditioning] your mind." She then understood the true purpose of mindfulness.

Acknowledgements I am grateful to Drs. Lynette Monteiro, Glenn Bilsborrow, and Andrea and Nick Grabovac for their useful suggestions.

References

Abroms, B. D., Fillmore, M. T., & Marczinski, C. A. (2003). Alcohol-induced impairment of behavioral control: Effects on the alteration and suppression of prepotent responses. *Journal on Studies of Alcohol, 64*, 687–695.

Apkarian, A. V. (2008). Pain in relation to emotional learning. *Current Opinion in Neurobiology, 18*, 464–468.

Baer, R. A. (2015). Ethics, values, virtues, and character strengths in mindfulness-based interventions: A psychological science perspective. *Mindfulness*. https://doi.org/10.1007/s12671-015-0419-2

Bahrani, S., Zargar, F., Yousefipour, G., & Akbari, H. (2017). The effectiveness of mindfulness-integrated cognitive behavior therapy on depression, anxiety, and stress in females with multiple sclerosis: A single blind randomized controlled trial. *Iranian Red Crescent Medical Journal*, e44566. https://doi.org/10.5812/ircmj.44566

Baliki, M. N., Geha, P. Y., Apkarian, A. V., & Chialvo, D. R. (2008). Beyond feeling: Chronic pain hurts the brain, disrupting the default-mode network dynamics. *The Journal of Neuroscience*, 28, 1398–1403.

Baliki, M. N., Petre, B., Torbey, S., Herrmann, K. M., Huang, L., Schnitzer, T. J., … Apkarian, A. V. (2012). Corticostriatal functional connectivity predicts transition to chronic back pain. *Nature Neuroscience*, 15, 1117–1119.

Bishop, S. R., Lau, M., Shapiro, S., Carlson, L., Anderson, N. D., Carmody, J., … Devins, G. (2004). Mindfulness: A proposed operational definition. *Clinical Psychology: Science and Practice*, 11, 230–241.

Bodhi, B. (2000). *The connected discourses of the Buddha: A translation of the Samyutta Nikaya*. Boston: Wisdom Publications.

Bowen, S., Chawla, N., & Marlatt, G. A. (2010). *Mindfulness-based relapse prevention for addictive behaviors: A Clinician's Guide*. New York: Guilford Press.

Bowen, S., Witkiewitz, K., Dillworth, T. M., Chawla, N., Simpson, T. L., Ostafin, B. D., … Marlatt, G. A. (2006). Mindfulness meditation and substance use in an incarcerated population. *Psychology of Addictive Behaviors*, 20, 343–347. https://doi.org/10.1037/0893-164X.20.3.343

Brewer, J. A., Worhunskya, P. D., Gray, J. R., Tang, Y., Weberd, J., & Kobera, H. (2011). Meditation experience is associated with differences in default mode network activity and connectivity. *Proceedings of the National Academy of Sciences USA*. https://doi.org/10.1073/pnas.1112029108

Buckner, R., Andrews-Hanna, J., & Schacter, D. (2008). The brain's default network: Anatomy, function, and relevance to disease. *New York Academy of Sciences*, 1124, 1–38.

Cayoun, B. A. (2010). *The dynamics of bimanual coordination in ADHD: Processing speed, inhibition and cognitive flexibility*. Saarbrücken, Germany: Lambert Academic Publishing.

Cayoun, B. A. (2011). *Mindfulness-integrated CBT: Principles and practice*. Chichester: Wiley.

Cayoun, B. A. (2015). *Mindfulness-integrated CBT for wellbeing and personal growth: Four steps to enhance inner calm, self-confidence and relationships*. Chichester: Wiley.

Cayoun, B. A., Francis, S. E., & Shires, A. (2017). *The Clinician's Guide to Mindfulness-integrated CBT: A step-by-step workbook and resource for therapists*. Manuscript in preparation.

Cayoun, B. A., Simmons, A., & Shires, A. (2017). *Immediate and lasting chronic pain reduction following a brief self-implemented mindfulness-based interoceptive exposure task: A preliminary open trial*. Manuscript submitted for publication.

Cramer, S. C., Sur, M., Dobkin, B. H., O'Brien, C., Sanger, T. D., Trojanowski, J. Q., … Vinogradov, S. (2011). Harnessing neuroplasticity for clinical applications. *Brain*, 134, 1591–1609. https://doi.org/10.1093/brain/awr039

Crane, R. S. (2016). Implementing mindfulness in the mainstream: Making the path by walking it. *Mindfulness*. https://doi.org/10.1007/s12671-016-0632-7

Desbordes, G., Gard, T., Hoge, E. A., Hölzel, B. K., Kerr, C., Lazar, S. W., … Vago, D. R. (2015). Moving beyond mindfulness: Defining equanimity as an outcome measure in meditation and contemplative research. *Mindfulness*, 6, 356–372. https://doi.org/10.1007/s12671-013-0269-8

Dimyan, M. A., & Cohen, L. G. (2011). Neuroplasticity in the context of motor rehabilitation after stroke. *Nature Reviews Neurology*, 7, 76–85. https://doi.org/10.1038/nrneurol.2010.200

Dreyfus, G. (2011). Is mindfulness present-centered and non-judgmental? A discussion of the cognitive dimensions of mindfulness. *Contemporary Buddhism*, 12, 41–54. https://doi.org/10.1080/14639947.2011.564815

Farb, N. A. S., Anderson, A. K., Mayberg, H., Bean, J., Mckeon, D., & Segal, Z. V. (2010). Minding one's emotion: Mindfulness training alters the neural expression of sadness. *Emotion*, *10*, 25–33.

Farb, N., Daubenmier, J., Price, C. J., Gard, T., Kerr, C., Dunn, B. D., … Mehling, W. E. (2015). Interoception, contemplative practice, and health. *Frontiers in Psychology*, *6*, 763. https://doi.org/10.3389/fpsyg.2015.00763

Farb, N. A. S., Segal, Z. V., & Anderson, A. K. (2013). Attentional modulation of primary interoceptive and exteroceptive cortices. *Cerebral Cortex*, *23*, 114–126. https://doi.org/10.1093/cercor/bhr385

Farb, N. A. S., Segal, Z. V., Mayberg, H., Bean, J., McKeon, D., Fatima, Z., & Anderson, A. K. (2007). Attending to the present: Mindfulness meditation reveals distinct neural modes of self-reference. *Social Cognitive and Affective Neuroscience*, *2*, 313–322.

Farzinrad, B., & Nazari, K. M. (2013). Comparison between Effectiveness of mindfulness integrated cognitive behavioral therapy (MiCBT) and rational emotional behavior therapy (REBT) on procrastination, perfectionism and worry in students. Dissertation, Tabtiz University of Medical Sciences, Iran.

Fox, M. D., Snyder, A., Vincent, J., Corbetta, M., Van Essen, D., & Raichle, M. E. (2005). The human brain is intrinsically organized into dynamic, anticorrelated functional networks. *PNAS*, *102*, 9673–9678.

Gard, T., Hölzel, B., Sack, A. T., Hempel, H., Lazar, S. W., Vaitl, D., & Ott, U. (2011). Pain attenuation through mindfulness is associated with decreased cognitive control and increased sensory processing in the brain. *Cerebral Cortex*, *191*, 36–43. https://doi.org/10.1093/cercor/bhr352

Gethin, R. (1998). *The foundations of Buddhism*. Oxford: Oxford University Press.

Goenka, S. N. (1998). *Satipatthana Sutta Discourses: Talks from a course in Maha-satipatthana Sutta*. Seattle, WA: Vipassana Research Publications.

Grant, J. A., Courtemanche, J., & Rainville, P. (2011). A non-evaluative mental stance and decoupling of executive and pain-related cortices predicts low pain sensitivity in Zen meditators. *Pain*, *152*, 150–156.

Grossman, P. (2015). Mindfulness: Awareness informed by an embodied ethic. *Mindfulness*, *6*, 17–22. https://doi.org/10.1007/s12671-014-0372-5

Hakamata, Y., Lissek, S., Bar-Haim, Y., Britton, J. C., Fox, N. A., Leibenluft, E., … Pine, D. S. (2010). Attention bias modification treatment: A meta-analysis toward the establishment of novel treatment for anxiety. *Biological Psychiatry*, *68*, 982–990. https://doi.org/10.1016/j.biopsych.2010.07.021

Hart, W. (1987). *The art of living: Vipassana meditation as taught by S. N. Goenka*. New York: Harper Collins.

Hawley, L. L., Schwartz, D., Bieling, P. J., Irving, J., Corcoran, K., Farb, N. A. S., … Segal, Z. V. (2014). Mindfulness practice, rumination and clinical outcome in mindfulness-based treatment. *Cognitive Therapy and Research*, *38*, 1–9.

Hölzel, B. K., Brunsch, V., Gard, T., Greve, D. N., Koch, K., Sorg, C., … Milad, M. R. (2016). Mindfulness-Based Stress Reduction, fear conditioning, and the uncinate fasciculus: A pilot study. *Frontiers in Behavioral Neuroscience*, *10*, 124. https://doi.org/10.3389/fnbeh.2016.00124

Hölzel, B. K., Carmody, J., Evans, K. C., Hoge, E. A., Dusek, J. A., Morgan, L., … Lazar, S. W. (2010). Stress reduction correlates with structural changes in the amygdala. *Social Cognitive and Affective Neuroscience*, *5*, 11–17.

Hutcherson, C. A., Seppala, E. M., & Gross, J. J. (2008). Loving kindness meditation increases social connectedness. *Emotion*, *8*, 720–724.

Ingram, R. E., Atchley, R. A., & Segal, Z. V. (2011). *Vulnerability to depression: From cognitive neuroscience to prevention and treatment*. New York: Guilford Press.

Jääskeläinen, I. P., Schröger, E., & Näätänen, R. (1999). Electrophysiological indices of acute effects of ethanol on involuntary attention shifting. *Psychopharmacology*, *141*, 16–21.

Jayasaro, A. (2011). *Mindfulness, precepts and crashing in the same car*. Bangkok, Thailand: Panyaprateep Foundation.

Jayasaro, A. (2013). *Without and Within: Questions and answers on the teachings of Theravāda Buddhism.* Buddhadasa Indapanno Archives, Bangkok: Panyaprateep Foundation. Retrieved from http://cdn.amaravati.org/wp content/uploads/2014/10/11/Without-and-Within-by-Ajahn-Jayasaro.pdf.

Jazaieri, H., Jinpa, G. T., McGonigal, K., Rosenberg, E. L., Finkelstein, J., Simon-Thomas, E., … Goldin, P. R. (2012). Enhancing compassion: A randomized controlled trial of a compassion cultivation training program. *Journal of Happiness Studies, 14,* 1113. https://doi.org/10.1007/s10902-012-9373-z

Kabat-Zinn, J. (1994). *Wherever you go, there you are.* New York: Hyperion.

Kabat-Zinn, J. (2005). *Coming to our senses: Healing ourselves and the world through mindfulness.* London: Piatkus.

Kirk, U., Downar, J., & Montague, P. R. (2011). Interoception drives increased rational decision-making in meditators playing the ultimatum game. *Frontiers in Neuroscience, 5.* https://doi.org/10.3389/fnins.2011.00049

Koelega, H. S. (1995). Alcohol and vigilance performance: A review. *Psychopharmacology, 118,* 233–249.

Kramer, G. (2007). *Insight Dialogue: The interpersonal path to freedom.* Boston, MA: Shambhala Publications.

Kumar, A., Sharma, M. P., Narayanaswamy, J. C., Kandavel, T., & Reddy, Y. C. J. (2016). Efficacy of mindfulness-integrated cognitive behavior therapy in patients with predominant obsessions. *Indian Journal of Psychiatry, 58,* 366–371. https://doi.org/10.4103/0019-5545.196723

Lackner, R. J., & Fresco, D. M. (2016). Interaction effect of brooding rumination and interoceptive awareness on depression and anxiety symptoms. *Behaviour Research and Therapy.* https://doi.org/10.1016/j.brat.2016.08.007

Leary, M. R., Tate, E. B., Adams, C. E., Batts Allen, A., & Hancock, J. (2007). Self-compassion and reactions to unpleasant self-relevant events: The implications of treating oneself kindly. *Journal of Personality and Social Psychology, 92,* 887–904.

Lokopalo, B. (2010). Importance of *vedana* and *sampajanna* in the Vipassana (Insight) system of meditation. Igatpuri, India: Vipassana Research Institute. Retrieved from http://www.vridhamma.org/Vedana-and-Sampajanna-in-the-Vipassana-Insight

Lutz, A., Brefczynski-Lewis, J., Johnstone, T., & Davidson, R. J. (2008). Regulation of the neural circuitry of emotion by compassion meditation: Effects of meditative practice. *PloS One, 3,* e1897.

Mansour, A. R., Farmer, M. A., Baliki, M. N., & Apkarian, A. V. (2014). Chronic pain: The role of learning and brain plasticity. *Restorative Neurology and Neuroscience, 32,* 129–139. https://doi.org/10.3233/RNN-139003

Marczinski, C. A., & Fillmore, M. T. (2003). Preresponse cues reduce the impairing effects of alcohol on the execution and suppression of responses. *Experimental and Clinical Psychopharmacology, 11,* 110–117.

Marinkovic, K., Rickenbacher, E., & Azma, S. (2012). Effects of alcohol intoxication on response conflict in a flanker task. *Journal of Addiction Research and Therapy, S3,* 002. https://doi.org/10.4172/2155-6105.S3-002

McDonald, J., Schleifer, L., Richards, J. B., & de Wit, H. (2003). Effects of THC on behavioral measures of impulsivity in humans. *Neuropsychopharmacology, 28,* 1356–1365.

Monteiro, L. (2016). Implicit ethics and mindfulness: Subtle assumptions that MBIs are values-neutral. *International Journal of Psychotherapy, 20,* 210–224.

Monteiro, L., & Musten, F. (2013). *Mindfulness starts here: An eight-week guide to skillful living.* BC, Canada: Friesen Press.

Monteiro, L., Musten, R. F., & Compson, J. (2014). Traditional and contemporary mindfulness: Finding the middle path in the tangle of concerns. *Mindfulness, 6,* 1–13. https://doi.org/10.1007/s12671-014-0301-7

Monteiro, L., Nuttall, S., & Musten, R. F. (2010). Five skilful habits: An ethics-based mindfulness intervention. *Counseling et Spiritualité, 29,* 91–104.

Narada, M. (1968). *A manual of Abhidhamma*. Kandy, Sri Lanka: Buddhist Publication Society.

Neff, K. (2004). Self-compassion and psychological wellbeing. *Constructivism in the Human Sciences*, *9*, 27–37.

Neff, K. D., Kirkpatrick, K. L., & Rude, S. S. (2007). Self-compassion and adaptive psychological functioning. *Journal of Research in Personality*, *41*, 139–154.

Oscar-Berman, M., & Marinkovic, K. (2007). Alcohol: Effects on neurobehavioral functions and the brain. *Neuropsychology Review*, *17*, 239–257. https://doi.org/10.1007/s11065-007-9038-6

Peters, J. R., Geiver, P. J., Smart, L. M., & Baer, R. A. (2014). Shame and borderline personality features: The potential mediating role of anger and anger rumination. *Personality Disorders: Theory, Research, and Treatment*, *5*, 1–9.

Roubos, L. (2011). *A comparison of group-enhanced and individual implementations of Mindfulness-integrated Cognitive Behaviour Therapy (MiCBT): An effectiveness study.* Unpublished master dissertation, James Cook University, Cairns, Australia.

Salzberg, S. (1995). *Loving-kindness: The revolutionary art of happiness*. Boston, MA: Shambala.

Schwartz, J., & Gladding, R. (2011). *You are not your brain: The 4-step solution for changing bad habits, ending unhealthy thinking and taking control of your life*. New York: Penguin.

Scott-Hamilton, J., & Schutte, N. S. (2016). The role of adherence in the effects of a mindfulness intervention for competitive athletes: Changes in mindfulness, flow, pessimism and anxiety. *Journal of Clinical Sport Psychology*, *10*, 99–117. https://doi.org/10.1123/jcsp.2015-0020

Scott-Hamilton, J., Schutte, N. S., & Brown, R. F. (2016). Effects of a mindfulness intervention on sports-anxiety, pessimism, and flow in competitive cyclists. *Applied Psychology: Health and Well-Being*, *8*, 85–103. https://doi.org/10.1111/aphw.12063

Segal, Z. V., Williams, J. M. G., & Teasdale, J. D. (2002). *Mindfulness-based cognitive therapy for depression: A new approach to preventing relapse*. New York: Guilford.

Senderey, E. (2017). Mindfulness and group cognitive behavioural therapy to address problematic perfectionism. *Athens Journal of Social Sciences*, *4*, 49–66.

Sharf, R. (2014). Mindfulness and mindlessness in early Chan. *Philosophy Est & West*, *64*, 933–964. https://doi.org/10.1353/pew.2014.0074

Shonin, E., van Gordon, W., & Griffiths, M. D. (2015). Teaching ethics in mindfulness-based interventions. *Mindfulness*. https://doi.org/10.1007/s12671-015-0429-0

Siegle, G. J., Thompson, W., Carter, C. S., Steinhauer, S. R., & Thase, M. E. (2007). Increased amygdala and decreased dorsolateral prefrontal BOLD responses in unipolar depression: Related and independent features. *Biological Psychiatry*, *61*, 198–209.

Starr, C. J., Sawaki, L., Wittenberg, G. F., Burdette, J. H., Oshiro, Y., Quevedo, A. S., & Coghill, R. C. (2009). Roles of the insular cortex in the modulation of pain: Insights from brain lesions. *The Journal of Neuroscience*, *29*, 2684–2694. https://doi.org/10.1523/JNEUROSCI.5173-08.2009

Taylor, V. A., Grant, J., Daneault, V., Scavone, G., Breton, E., Roffe-Vidal, S., … Beauregard, M. (2011). Impact of mindfulness on the neural responses to emotional pictures in experienced and beginner meditators. *NeuroImage*, *57*, 1524–1533.

Walshe, M. (2012). *The long discourses of the Buddha: A translation of the Digha Nikaya*. Boston: Wisdom Publications.

Yazdanimehr, R., Omidi, A., Sadat, Z., & Akbari, H. (2016). The effect of mindfulness-integrated cognitive behavior therapy on depression and anxiety among pregnant women: A randomized clinical trial. *Journal of Caring Sciences*, *5*, 195–204. 10.15171/jcs.2016.021

Zeidan, F., & Vago, D. R. (2016). Mindfulness meditation-based pain relief: A mechanistic account. *Annals of the New York Academy of Sciences*, *1373*, 114–127. https://doi.org/10.1111/nyas.13153

Zhang, S., Wu, W., Huang, G., Liu, Z., Guo, S., Yang, J., & Wang, K. (2014). Resting-state connectivity in the default mode network and insula during experimental low back pain. *Neural Regeneration Research*, *9*, 135–142. https://doi.org/10.4103/1673-5374.125341

Chapter 8
Mindfulness-Based Symptom Management: Mindfulness as Applied Ethics

Lynette M. Monteiro and Frank Musten

Introduction

The principles of mindfulness-based stress reduction (MBSR; Kabat-Zinn, 2013) and mindfulness-based cognitive therapy (MBCT; Segal, Williams, & Teasdale, 2012) present a challenge to teleological, conceptual, and relational aspects of Western concepts of health care. The directional aim of health care was, and likely still is, predominantly about reversing or excising the causes of illness with wellness left to evolve as it may. Conceptually, the targets of interventions are categorized as physical (focused on the body) *or* psychological (focused on the mind) with the intent of reducing symptoms and the discomfort they produce. Not only are body and mind seen through a lens of dualism, the concepts of illness and wellness are dichotomized, with wellness defined as the absence of illness and illness as a circumscribed event ranging from acute to chronic. Relationally, traditional models of care are portrayed with the health care provider holding unique expertise and the patient as the recipient of that expertise. The relationship is hierarchical with primacy given to knowledge and its flow from the professional to the patient.

With the advent of MBSR and MBCT, three important shifts in the teleological, conceptual, and relational aspects of health care entered the mainstream. First, the idea of "fixing" the problem of illness is being accepted as unrealistic because of a more interconnected view of illness and well-being. This gave way to an understanding of the biopsychosocial system as subject to all manner of change that is only partially in our control. Second, reinhabiting the connection between mind and body has been introduced as the path to experiential awareness. Finally, the source

L.M. Monteiro, PhD (✉) • F. Musten, PhD
Ottawa Mindfulness Clinic, 595 Montreal Road, Suite 301, Ottawa, ON, Canada, K1K 4L2
e-mail: lynette.monteiro@gmail.com; frank.musten@gmail.com

© Springer International Publishing AG 2017   193
L.M. Monteiro et al. (eds.), *Practitioner's Guide to Ethics and Mindfulness-Based Interventions*, Mindfulness in Behavioral Health,
DOI 10.1007/978-3-319-64924-5_8

of wisdom and healing has shifted to a relationship that is co-created between the individual who is suffering and the health care professional where wisdom arises from knowledge and insight. In addition, the means of addressing the individual's suffering is seen as lying in the relationship between their state of mind and the event they are experiencing.

Now, almost 40 years later, the efficacy of mindfulness-based interventions (MBIs) has become better researched (Baer, 2003; Brown & Ryan, 2003; Fjorback, Arendt, Ornbol, Fink, & Walach, 2011; Goyal, Singh, & Sibinga, 2014). The rapidity and sheer volume of research also has given rise to calls for caution against the overly positive tone of the studies and the uncritical swell of popularity (Eberth & Sedlmeier, 2012; Khoury et al., 2013); that in turn raises concerns of mindfulness becoming increasingly presented as a panacea (Hanley, Abell, Osborn, Roehrig, & Canto, 2016; Purser & Loy, 2013). However, MBIs have enjoyed a growing acceptance through work on defining the psychological nature of mindfulness (Brown, Creswell, & Ryan, 2015; Brown & Ryan, 2004; Coffey, Hartman, & Fredrickson, 2010), investigations into its mechanisms (Coffey et al., 2010; Grabovac, Lau, & Willett, 2011), and models of understanding efficacy studies (Dimidjian & Segal, 2015). Further, as the chapters in this book exemplify, MBIs have branched out from MBSR and MBCT in unique ways that offer a variety of approaches and serve many vulnerable populations, indicating the term "mindfulness-based programs" (MBPs) may better reflect their scope beyond the psychotherapeutic. The growth of these "second generation" mindfulness programs (Van Gordon, Shonin, & Griffiths, 2015) also offers an opportunity to address one of the key concerns raised about MBSR and MBCT: the multilayered ethics involved in translating mindfulness from Buddhism to a Western psychological and secular intervention (Monteiro, Musten, & Compson, 2015).

There are two important issues of ethics for health care professionals to consider in relation to the issue of ethics and mindfulness. The first is the ethics *of* mindfulness, which comprises the complexity and implications of migrating Eastern philosophical approaches into a secular Western framework. Specifically, it poses the following questions: What are the ethical implications of reconstructing a spiritual process as a secular intervention? How does this impact issues such as informed consent and sufficient training in the new interventions. An auxiliary concern relates to the question of who can or should be taught mindfulness; this raises questions about the potential for misguided or outright misuse of mindfulness practice, for subverting social justice by maintaining an unconscionable status quo for vulnerable populations, or by giving military and police members the capacity to suppress compassion and care in order to commit acts of violence and killing (Stanley, 2013).

The second issue is ethics *in* mindfulness and comprises how the content of MBIs embodies or conveys the practice and cultivation of morality and virtues. It prompts the following questions: Can a secular program hold to the same teleological path of mindfulness as described and practiced in Buddhism (Davis, 2015; Greenberg & Mitra, 2015; Lindahl, 2015); in fact, does it need to? Given morality and the cultivation of virtues is central to Buddhist teachings of mindfulness, how can this migrate to secular programs with sensitivity to multicultural perspectives of how values are lived? Critics of secular mindfulness point out that the definition of mindfulness in secular terms is stripped down to bare essentials and loses the Buddhist intention for a wider and deeper practice of growth (Purser, 2015; Purser & Loy, 2013; Titmuss, 2013). In Buddhism, mindfulness is part of a tightly interwoven series of practices whose ultimate purpose is the cultivation of virtues with the intention of full liberation from the suffering generated by our misperceptions (Olendzki, 2008, 2011). Reduced to an eight-session protocol, can secularized mindfulness be effective as a highly truncated version of a key Buddhist practice or does it become symptom-focused? That in turn questions whether it is also individualistic and therefore inconsistent with the Buddhist intention of mindfulness as a wholistic process (Amaro, 2015), which McCown (2016) appropriately describes as a relational process. Moreover, McCown (2014) argues that the current focus on studying the individual responses to MBIs in service of establishing treatment efficacies has misdirected the practice away from its relational component.

These concerns foretell a common process and outcome: The secularized practice risks cultivating a form of awareness that is antithetical to Buddhist philosophy and therefore destined to do harm. In Buddhism, all practices have a moral arc of cultivating virtues that result in wisdom and therefore moral action, not only for self, but also for others and the world (Bodhi, 2011, 2013). The development of MBSM sought to find a path through this complex world of spiritual and secular principles and practices. In the sections that follow, we describe the issues that influenced both ethics *in* and in later sections we describe our approach to ethics *of* mindfulness in MBSM.

Roots of Mindfulness-Based Symptom Management

History

In developing Mindfulness-Based Symptom Management (MBSM), we were especially concerned about the issues of how to communicate Buddhist concepts clearly, ensuring the issues of ethics *in* and ethics *of* mindfulness were embodied in the co-created relationships and embedded in the program delivery, respectively. Although we held both aspects of ethics and mindfulness as equally important, how to convey the concept and practice of ethics in the curriculum and embody it in our role as teachers was our initial focus. We sought to translate the Buddhist model of alleviating suffering, seen as an arc of moral development, into a language that was accessible to participants while standing on a base of psychological models that supported mindfulness as a treatment protocol. Further, we viewed the intention of the intervention and the practice of mindfulness itself as an arc of (relational) moral development. Thus, we worked to keep the role of ethics as action-guides (Gombrich, 2009/2013; Harvey, 2013) and values-clarification front and center in our vision of a mindfulness program that offered more than alleviation of the distressing symptoms of depression, anxiety, and reactions to physical pain. In fact, we struggled over naming the program, finally settling on "symptom management," which reflected the reality of our clinical population. In other words, we are always symptomatic of some aspect of suffering and its impact on our actions, thoughts, and values could only be managed through diligent and ardent practice of wise choices. Finally, if the intent in our programs was to facilitate symptom management rather than simply symptom reduction or symptom elimination, then it followed that the program had to cultivate an ongoing presence to the complete experience of well-being *and* suffering, the values we live well by *and* those we are distanced from.

Antonio Machado's poem "Campos de castilla" (Machado, 2002) is frequently quoted by mindfulness scholars and teachers; it stands as a guiding wisdom of what it means to practice mindfulness: *Wanderer, your footsteps are the road, and nothing more; wanderer, there is no road, the road is made by walking.* Developing mindfulness programs is a process of constantly revisiting and refining its intention. Dimidjian and Segal (2015) described a stage model developed by the National Institutes of Health (NIH) "from an interest in shaping the training of future generations of clinical scientists by providing a well-articulated view of the goals and process of clinical psychological science" (p. 593). Using the stages as defined by the NIH, Dimidjian and Segal (quoting Onken, Carroll, Shoham, Cuthbert, & Riddle, 2014) describe Stage I as the process of creating a new intervention or the adaptation of an existing one (Stage IA); this definition would include most mindfulness-based programs that emerged immediately after MBSR/MBCT gained traction in the health care community. Feasibility and pilot studies were defined as Stage IB, which included the development of training and supervision. Stage II involves testing treatment protocols in research settings using research, and in Stage III, testing is conducted in community settings using community facilitators.

While the model clearly organizes a way forward and is important to the work of clinical psychological science, it is vague in its reference to "all activities related to the creation of a new intervention, or the modification, adaptation, or refinement of an existing intervention." With Stage I set as part of an empirical process or evidence-based model, the implication is that the development of a new intervention is de facto evidence-based. In fact, part of the development of a new or adapted intervention can include and benefits from practice-based evidence, an iterative approach that is relational with respect to the community and which inquires into the relevance of the protocols to the population treated (Barkham & Mellor-Clark, 2003; Holmqvist, Philips, & Barkham, 2015).

As clinical psychologists, informed by both our clinical training and the constant need to modify, adapt, or refine treatment protocols for our individual clients, we approached the development of MBSM with a close eye to our own development, how the inclusion of an explicit values-based approach served the real-life situations of the participants, and the adaptations that were made for different populations. As teachers of mindfulness protocols, this required an iterative process of being in conversation with participants in the program and refining what and how we delivered the teachings; it grew in parallel to the thematic structure of the program itself. It began with the struggle of integrating seemingly disparate ways of knowing in the Buddhist and Western approaches to awareness (essentially the early stage participants encounter in an 8-week program). For example, our cognitive and behaviorist inclinations would seek to change thoughts and actions while observing for concomitant changes in emotions; the frame of mindfulness required a shift to an open and invitational stance to our experience and that of our participants. This different way of being in relationship with participants and working with the discomfort of uncertainty that is the mark of all relationships required attention to our own ways of being with our difficult and unwanted experiences. In turn, this highlighted the subtle values we were bringing into the room, the main one being a primacy of the thinking function.

With the inclusion of a values-based practice that explicitly addressed the ethics, MBSM stands in counterbalance to the tenet of MBSR that ethics remain implicit (Kabat-Zinn, 2011); thus we did not view MBSM as a modification or adaptation of MBSR/MBCT. Instead it was envisioned as what is now called a "second generation" mindfulness programs that directly addresses the issues of attention cultivation, spiritual roots, and ethics in the pedagogy (Van Gordon et al., 2015). Navigating the complex territory of ethics in general also presented challenges in differentiating ethics *of* mindfulness (transparency, informed consent) from ethics *in* mindfulness (inclusion of cultivating virtues in the curriculum). And finally, we were faced with making a deep discernment of how to take the program into the marketplace. Could we offer mindfulness to individuals and organizations whose vision and mission would be antithetical to cultivating compassion, the highest ethic of practice? Throughout this process, we were informed and inspired by Buddhist and psychological teachings in how to meet and be with our experience. These are explored in the next two sections followed by an examination of the complexity of ethics and mindfulness programs.

Buddhist Roots

Foundational Teachings Relevant to Secular Mindfulness The Buddha is said to have described what he taught as only a handful of leaves compared to all the leaves in the forest (Thanissaro, 1997b). However, the teachings are of sufficient depth to effect change. By focusing on the nature of suffering and its cessation, they are a self-administered treatment that eliminates the roots of suffering and cultivates an ethical, values-based life for the good of all beings (Thanissaro, 2012). Although one would argue that understanding and practicing with all the teachings is essential to liberation, much like any religious or philosophical system, some Buddhist teachings are more immediate in their helpfulness and more readily accessible to the everyday person (known as a householder in the Buddha's times). Space precludes examination of the many relevant teachings. However, Monteiro (2015) has explored the various teachings that inform secular mindfulness programs and Cayoun (2011) offered a detailed examination of Buddhist psychology as applied to secular mindfulness. For the purposes of this chapter, we will focus on three core Buddhist teachings that we incorporated into the MBSM curriculum: suffering, mindfulness, and ethics.

Suffering The first core teaching is the meaning of suffering or *dukkha*. The idea that we suffer is difficult to grasp because the conventional use of the term is typically in the context of profound tragedy, loss, or some life-rending event beyond the pale of our cultural experience (Batchelor, 2017; Epstein, 2013, 2014). In Buddhist terms, suffering or *dukkha* refers to the essential dissatisfaction we feel when we don't want what we have (objects, experiences), want what we don't have, or are generally confused about what we want or what our experience is (Bodhi, 2008; Gunaratana, 2001). These three stances to our experience are referred to as the three poisons: aversion (aversive type), clinging/grasping (greedy type), and delusion (misperceiving type). The presumptive idea in this teaching is that we cannot avoid things happening to us; we are, without exception, heir to illness, death, injury, and loss. Suffering then is defined as our stance to or how we meet these experiences. The Sallatha Sutta (Thanissaro, 1997a), one of the many teachings of the Buddha, uses the metaphor of being struck by two arrows showing suffering as both physical (the initial event) and mental (reactivity). For example, when we are injured, we feel the physical pain, which is then accompanied by a mental proliferation, or what it means to have been injured ("I'm never going to walk again!" "This is unfair." "How am I going to get to work?" or "I can't afford not to work."). In another Buddhist teaching, our resistance to treat our suffering is compared to a person struck by a poison arrow and who is refusing to remove it until they understand why and how it happened, by whose hand, and the meaningfulness of the act (Thanissaro, 1998).

Becoming aware of the vulnerability of our mind to aversion, greed, and delusion requires diligent practice. For most of us, "practice" carries a sense of working towards a specific outcome; it is something one does, driven by internal and external factors, with the intention of achieving a goal. Once the goal is achieved, the drive reduces or extinguishes and is typically replaced by another drive. This perspective is also consistent with the idea of attaining milestones developmentally. As adults in a hedonic culture, we check off most of the achievements: home, family, education, relationships, career, etc. The idea of practice without a driven quality to it and as something continuous is a personal paradigm shift. It also brings into high relief the suffering we create by our aversion, grasping, and delusion. The teachings of Zen master Thich Nhat Hanh (1999, 2007, 2009, 2011) are invaluable in understanding what it means to practice continuously; his talks, retreats, and books compassionately introduce the practice of non-attaining and mindfulness as a continuous engagement with every moment.

Mindfulness The second core teaching is the cultivation of mindfulness itself. Although efficiently defined by Kabat-Zinn (2003) as "the awareness that emerges through paying attention on purpose, in the present moment, and nonjudgmentally to the unfolding of experience moment by moment" (p. 145), understanding the term "mindfulness" remains complex and discussion among mindfulness researchers and Buddhists of different traditions offers insight to that complexity (P. Grossman & Van Dam, 2011; Williams & Kabat-Zinn, 2013). Despite these differences in interpreting mindfulness, there is consensus that the teachings on establishing mindfulness and the practice of breath awareness underlies and informs, implicitly or explicitly, secular mindfulness programs (e.g., MBSR training includes attending silent retreats that teach in the context of the four foundations of mindfulness). The formal process is described in the Satipaṭṭhāna (Four Foundations of Mindfulness) and Ānāpānasati (teaching on Awareness of Breathing) Suttas (Analayo, 2003, 2013; Goldstein, 2013); the practice cultivates sustained attention, awareness of experiential processes, and development of virtues necessary for liberation from suffering.

The Satipaṭṭhāna and Ānāpānasati Suttas work in unison with the former offering the framework for practice and the latter the meditative component that supports practice (Gunaratana, 2012; Hanh, 2006). The practitioner begins with stabilizing attention using the breath as an object of meditation. When attention is disciplined and steady, the focus shifts to awareness of the body, feeling tones (pleasant, unpleasant, and neutral), the mind, and the nature of all phenomena. Although the text implies a sequential process, it is far from sequential and progressive (Analayo, 2013). As with all practices that build capacity, meditation is an iterative process, returning repeatedly to the object of meditation (the breath) and approaching the experiences that arise with an observer's stance or without reactivity.

As attention and awareness develop, phenomena are experienced as impermanent; they are observed as rising, enduring, and dissipating over and over. With continuous practice, insight develops into seeing the nature of suffering as being clearly rooted in the three poisons, and how we have the tendency to misidentify with our experience. The cultivation of mindfulness continues with a systematic practice in the Eightfold Noble Path (right view, right thinking, right action, right livelihood, right speech, right mindfulness, right effort, and right concentration; Gethin, 1998; Harvey, 2013); with further practice the factors of awakening (mental states of mindfulness, investigation, energy, joy, tranquility, concentration, and equanimity) develop. Monteiro et al. (2015) discussed the depth to which these two specific components of the Satipaṭṭhāna extend into secular mindfulness programs, concluding that while the programs focus on attention and open awareness, they may fall short of fully cultivating the depth of wisdom possible through the wisdom aspects of practice. Arguably, it may be possible that the cultivation of attention, awareness, and initial insight into the nature of phenomena is sufficient for addressing acute experiences of the second arrow of suffering (our reactivity). However, this is also the equivalent of not completing the full course of treatment that can provide deeper resilience to the three poisons of anger, greed, and delusion.

Ethics   The third core teaching is ethics or sīla, a critical aspect of practice often left unaddressed and therefore resulting in a major criticism of secular mindfulness programs (Senauke, 2013; Titmuss, 2013). Buddhist ethics or sīla are defined variously as an action-guide, a cultivation of virtues, or the taking up of vows; they form the fundamental rationale for practice (Aitken, 1991; Anderson, 2001; Harvey, 2000; Keown, 2001, 2005). The virtues of kindness, generosity, and wisdom comprise the antidotes to the three poisons of aversion, grasping, and delusion and are practiced through wise action, speech, and livelihood, the relational (interconnected) aspect of the Eightfold Noble Path. Ethics is conveyed through a set of precepts, the number of which depends on the role of the individual whether they are householder or monastic. For the householder or non-monastic, there are typically five precepts of restraint: do not kill, do not take what is not given, do not engage in inappropriate sexual activities, do not engage in false speech, and do not use intoxicants. Zen teacher Robert Aitken (1984) describes the precepts as both restraint (the putting down of harmful thoughts, speech, and action) and enacted (the taking up of compassionate thoughts, speech, and action). Thich Nhat Hanh (1998, 2007) formulated the five precepts as action-guides called the Five Mindfulness Trainings: reverence for life, generosity, responsible sexual desire/conduct, mindful speech, and mindful consumption. Both Aitken and Thich Nhat Hanh extend the concept of each precept beyond the concrete definition of physically taking a life. For example, we can engage in "killing" speech, act in ways that "kill" a relationship, or hold thoughts that "kill" our compassion for others. Thich Nhat Hanh also extends mindful consumption beyond the physical act of ingesting food or substances. In his conceptualization, consumption includes messages we send out and take in from the media and in relationships. The Five Mindfulness Trainings ultimately relate to stewardship of communities and the environment. This particular formulation of vows or principles offers the opportunity to explore and engage, beyond the idea of restraint, through action-oriented ways of being. The Five Mindfulness Trainings also provide the opportunity to generate a set of actionable behaviors that reflect a values-based approach to practice grounded in the individual lived experience. Both Aitken and Thich Nhat Hanh's approach to the precepts are important because they present the concept of ethics as a balance between inhibition and activation, between an avoidance- and approach-based moral regulation (see Janoff-Bulman, Sheikh, & Hepp, 2009, for a discussion of proscriptive and prescriptive ethics and moral regulation).

Not Getting Lost in Translation The vastness of Buddhist philosophy and psychology is daunting even to scholars. Still, carving away sections for specific use in a culture and context that is very different from that in which the original teachings were delivered has been discouraged by Buddhist scholars and teachers (Amaro, 2015; Bodhi, 2011, 2013). And certainly, cannibalizing Buddhist practice is no more justifiable than excising Catholic spiritual practices such as praying the rosary or novenas and repackaging them as stand-alone psychological interventions. Like other religious communities, the practice of Buddhism is a slowly unfolding process that allows it to take hold and transformation to be more likely; further, growth and adherence to the process is individual. In that context, it is possible to see secular mindfulness as having a similar influence through a paced process with respect for individually determined trajectories (Compson & Monteiro, 2015). However, because our program is offered to people who typically are not Buddhists and who have a Western mind-set with regard to psychological interventions, we needed to ensure there was support in current psychological science mindfulness. The psychological concepts that influenced MBSM are explored in the next section.

Psychological Roots

Convergence of Concepts In developing MBSM, we were informed by three psychotherapeutic theories and approaches, some of which echoed Buddhist thought: Cognitive Behavioral Therapy (CBT) with its emphasis on examining and challenging negative mind states resonates philosophically with both Buddhism and the Greek Stoics (Tirch, Silberstein, & Kolts, 2016); somatic awareness therapies (Levine, 1997) invite cultivation of awareness of body-mind in tune with the Satipaṭṭhāna and Ānāpānasati suttas; and the Polyvagal Theory (Porges, 2007, 2011), as a physiological theory, contributes significantly to understanding the issues of emotional dysregulation and reactivity. A detailed exploration of each modality is beyond the scope of this chapter; thus, we take a conceptual approach below to the way psychological concepts have informed MBSM and indicate the overlap with Buddhist concepts.

Underlying the approaches from different psychological lineages is the interplay of three Western psychological concepts (Monteiro, 2015): identity, emotion regulation, and stress. In Western psychology, the concept of self contains a sense of agency and the presence of an agent, a doer of deeds, thinker of thoughts (Baumeister, 1999, 2011). In contrast, Buddhist thought differs and holds the view that there is no agent, no lasting, substantive "self," although Tuske (2013) notes this concept is not without its difficulties. Buddhist and Western psychology, however, share an overlapping idea of a constantly changing perception of who we are based on cultural, emotional, and situational influences, that is, an emergent and embodied self (Varela, Thompson, & Rosch, 2017). Cognitive theories and therapies (Beck, Rush, Shaw, & Emery, 1987; Riso, du Toit, Stein, & Young, 2007) view identity as schemas or aggregates of characteristics, relationships with others, and aspirations in the world. A schema can be challenged by lived experiences especially if the schema holds or is close to an aspect of self that is valued. Traditionally, psychological distress is viewed as our response to these challenges, typically framed as a response to a threat to self-constructs (R. S. Lazarus & Folkman, 1984).

Emotion regulation and the role of mindfulness training is perhaps the central focus of contemplative approaches in psychology and thus occupy a larger space for discussion here. Holzel et al. (2011) outlined a set of mechanisms that interact to produce self-regulation and Roeser et al. (2014) described the intricate research connecting emotion regulation and sensory perception in developing ethical action. Emotions, while not specified in the Buddhist view, are linked to sensations, ephemeral arisings from the process of contact with the world and one's interpretation of that experience. From the Western perspective, Ekman and Davidson (1994) conceptualized emotions as arising from a confluence of cognitive, behavioral, and physiological responses to an external or internal event. R. S. Lazarus and Folkman (1984) proposed that cognitive appraisal of an event activates the stress response system. A. Lazarus (1989, 2006) placed emotions (affect) as part of a multimodal determination of experience involving behavior, affect (emotion), sensations, imagery, and cognition (BASIC). Emotion regulation is central in Western psychological theories of psychotherapy and is often one of the core intentions in psychotherapy. Thus, although emotions are not a specific concept in Buddhism, becoming dysregulated can be seen to arise from a fixed idea of who we are, which is itself a manifestation of the three poisons of aversion, clinging, and/or confusion.

Porges (2011) proposed in the polyvagal theory that the brain is a risk assessor, through an unconscious automatic process he refers to as neuroception. For most of us, our neuroceptors are activated periodically throughout the day. But once it has been determined that there is no threat, we settle back into what we had been doing. That process of resettling involves the vagus nerve, the primary nerve activating the parasympathetic system that, as part of the autonomic nervous system, lowers arousal and returns a complex set of physiological processes back to homeostasis. This change can be measured in terms of heart rate variability that is referred to as vagal tone and means that an individual can quickly return to resting heart rate, and equilibrium, after determining that an event was not a threat. However, because of historical or current experience with stress some individuals have poor vagal tone and are not able to reset to equilibrium.

Further, Porges (2011) relates the breath to vagal tone and specifically notes that the aspiration (out-breath) puts a cap on the heart rate. This relationship between breath and heart rate is taught as breathing exercises in, for example, the tactical breathing techniques taught to soldiers (G. Grossman, 2009). The meditation instructions in mindfulness programs invite participants to let the breath breathe itself. Through repeated practice the breath tends to fall into a natural rhythm of slower, deeper in-breaths and longer out-breaths effectively increasing vagal tone. Porges indicates that as vagal tone increases, there is less emotional dysregulation along with related greater cognitive capacity. Eisenberg and Eggum (2008) reported that good vagal tone is associated with improved prosocial behavior in children. Keltner (2009), as quoted in Narvaez (2014), has noted that good vagal tone was correlated with compassion and open heartedness towards others suggesting that good vagal tone also promotes moral behavior.

Finally, stress models have a favored position in the work of general psychology and mindfulness interventions. Endocrinologist Hans Selye (1974) was among the first to investigate and define stress (he later noted it was better referred to as "strain") as the physiological response regardless of the positive or negative nature of the stimulus and that pathological outcomes occur when the stress is unremitting. Later models include Bruce McEwen's model of allostatic load which more closely aligns with the idea that strain on an existing biological system results in its eventual breakdown (McEwen, 2002). As discussed above, Porges' polyvagal theory posits a complex model of neural regulation of the autonomic system (Porges, 2011). According to Porges (2007), external events and intentionality in social contexts are appraised via neuroception and discerned for their threat value, which activates the appropriate response, defense, or engagement. Evolved to be adaptive to both low and high threat environments, the neural system is staged to appraise the degree of safety in a hierarchical manner with the higher cognitive functions able to override lower "primitive" systems in responses to threat. Under prolonged stress, the lower appraisal system is reinforced to be highly active and the feedback provides what can be seen as misperceived levels of threat. Under such conditions, moral decision-making may be biased towards individual survival. Thus, regulation of the nervous system, when under stress or threat while activating the downregulation to reestablish homeostasis, relies on a well-functioning feedback system and plays an important role in developing ethical actions.

Our intent is not to claim there is nothing new under the sun, rather an interweaving of several strands of psychological and spiritual lineages. Baer (2015) and Harrington and Dunne (2015) both describe how psychological science and the interweaving of psychology with Buddhist practices, respectively, have contributed to an understanding of contemplative practices. In our perspective, there is a constantly emerging wisdom that has always been in the service of meeting and transforming suffering so that one could flourish as a human being. By grounding MBSM in current psychological science, we sought a manner of communicating mindfulness that is authentic in the current culture and language, which becomes important when communicating the concepts of mindfulness to a clinical population. Humanist approaches and psychotherapies such as those developed by Carl Rogers (Rogers, 2003; Rogers & Kramer, 1995) and the concepts of human potential developed by Maslow (2014) laid down the path to what became Positive Psychology, an approach focused on developing conditions for flourishing. Defined by Seligman's Wellness Theory as comprised of positive emotions, engagement, positive relationships, meaning, and accomplishment (PERMA; Seligman, 2012), it includes the development of virtues, which Seligman defines as a core characteristic that is universally valued. The six virtues are wisdom, courage, humanity, justice, temperance, and transcendence. Its contribution to the integration of ethics, values, and secular mindfulness is Seligman's view that seeking personal happiness independent of relationships and meaning makes a poor moral guide for caring behavior. We now examine what constitutes a moral guide or moral decision-making.

Moral Development and the Ethic of Care Because we conceptualized mindfulness practice as a process of moral development consistent with Buddhist views of mindfulness as cultivation of virtues through ethical actions, it was important to explore how moral decisions are made and what is important in guiding those decisions. S.L. Shapiro, Jazaieri, and Goldin (2012) reported that there are few studies linking mindfulness with moral reasoning and that moral reasoning in their study was not impacted by MBSR post-intervention, although it did improve at a 2-month follow-up. Shapiro and her colleagues posited that moral reasoning like mindfulness might require time to coalesce and strengthen. It is however important to note that the measure used in this study was a traditional format of posing a moral dilemma requiring a selection of a single response from participants. Moral reasoning and its investigation are complex and may require a different approach, one that is more relational and exploratory of the individual's own process of making moral decisions.

The study of moral development began with Kohlberg (1976) and a turning point in the study of the complex nature of moral guides, or how we make moral decisions, occurred with the work of Carol Gilligan (1993). Her book, *In a Different*

Voice (Gilligan, 1993), broke ground for a deeper understanding of moral decision-making; choices in real life are not just made as means of securing justice but as an expression of care. Flanagan (1993) explored the important differences between Kohlberg's and Gilligan's concepts of moral development and others have discussed the contrasting models and issues in justice and care (Giammarco, 2016; Larabee, 1993). In subsequent work extending the understanding of her model (Gilligan & Attanucci, 1988) and recent exploration of a "human voice" that arises from moral injury (Gilligan, 2014), she refined the theoretical concepts of justice and care orientations. The relevance of Gilligan's work to mindfulness lies in her conceptualization of morality as care and responsibility in the context of relationships. Blum (1993) describes it as "genuinely distinct from impartiality" (p. 50) and consisting of "attention to, understanding of, and emotional responsiveness toward the individuals with whom one stands in these relationships" (p. 50). He is also careful to point out that care is not a replacement of impartiality or a theory of everything in moral development; instead it offers a broader landscape within which moral decisions are made, specifically one that includes the role of personal integrity.

The concept of an ethic of care, mentioned in a reflection on key ideas in her body of work (Gilligan, 2011), draws from Tronto (1993) who challenged the association of care with "women's morality." The expanse of the discourse of the ethics of care is beyond the scope of this chapter; however, the potential for secular mindfulness to benefit from Tronto's arguments is compelling (see B. Fisher & Tronto, 1990; van Nistelrooij, Schaafsma, & Tronto, 2014, for details of Tronto's perspectives of an ethic of care). Not only does she challenge the feminist localizing of care in the domain of being female, but also, quoting Walker (2007), she argues instead for "an ethics of responsibility," which "as a normative moral view would try to put people and responsibilities in the right places with respect to each other" (in van Nistelrooij et al., 2014). Care, therefore, is a moral activity that is both contextual and relational; it is embedded in a negotiated relationship among equals but does not presume a commonality of cultural or psychological experiences. It is embodied in practitioners and located in the world. These tenets fall close to the intentions of MBIs, which are to cultivate values that result in care, or responsibility, for self, and others. In other words, the resting place of mindfulness is compassion for self and others. Whereas it is hoped that including ethics explicitly in MBSM can cultivate an ethic of care in the individual for themselves and their relationships, there are challenges, which are explored in the next section.

The Ethos of Ethics in MBIs

In the Thick and Thin of Ethics The contentious nature of ethics in MBIs may not be easily resolved in the context of a debate about whether and what ethics should be implicit or explicit in a program because, in any relational process, both processes exist. In MBIs, ethics *in* mindfulness emerges through the teacher's professional conduct and is embodied in the relational aspects of delivering the teaching points while interacting with the participants. While the former bridges into ethics *of* mindfulness, that is, the procedural aspects of an MBI, both address a deep exploration of the intangible aspects of an MBI such as teacher and participant characteristics, their intentions, and the meaning they give to the relational and pedagogical process. However, McCown (2013) discovered that an online search of "the terms 'mindfulness' and 'ethics' was actually the concept of 'ethical mindfulness': a vital awareness of the ethical implications of a situation" (p. 40). In other words, the online search tapped into what we are calling the "ethics *of* mindfulness," which is related to the procedural aspects and asks questions about the "right" and "wrong" of MBIs. What remains to be explored are "ethics *in* mindfulness" that asks about the process of connecting and being in relationship.

In ethnographic terms, procedural issues are called a "thin description," an evaluative statement (Kurchin, 2013) which is related to culture and interpretation (Geertz, 1973). Gilligan's work discussed above, for example, constitutes a "thick description" of moral development (Blum, 1993). An example of a thick description is distinguishing among a variety of possible deeper descriptions for someone who winks. A thin description is to say that there was a wink. A thick description is to explore not just the contraction of an eyelid but also the ways it was done and the reasons for it being done (Geertz, 1973; Kurchin, 2013). In the context of mindfulness, thin descriptions arise when we ask whether ethics should be implicit or explicit in MBIs. This classification leads to a description of procedural ethics and while important, belies the more complex issue of ethics in mindfulness, which requires "thick descriptions." That is, thick descriptions allow for an exploration of the cultural and deeper aspects of relational components and of the development of virtues that underlie the more evaluative terms of ethics being right/wrong or good/ bad.

In what might be read as a call for thick descriptions of ethics in mindfulness, McCown (2013, 2016) asks, "How are teachers and participants to be together ethically?" A transection of this question exposes several layers of relational components that run through an MBI. For example, as a thick concept in the framework of ethics in mindfulness, we would want to know what implicit and explicit values teachers and participants bring to the room that will influence the relationship. In the sections that follow, we explore the debate around implicit/explicit ethics, resistance to including explicit ethics in MBIs, the issue of presumed values-neutrality, and the complex relational processes in an MBI.

Implicit and/or Explicit Ethics The issue of ethics and MBIs remains a central and often contentious topic in Buddhist and secular mindfulness circles. Buddhist teachers and scholars argue that the absence or high opacity of ethics in secular mindfulness renders the programs inauthentic and likely to do harm (Purser & Loy, 2013; Rosenbaum & Magrid, 2016; Titmuss, 2013). Recent responses from Buddhist and secular mindfulness teachers to Monteiro et al. (2015) explored the complexities of integrating Buddhist ethics as action-guides into contemporary mindfulness programs including the issue of explicit versus implicit ethics (Amaro, 2015; Baer, 2015; Greenberg & Mitra, 2015; P. Grossman, 2015; Lindahl, 2015; Mikulas, 2015).

Critics of implicit ethics (sometimes confounded with the assumption of an absence of ethics) suggest that the exclusion of explicit teachings of Buddhist ethics uncouples the core elements of mindfulness from its roots. Amaro (2015) noted that Kabat-Zinn's (2011) rationale for such an approach is "vague" and lends itself to a "dubious principle upon which to structure a pedagogical approach" (p. 67). Monteiro et al. (2015) indicated that regardless of the intention not to impose extraneous values, the very act of teaching a philosophy derived from an Eastern spiritually oriented practice has led into that arena. That is, the challenge is not simply what and how to teach in a curriculum but to address higher-order ethical issues (see also Chap. 3—Dr. Gunther Brown) such as the value-infused therapeutic relationship and the complex container of the teacher, teachings, and who is taught. These three categories are examined in the sections below.

Secular practitioners argue that making ethics explicit would itself result in ethical difficulties. Cullen (2011) noted that the implicit form is consistent with the Buddha's pedagogy of discovering for oneself how unethical actions lead to suffering; the implication being the inclusion of explicit ethics would alter the intent of the Buddha's teachings. Kabat-Zinn (2011) stated that ethics are implicit and embodied in the presence of the teachers of MBIs through their personal practice and the guidelines of their professional ethics. In other words, ethics are best expressed in MBSR by its embodiment by teachers without turning it into an "ideal" or carry it as a "burden" (p. 295). Cullen (2011) suggested that ethics and mindfulness support each other and that an insight arising from personal experience of the connection between unethical action and one's suffering could be more transformative than "imposed edicts." In both cases, while not explicitly stated as such, the argument for implicit ethics is set up as a desire to avoid proscriptive ethics, which are restraining and avoids the negative, and incline to prescriptive ethics, which are action-based and engages in the positive (see Janoff-Bulman et al., 2009, for a discussion on the need for balance between these two modes of moral regulation).

Taking a vastly different stance, McCown (2013) argues for making ethics explicit in MBIs by which he means the qualities or virtues that are developed relationally between participant and teacher. According to McCown, ethics lies in the pedagogy and emerges out of community where qualities of corporeality, contingency, friendliness, and cosmopolitanism or openness to possibility inform the participant's experience. Experiencing the curriculum creates the ethical space without imposition through interpretation or ascribing meaning on the participant's experience.

Values-Neutrality in Psychotherapy From the Buddhist perspective, mindfulness and ethics are inseparable; they are embedded in the teachings and embodied in practice. It is possible that the resistance to make ethics explicit in secular mindfulness is a holdover of an historical idea that therapeutic interventions must be values-neutral (Monteiro, 2016). The assumption that therapies and interventions are or should be values-neutral represents an historical division in psychology away from a study of character and towards an objective, actuarial science with a focus on measures of personality. This view of values-neutrality may continue in subtle ways despite evidence that the clinician and client bring their unique patterns of values into the therapeutic space (Jackson, Hansen, & Cook-Ly, 2013; Patterson, 1959). In fact, there is sufficient evidence currently that no therapeutic approach is values-neutral (Hathaway, 2011).

Alan Tjeltveit (1999) suggests that the adherence to values-neutrality arose from viewing therapy as a scientific endeavor. He also presents strong arguments that psychologists' resistance to philosophical reflection (as opposed to relying on scientific findings) has been a primary obstacle to understanding ethics and values in psychotherapy. Tjeltveit organizes the examination of ethics into six intertwined dimensions of professional ethics, theoretical ethics, virtue ethics, social ethics, clinical ethics, and cultural ethics.

Typically, in debates around the need to include ethics in MBIs, the dimensions of professional and clinical ethics are appealed to as proof that the ethical component does not need to be explicit in the teachings because they are implicit in those values. For example, Kabat-Zinn (2011) claims the Hippocratic oath is sufficient for ensuring ethics are upheld in MBSR because all teachers adhere to this oath. While this may be necessary to galvanize a commitment to do no harm, it is certainly not sufficient; this is more so where mindfulness is offered by persons or organizations with no training or conduct oversight from regulatory and disciplinary associations. It also does not ensure that individual or organizational values will not influence and shift the application of ethics, changing what it means to do no harm.

Teacher, Teachings, and Who Is Taught The abovementioned implications of implicit/explicit values conveyed in therapy are not the sole bête noir of MBIs. Amaro (2015) noted that it is equally important to investigate the "subtle influences that are already with us, in the Judeo-Christian conditioning of the West, particularly in relation to such issues as the concepts of right and wrong as well as the broader topic of ethics" (p. 64). These points are consistent with the explorations of the fallacy of values-neutrality in therapy and the implicit ethics and values embodied by the therapist and therapeutic models (Burns, Goodman, & Orman, 2013; Hamilton, 2013).

As mentioned above, it appears that much of the debate about explicit or implicit ethics in MBIs is rooted in the historic aim of medicine and psychology to be objective and scientific. If therapies are viewed as moral encounters (Burns et al., 2013), the process of treatment lies in the client's examination of disconnection between ideal and actual values, a state that leads to distress (J. W. Fisher, 2011; Jackson et al., 2013; Leiter, Jackson, & Shaughnessy, 2009). Influenced by the assumption of values-neutrality as a form of respect for the client's own values, therapies have adopted a putative stance of objectivity and neutrality to avoid unduly influencing or detracting from these values. It is understandable, therefore, that the desire to avoid an overt ethical framework in MBIs arises from this historic paradigm of therapy as being values-neutral of necessity to not interfere with or negate the participants' own values.

Nevertheless, having noted the fallacy of values-neutrality, it is important to examine the role of ethics and values in mindfulness-based programs. These are present in three dimensions (Monteiro et al., 2015). First, ethics is contained, explicitly or implicitly, in the content of a mindfulness program. While Buddhists precepts may not be formally referenced in an MBI, the theme of restraint by not doing harm to self and others, found in many traditions, is implicit in the process of cultivating awareness of one's actions and their consequences (Mikulas, 2015). Recent debates have focused on the consequences of implicitly conveying ethics in MBIs and, given the commonality of ethics among faith traditions, whether it is appropriate to assume Buddhist ethics are the only ones conveyed in an MBI (Amaro, 2015; Davis, 2015; Lindahl, 2015).

Second, ethics is modeled or embodied in the person of the MBI teacher (Evans et al., 2014; P. Grossman, 2015; McCown, 2013; van Aalderen, Breukers, Reuzel, & Speckens, 2014). There are many MBI training programs and they typically require pre-existing meditation practice, attendance at (usually Buddhist) retreats, and an ongoing personal contemplative practice (Crane, Kuyken, Hastings, Rothwell, & Williams, 2010; Crane et al., 2011). The primary aim in teacher training is to cultivate an embodiment of the principles, including ethics (P. Grossman, 2015) that support the cultivation of character, or what is called in Buddhism, the "Noble Person" (Harvey, 2000, 2013). Health care professionals such as physicians, psychologists, social workers, and nurses who train as MBI teachers would carry these principles along with the additional, though not contradictory, set of ethical guidelines of their specific professional practice.

The third dimension is related to those who are taught, who seek out a mindfulness program. One of the major concerns of Buddhist practitioners and scholars of contemporary mindfulness applications is that it may be misappropriated by agencies such as police and military institutions as well as profit-focused business corporations whose mission-related ethics may be questionable (Senauke, 2013; Titmuss, 2013). In this regard, the issue of ethics is a crucial one, not only as it relates to the teacher's own ethics, but the intention of the program and oversight of its eventual use. However, it is important to remember that even in an 8-week program the participants present with their own system of desires and intentions that can lead to misunderstanding and misuse of mindfulness practices (see Thanissaro, 2004, for a simile that addresses the potential consequences of misunderstanding or misusing teachings).

Each of these dimensions—teachings, teacher, and who is taught—is fertile ground for the cultivation of what Amaro (2015) called a holistic mindfulness. McCown (2013) describes this as a co-created ethical space, within which transformation arises; he acknowledges that ethics in MBIs are implicit but also important that they are made explicit. Present in that ethical space are the values brought by the teacher and the participant; the personal preferences, perspectives of well-being, and the subtle influences of the values of the teacher are entwined immediately in the delivery of the curriculum. It is a rarely considered reality, but crucial nevertheless; each participant and teacher comes to mindfulness with their own set of ethics, values, and perspectives of well-being. Neither arrives *tabula rasa*; their ethics and values enter the space in the first session, if not in the moment they decided to seek out the potential of mindfulness.

While the analysis of secularized mindfulness has focused on the content of MBIs (i.e., the debate around implicit and explicit ethics as a dichotomy), a far more complicated picture emerges when teachings, teacher, and who is taught are taken as a three-fold interaction of already existing implicitly and explicitly expressed values and ethics. Perhaps the allure of claiming that implicit ethics are best practice is simply an historic artifact of the fallacy of values-neutral therapy; it may even be a misguided effort to maintain respect for the client by inadvertently shifting from client to protocol. However, actual respect for the client's values and ethics lies not in the red herring of values-neutrality, but rather in the more challenging process of how to cultivate well-being as an aspect of character. That is, the roots of the intervention, its spiritual framework, and the teacher's values as informed by those roots all must be transparent in relationship. To do less is to circle back, negate the non-hierarchical relationship in healing, sustain the fallacy of a values-neutral system, and maintain the split between personality factors and character. In our terms, the ethics *in* mindfulness and the ethics *of* mindfulness serve and support each other through the relationship of the teacher and the participants of an MBI.

Viewed through the lens of cultivating character, mindfulness is consistent with the Buddhist intention of mindfulness practice as the cultivation of the Noble Person (Harvey, 2013). In Western psychology, for researchers and clinicians the dominant paradigm of best practice is supported by scientific psychology and an actuarial measure of personality, which has eclipsed the development of character as a goal in therapy. Therefore, if MBIs are to contribute to the well-being of its participants, it is important to acknowledge the ways in which ethics and values unfold in MBIs.

The Arc of Moral Development   If an MBI is viewed as an arc of moral development, then flourishing as the cultivation of the Noble Person is consistent with the Buddhist paradigm. Participants begin in the clutches of their delusion, craving, and anger; as the program progresses, they and the teachers are faced with choice point after choice point to turn towards and transform suffering or to continue to simmer in the anger, greed, and ignorance. As their practice grows in the relational container of the program, and their capacity to meet difficult and unwanted experiences strengthens, they begin to take cognitive and experiential responsibility for their well-being and to trust in their capacity for insight in how their ethics and values guide them. In fact, Kabat-Zinn's paradigm shift towards the wholeness of the person points to the process of growth as both *intra-* and inter-relational. McCown (2013) suggests the relationship that is co-created between teacher and participant (actually both are participants and a more appropriate term may need to evolve) is both necessary for transformation and the heart of ethics in mindfulness. Mindfulness practice as an intrapersonal cultivation of well-being is intricately bound with the cultivation of character through values awareness and clarification. While there is concern that introducing character invites historic beliefs that connect illness to moral weakness, the holistic view of the individual and relationships mitigates that fear by creating an environment where strengths and weaknesses become the source materials to develop insight. It is also important to note that, in Buddhist practice, insight arises through mindfulness by calling to mind past actions and their consequences, and to foster skillfulness (Goldstein, 2013). In other words, insight arises through an awareness of incongruence between one's values and actions, with the precepts offering an opportunity to clarify and reset. Finally, because values and the desire to live well are in and of the world, the practice of mindfulness offers a larger vision than changing individual suffering. It can be seen as cultivating the character of the Noble Person whose interest is the welfare of all beings, that is, clarifying what it means to "live well" in the world. Secular mindfulness therefore cannot be limited to symptomatic relief and must encompass the welfare of society by also healing the conceptual and structural divisions within it.

Walking the Path Continuously

Mindfulness-Based Symptom Management

Communicating Mindfulness The primary issue of ethics *of* mindfulness is being transparent and striving for informed consent to take part in MBSM. In 2003, when the program was first offered, a significant amount of time was spent individually meeting with participants and creating space for questions about the roots of mindfulness. Questions tended to focus on the concerns that this would be a religious inculcation or that some type of conversion to Buddhism would be attempted. With the rapid increase of mindfulness in the media and the scientific literature, these questions have taken a different slant. Participants are more concerned with not having meditation experience or even a concern that the practices in the program may interfere with their current meditation practice. Nevertheless, effort is made to be clear that the program is derived from a spiritual tradition, is a secular translation, and that it includes a practice of clarifying and cultivating one's values so that actions foster well-being.

Infrastructure MBSM was designed through an iterative process of delivering the curriculum and recalibrating it after feedback from participants. It is an 8-week program held once a week for 2 to 2 ½ h with a 5-h. session ("all-day") held about halfway through the program. The all-day session is ideally set after the fourth session but no earlier than the third or later than the fifth sessions. The rationale for the timing of the all-day is important as it relies on practice in the meditations having been sufficiently strengthened by this point in the program. It also serves as a check-in and is often a pivotal point for the participants' felt experience and realization of the impact of continuous practice. The program is delivered in small-group format (8–14 participants) and typically led by two teachers trained in the MBSM curriculum. Contact with the teachers is made available throughout the program either via email, telephone, or individual meetings if necessary. Halfway through the week, a summary called "Session Essentials" is emailed to the participants; these summarize the core practices of the session, repeat links to the meditation for that week, and give a brief description of any specific topic that was part of the session (practice obstacles, expectations, frustration, helpful insights). Specific sharings from the group process are not included in the "essentials." Each session begins with the meditation (Body Scan, awareness of breath, BEST, compassion/loving-kindness, or silence) appropriate to the session (see Monteiro & Musten, 2013, for practice details).

Session Themes and Formal Practices The eight sessions unfold as building blocks with each session adding to or extending the previous session. The core structure of MBSM includes meditation practices such as the Body Scan, awareness of breath, BEST (a guided meditation exploring body, emotions, sensations, and thoughts), loving-kindness or compassion meditation, and a silent meditation at the last session. Thematically, session one introduces the concept of mindfulness practice and session two explores the challenges of folding practice into a busy and harried life. Sessions three to six explore the various ways of reconnecting body and mind. Session seven introduces compassion and session eight prepares for the "ninth session," the rest of our life.

The overarching template for the MBSM protocol draws from S.L Shapiro, Carlson, Astin, and Freedman (2009) who describe the mechanisms of mindfulness as Intention, Attention and Attitude (IAA model). Each class is structured so that these three components are embedded in the class exercises, in the didactic material covered in class, and in the formal and informal practices (see below) throughout the week. The core practices of MBSM sessions, like most 8-week MBIs, are derived from the original mindfulness-based stress reduction (MBSR) program designed by Kabat-Zinn (2013). Thus, for example, in the first class, participants are introduced to the now-iconic Raisin Exercise as their first practice of IAA. They are asked to *intentionally* use one sensory system at a time—vision, touch, etc.—to observe the raisin. They are then asked to find one word that describes what they noticed when they *attended* to the raisin using, for instance, the vision sense. Typically, some participants will find themselves slipping away from the intention of the exercise into stories about the raisin (e.g., "It reminds me of my mother's raisin pie," "I always had raisins in my lunch box at school and I hated them"). When that happens, the participant is invited through the inquiry (see Monteiro in this book and Crane, 2009) to adopt an *attitude* of curiosity, noticing the mind's natural tendency to create stories that take us away from the actual experience. Participants are encouraged to take this attitudinal stance into their everyday life events, noticing the multidimensional nature of their experience as well as the quality of mind they bring to the experience.

Similarly, the meditations cultivate the intention to pay attention to the object of attention associated with the particular meditation. The Body Scan, the first meditation in the program, asks participants to intentionally bring their attention of a specific part of the body as they are progressively led from the tips of the toes to the top of the head. Participants again are invited to be curious about their experience, notice the mind's propensity to prefer one experience over another and remember that the practice **is** in the noticing. This basic practice protocol unfolds across the eight sessions and provides participants with a constant framework they can use as they confirm their mindfulness skills in the classroom.

Informal Practices Beginning with the first class, participants are introduced to practices called Mindful Bells and Brief Ordinary Tasks. Mindful Bells are ambient events in a participant's day-to-day environment that signal for a pause, take three or four conscious breaths, and intentionally bring attention to what is unfolding in that moment. This cultivates awareness of attitudinal stances as they engage with events in brief practices (informal practices) intended to promote a mindful way of being in everyday life. Thus, for instance, a participant reported that she used her telephone ringing at work as a "Mindful Bell" reminding her to take a conscious breath or two as she created an intention to turn away from her computer. She then intentionally shifted her attention to the telephone, noticing from call display that it was her boss calling and also noticing that she was holding her breath. Without spinning off into a story about why, she brought her awareness back to her breath, returning her attention to answering the phone while letting go of expectations of what the call is about. In Shapiro and Carlson's terms (2009), this may be viewed as an attitude of openness or beginner's mind. It may also, in a Buddhist teacher's terms, be viewed as skillful means. Thus, when session eight begins with a silent meditation, participants can more easily and intentionally bring their attention to the breath, becoming aware of the changing nature of experience, and adopting an attitude of nonjudgmental awareness of their experience while letting the experience be what it is. Brief Ordinary Tasks are ones that participants can chose to make an intentional focus of their attention. Brushing teeth, drinking a cup of tea or coffee, washing dishes, etc. are opportunities to intentionally attend to a mundane part of life and observe with an attitude of curiosity how hard it can be to hold one's attention on brief, simple tasks. These two tasks are regular weekly practices over the 8 weeks. Other home practices include Pleasant Event (Week 2) and Unpleasant Event (Week 3) logs (Kabat-Zinn, 2013).

Curriculum MBSM is unique in its building-block approach to teaching themes and specific practices that frame and encourage the experiential connection of body-mind and to clarify and cultivate the values important to the participants. Although it shares the infrastructure of MBSR, its curriculum has been developed as a progression in cultivating intention, attention, and an awareness of mental states, as well as a behavioral-focused practice of values awareness and clarification. These are the BEST model and the Five Skillful Habits described below.

Body, Emotions, Sensations, Thinking (BEST) The curriculum of MBSM was adapted from the core teachings of the Satipaṭṭhāna, which is taught as mindfulness of the body, feelings (pleasant, unpleasant, neutral), mind, and all phenomena (Analayo, 2003; Goldstein, 2013; Hanh, 2006). Because the majority of participants who attend are not versed in Buddhist terminology or teachings, the four ways to establish mindfulness were adapted as mindfulness of the body, emotions, sensations, and thoughts (BEST) to reflect a set of themes that would resonate with them.

From the first session onwards, participants practice noticing how their storylines hijack them and lead to emotional distress and painful, often ruminative, thought patterns; the metaphor of heedlessly getting on a train resonates with participants. Being taken away from our intended practice is likened to standing at a train station intending to get on a particular train but, because of lack of attention, automatically getting on the wrong (typically negative) train that is often bound for a dark neighborhood. It offers an image that is very likely to have happened to most of them (e.g., getting off on the wrong floor of their office, taking the wrong exit on the highway, getting on the wrong bus). The working principle in the metaphor is not about never getting on these trains; we are all born with tickets and will keep getting on trains. The practice is to notice as soon as we can that we are not headed in a direction we intended (emotionally or in our thinking patterns) and, without analyzing what is happening, getting off the train. The exercise has a cognitive overlay of noticing, disrupting the forward momentum of unintended practice, and by doing so, slowing down its unintended consequences. The impact of the practice is to connect with the internal reactivity, creating a space between stimulus and the string of reactions. In that pause, changing the trajectory of the experience becomes more possible.

Starting with the third session, awareness of BEST (Body, Emotions, Sensations, Thoughts) is introduced with their accompanying practices. Mindfulness of the body resonated with the clinical population because they tended to present with physical health issues such as cancer, diabetes, and injuries. They also report stress-related illnesses such as tension and physical symptoms of insomnia, hypervigilance, and agitation. Their stance to their body is typically one of benign or deliberate neglect; in cases of trauma or injury their reaction is woven with shame and deep fear. In general, their stance is that the body had failed them and they felt betrayed, let down, fearing the future, and angry because of the limitations imposed by what they perceived as a mechanical breakdown. To be invited into intimate connection with the body in these circumstances proves a challenge and necessitates slow, deliberate steps. Returning to awareness of the body while lying down, sitting, moving when walking, or engaged in daily activities typically resulted in a capacity to befriend themselves.

Nuttall (2009) examined the effect of participating in an MBSM program on the number of symptoms endorsed (positive symptom total, PTS) and the degree of distress associated with the symptoms (positive symptom distress index, PSDI) using the Symptom Checklist (SCL-90-R; Derogatis, 1994). The impact of psychological symptoms on daily functioning (effects on daily functioning, EDF) was measured using an in-house psychometric scale developed for assessing personal injury history and daily functioning (Self-Administered Psychosocial Survey, SELAPS; Musten, Monteiro, & Hollands, 2007). The results indicated gender differences and the data were presented separately by gender. Both genders reported reduced number of symptoms (Cohen's d: Female, 0.53; Male, 0.34) and lower distress about the symptoms (Cohen's d: Female, 0.94; Male, 0.55); the former result was contrary to the hypothesis which proposed that mindfulness would shift the attitude or mental distress about symptoms and therefore not impact the actual number of symptoms themselves. However, it is likely that with increased awareness of sensations, participants were more discerning between acute and chronic symptoms. Daily functioning improved for both genders with lower impact of symptoms reported post-intervention (Cohen's d: Female, 0.57; Male, 0.55).

Mindfulness of feelings (tones) was expanded to include emotions for obvious reasons. The dominant language in clinical settings is of the emotional states and, perhaps because they feel disconnected from the body, most difficulties are presented through the language of emotions. Participants speak of feeling angry, frustrated, shame or shamed, depressed, anxious, and afraid. This shift to conventional psychological concepts and language gave a space for deeply felt experiences that often could not be voiced elsewhere. Awareness of emotions exposes difficult and unwanted emotions that have been silenced or suppressed, needs that have not been met, and comfort that has not been received. The result is typically a resurgence of emotion avoidance strategies because of the often-intense states of feeling dysregulated (see Holzel et al., 2011, for discussion of emotion regulation). However, practice provides the opportunity to calm the reactivity and create space in which the arising, presence, and dissipation of the emotional state can be observed. Practice then leads to an awareness of emotions as aggregate terms, labels, or schema (e.g., I am an angry person) along with the feeling tone (pleasant, unpleasant, neutral) and sensations (e.g., tension in the gut, tightness in the shoulders) that coalesce as the emotion label.

Mindfulness of sensations extends the previous practice of feelings (emotion, tone, schema) and is informed by somatic experiencing approaches (see Levine, 1997, for description of somatic experiencing therapy related to trauma). This section takes a deconstructive stance to experience, investigating the underlying sensations of experience, noticing both the emotion label and the narrative that arises along with the experience. How labels are applied to experiences is explained as dependent on personal and cultural history of classifying aggregates of sensations. One example, inspired by an historic study by Schachter and Singer (1962) and the two-factor theory of emotions, is to imagine standing at the top of a mountain on skis, feeling sensations of shakiness, shortness of breath, knot in the stomach, etc. Someone exposed to skiing down mountains would label that as exhilaration whereas another might label it as terror. The central teaching point is that labels we provide for our experiences are multifactorial, arising from many causes and conditions, most of which may never be fully known.

Mindfulness of thoughts draws from cognitive behavior therapy. It explores the way thoughts can color mind states and how that impacts the body as well. Consistent with Buddhist teachings, this session also explores how we construct our reality through our assumptions and perceptions. The session includes a dedicated didactic section on the stress model and how trauma is registered in the body, and is also the first time in the 8 weeks that the participants are "allowed into the frontal lobe." That is, up to this session all interactions through their descriptions of weekly practice, events they experience, and emotions they felt have been gently guided back to their experience while noticing the story about the experience. Their language of sensations and feeling tones has developed over the previous sessions and the reliance on stories to validate their inner experience has uncovered the subtle ways of the mind. More than that, the supremacy we give to our thinking function has been challenged, and trust in the subtler ways the body speaks to the mind has developed. What also develops is the beginning of an ability to track physical sensations as the first markers of states of being that may lead to heightened emotions and consequent catastrophic thinking.

Session seven is unique in the challenges it presents and benefits from a specific description. It introduces compassion for self and others and the session begins with a loving-kindness practice as the meditation. Where the first six sessions were focused primarily on developing an inner steadiness in the face of physical and emotional challenges, the exploration of the responses to the meditation in session seven brings out the challenges of self-compassion (Germer, 2009; Neff, 2011), the aversion it evokes (selfish, not deserving, being criticized or diminished), and the fear that it will dull the edge of competitiveness participants feel is necessary to survive in their lives. The brahmaviharas or the four limitless contemplations (Gilbert & Choden, 2014) are introduced as four ways to engage in loving relationship: loving-kindness, resonant joy, compassion, and equanimity. The first two are described as practices we engage in to nourish and sustain relationships; the second two are necessary to meet and transform moments and periods of suffering. We liken these to prophylactic and curative measures, respectively. Both are necessary for a balanced stance in the constantly changing flow of being in relationship with others, the world, and ourselves.

Shaw (2012) studied the relationship of participating in MBSM and its impact on factors of burnout (MBI, Maslach Burnout Inventory; Maslach & Jackson, 1981) and self-compassion (SCS, Self-Compassion Scale; Neff, 2003). Results for the MBI indicated a significant reduction in only one subscale, Emotional Exhaustion ($p < 0.001$; Cohen's d: 0.46). The SCS obtained significant increases in all three subscales of Self-kindness ($p < 0.001$; Cohen's d: 0.66), Common Humanity ($p < 0.001$; Cohen's d: 0.53), and Mindfulness ($p < 0.001$; Cohen's d: 0.53). The counterparts to these subscales (Self-judgment, Isolation, and Over-identification) decreased significantly ($p < 0.001$; Cohen's d: 0.83, 0.44 & 0.59, respectively). At follow-up 3 months later, most gains measured by the MBI and SCS had been maintained; however, the MBI subscale of Cynicism had decreased further. Self-judgment increased reversing towards the pre-intervention levels. Informal practices of the 3-min breathing exercise and walking meditation were associated with maintaining post-intervention positive gains in self-kindness. In an interesting process, thought awareness practice and time spent in informal practices were related to decreases in self-judgment; recalling that self-judgment had increased at post-intervention, it appeared the informal practices had the effect of "slowing down" the reversal to preconditions. These results supported our approach to mindfulness as inherently a practice of self-compassion and continued to set the tone for conversation around perceived failure as well as cultivating trust in personal experience and in empathy with others.

This session also integrates the Five Skillful Habits as a central practice of compassion and highlights its application across the four platforms of mindfulness practiced in the previous weeks. The next section explores the Five Skillful Habits specifically.

Five Skillful Habits (5SH)   The arc of MBSM is the cultivation of skillfulness in living; that skillfulness is comprised of making wise decisions based on a clear understanding and connection with the values that underpin thought, speech, and action. Embodying the spirit of creating the path by walking, the 5SH are the framework of practice that breathes life into the abstraction of values and the virtues they represent. Its intersection with BEST is introduced in the third session.

Derived from Thich Nhat Hanh's Five Mindfulness Trainings, they are respect for mortality, generosity, respect for boundaries, compassionate speech, and mindful consumption (Hanh, 2007). We introduce them as daily practices early in MBSM because we believe there is a need for intentional practices; these practices also honor the idea that moral effort was a necessary condition for meditative practices to be effective (Whitehill, 2000). S.L. Shapiro and Carlson (2009) make a similar point when they suggest that, consistent with both Buddhist and Western approaches to moral psychology and philosophy, the Buddhist concepts of "right" or "wholesome" intentions are descriptive of a way of living that is intended to relieve suffering. And, importantly, they "believe that explicit teachings of these guidelines are critically important to mindfulness practice" (p. 10).

It was also apparent in our discussions with participants that the incongruence between their ideal state and actual lived state was experienced as the root of their suffering; that is, living with authenticity was important to them. Kernis and Goldman (2006) investigated the relationship between authenticity and mindfulness, noting "that an open and trusting stance toward one's self-aspects goes hand-in-hand with tendencies to observe internal and external stimuli, competence in describing one's internal states, ability to focus one's attention on the task at hand, and a nonjudgmental stance in general" (p. 312). Further, Smallenbroek, Zelenski, and Whelan (2017) reported that acting in congruence in one's values was related to state and trait authenticity, which they define as "generally understood as acting in accordance with core aspects of the self" (p.197).

Exploring whether participants attending MBSM presented with such incongruences of values, Monteiro (2012) examined the relationship between burnout factors (MBI, Maslach Burnout Inventory; Maslach, Jackson, & Leiter, 1996) and incongruence in spiritual values (SWBQ, Spiritual Well Being Questionnaire; J. W. Fisher, 2010) in a group of MBSM participants at pre-intervention. Significant differences were obtained between the ideal and actual scores of the SWBQ (used as a measure of incongruence) with ideal scores higher than actual scores. Personal incongruence was significantly different from the other three SWBQ factors (communal, environmental, and transcendental) suggesting participants entered the MBSM program with a sense of not feeling aligned with their ideal personal values. Correlations with the burnout factors and personal incongruence scores were significant for exhaustion ($p < 0.05$), cynicism ($p < 0.05$), and personal effectiveness ($p < 0.01$). Analysis of the effect of emotional exhaustion scores on personal incongruence indicated that, compared to those in the high emotional exhaustion group, participants in the low emotional exhaustion group reported lower incongruence on the personal values factor ($p = 0.016$; Cohen's d: 0.65). Participants with high personal effectiveness scores reported low personal incongruence ($p < 0.01$; Cohen's d: 0.72) compared to those in the group with low personal effectiveness scores. These results suggested participants present with an experience of incongruence in their personal values and indicated a connection between their burnout symptoms and the incongruence they experience.

In this context, the 5SH are viewed as guideposts that provide the framework for participants to develop an embodied ethical relationship to their lived lives. They provide the framework that first affords participants the opportunity to look at how they are living their lives and second provides the frame for them to introduce healthier, more compassionate ways of being with themselves. In the words of Thich Nhat Hanh, mindfulness is always mindfulness of something, be it the breath, speech, thought, or action. In other words, because we are always practicing something, it may as well be something congruent with our values.

Although mindfulness is usually taught as present-moment awareness, it is also a recollection of actions and their consequences, a nodal point at which a different choice is possible, and a recalling of what supports practice (Goldstein, 2013). In order to see the need for and to support choices that have a different outcome, action-guides are necessary. Held up against the template of who we wish to be (ideal) and the question of who we are in the moment (lived experience), the 5SH provide a way of directing or experimenting with change. These habits, in the service of well-being, are intended to cultivate behaviors that: (1) attend to physical health to reduce risks related to higher mortality; (2) develop appropriate generosity; (3) increase awareness of physical and emotional boundaries; (4) cultivate compassionate speech, and (5) increase discernment in consumption of physical and emotional nourishment, including use of necessary medication treatments. Table 8.1 shows interconnection of the four methods of establishing mindfulness (body, emotions, sensations, thinking) and the 5SH with examples of possible actions or attitudes to cultivate.

Making the Five Mindfulness Trainings congruent with Western approaches to cultivating wholesome living required sensitivity to intent and language. The intentions of the first, second, fourth, and fifth of Thich Nhat Hanh's Five Mindfulness Trainings with an emphasis on cultivating values-congruent behaviors fit well with Western values as noted by our participants. The third mindfulness training, however, presented unique issues because it was a prohibition against excessive sensual indulgence (Hanh, 2007) and refers specifically to sexual relations. This focus on sexuality was considered too narrow and perhaps likely to trigger feelings of being judged or being "sinful." We sought a broader and more applicable concept of sensual attachment that would connect with participants who felt challenged in knowing when their physical and emotional pain threshold had been exceeded. They described pushing themselves physically and emotionally beyond limits because of messages to "get through" or "breakthrough" their unpleasant experiences of depression, injuries, grief, and so on. Despite their vulnerable state, they often practiced a "no pain, no gain" philosophy which only served to exacerbate their condition or deplete their resources. Pushing the boundaries of physical and emotional tolerance was a form of overindulgence in physical or emotional sensations and a misguided attempt at symptom management. Given these parameters, it seemed appropriate to modify the third mindfulness training to reflect respect for physical and emotional boundaries.

Each week participants in the program are invited to focus on one aspect of their experience in the context of body, emotions, sensations, and thinking. We also are

Table 8.1 Examples of possible behaviors to cultivate in each domain of mindfulness

Five Skillful Habits	Behavioral examples
Respect for mortality (the life we have)	Body: Exercise, attend to treatment plans (medication, etc.).
	Emotions: Note how positive and negative experiences are connected to physical sensations.
	Sensations: Notice the sensation of your heart beat, muscles relaxing or aching, joint pain, heaviness, lightness, etc.
	Thoughts: Note positive and negative thoughts and connection to physical experiences.
Generosity	Body: Rest, sleep in, take frequent breaks.
	Emotions: Allow yourself to feel the range of emotions guilt, anger, happiness, etc.
	Sensations: Practice deep diaphragmatic breathing when you notice uncomfortable sensations. Incline towards experiences with kindness and compassion.
	Thoughts: Allow thoughts to come and go (allow yourself to hop off trains).
Respect of limits	Body: Note when fatigued, appropriate pain monitoring, say "No," manage expectations.
	Emotions: Note unpleasant emotions and be present to them as long as is comfortable for you. Note pleasant emotions and savor them.
	Sensations: Stay with sensations as long as is comfortable for you—play with that edge. Notice the arising, presence, and dissolving of sensations.
	Thoughts: Notice when your thoughts are dictating your limits rather than what your body really feels (e.g., I can't do this).
Compassionate speech	Body: Bring a flavor of kindness to whatever physical experience you are having.
	Emotions: Approach arising of emotions with an attitude of curiosity.
	Sensations: Notice when judging about sensations arises.
	Thoughts: See the thoughts as they are, just thoughts
Mindful consumption	Body: Take time for lunch, notice effect of media messages about body image
	Emotions: Note the sensation/emotional effects of what you are watching on television
	Sensations: Note sensations of satiation
	Thoughts: Note thoughts while eating: tone, language, etc. Also note how interactions are "consumed": joyful, kind, angry, tense, etc.

clear that experience is not categorical or orderly and the four frames of experience tend to flow together. Participants are invited to adopt an approach of holding one in the foreground while holding the others lightly in the background. Folded into these four ways to establish mindfulness, the 5SH form an intentional behavioral focus for the home practice and each week a different way to establish mindfulness is chosen until the four ways are integrated in the penultimate class on compassion and loving-kindness. At the end of each session, as part of the home practice discussion, participants are invited to identify specific behaviors, based on the 5SH themes, to which they can commit as their practice for the week; occasionally someone declines and this is typically because they wish to think further on the value or behavior that is salient for them. Table 8.2 summarizes responses by program

Table 8.2 Examples of behaviors selected by participants to practice in each method of establishing mindfulness

	Body	Emotions	Sensations	Thoughts
Respect for Life	Health-related (e.g., while eating, paying attention to body)	Attend to emotional suffering Established a formal gratitude practice	Observe ("tune in") Try not to avoid pain	Attend to underlying pain when thinking "violent" thoughts
Generosity	Exercise Rest	Nonviolent communication (speech/thoughts) to identify responsibility Charitable donations	Listening Eating slowly	Compassion, self-empathy, focusing Tapas acupressure technique
Boundaries	Saying "no" Taking time for self and others Taking breaks, not over-exerting self	Expressing emotions in ways not be harmful to self or others	Reduce and deal with negative events/ emotions	Expressing gratitude Noticing good in life
Speech	Being nonjudgmental about health-related choices	Express and allow emotions to exist Express self in non-harmful ways (choose words carefully and aware of intentions behind words)	Listening	Let go of negative thoughts Welcome thoughts but let them pass Watch "train" (thoughts) pass and refocus on now More sensitive to others, less critical
Consumption	Not eating foods that are hard to digest (healthy choices)	(no participants provided examples here)	Eating slowly	More relaxed More positive Accepting "this is me"

graduates on the behaviors chosen and insights that emerged when using the 5SH (Monteiro, Nuttall, & Musten, 2010; Nuttall, 2009).

In summary, MBSM, and the 5SH specifically, are an exploration of well-being as it is experienced by each participant personally; inevitably the inquiry and awareness that develop lead to understanding how they value their relationships with others and the world. The behavior participants chose to action their understanding of each 5SH represents what they value as a path to personal well-being. Respect for mortality (the life we have) investigates ways of living that undermine or enhance well-being in terms of body, emotions, sensations, and thinking. Generosity explores ways to give and receive so that there is a constant process of replenishing. Respect for limits experiments with the hard and soft edges of emotional and physical limits that signal the need for attention and recalibration. Compassionate speech brings awareness to the impact of the inner critic and an opportunity to become more skillful in how to encourage kindness. Mindful consumption cultivates awareness of the intake and "digestion" of all forms of toxic material from food to media messages. What each participant chooses to practice is individually determined; however, the intent is not to replace one behavior for another. Practice offers the opportunity to bring awareness of the dance between ideal and lived states; it is an inquiry into what is valued (the preciousness of life, kindness, etc.) and how that is lived, and to develop awareness of how it can be lived more skillfully. The richness of this practice is in the way participants discover the futility of perfectionistic approaches and the many simple ways their values can be upheld.

Conclusions

In this chapter, we have explored the development of a mindfulness-based intervention which we hoped would address the gaps we experienced in the seed programs of early mindfulness interventions. The process was challenging at professional and personal levels. We were constantly faced with the complex intersection of religion, spirituality, ethics, values, mental health issues, and our own concerns about the now-apparent iatrogenic effects of meditation. Along the way, we also had to examine issues of earning a living through the use of religious/spiritual practices, what in Buddhism is right livelihood, one of the three components of cultivating the moral aspect of a life well lived. The other two are right speech and right action, practices that became our touchstone as we struggled to ensure that what we offered respected the professional, spiritual, and local communities around us.

MBSM, we hoped and continue to hope, represents an easeful integration of what the Buddha intended in his teachings of 2600 years ago with our knowledge of how people in this century meet and manage their experiences of distress, joy, love, and care. Our concerns that mindfulness could become a mechanical technique or a topical application for quick relief have substance when we listen to our participants initially ask for a "quick fix" or "magic bullet." This desire is very understandable because the pain of change is hard to accept and the suffering that arises from being averse to, clinging to alternatives, or feeling doubt about managing feels overwhelming. Nevertheless, while MBSM offers that initial relief in the form of relaxation or calm, we aimed for a design that dug into the roots of our dissatisfaction—or at the very least offers an idea that such action was possible. And for us those roots are the values by which we try to live and from which we often felt disconnected.

However, MBSM is far from—and likely never will become—an intervention that is fixed and manualized. The essential truth is that nothing is permanent and everything is in constant state of change; it is both a spiritual claim of Buddhism and of physical science. But there is also a more immediate reason for the constant state of change: every program we offer is new simply because all those who come together are doing so for the very first time. In the space that each program is conducted, everything is happening for the first time. Even as teachers who have walked into that room hundreds of times over the years, we too are new because the relationship with everyone there creates us anew.

What we aspire to then is that the core values which drew us together in the first place—that value for a life lived well—become our North Star and together we learn again how to use our moral compass to navigate the waters we are in together.

References

Aitken, R. (1984). *The mind of clover: Essays in Zen Buddhist ethics*. New York: North Point Press.

Aitken, R. (1991). *The gateless barrier: The Wu-Men Kuan*. Berkeley, CA: North Point Press.

Amaro, A. (2015). A holistic mindfulness. *Mindfulness, 6*(1), 63–73. https://doi.org/10.1007/s12671-014-0382-3

Analayo. (2003). *Satipatthana: The direct path to realization*. Birmingham, AB: Windhorse Publications.

Analayo. (2013). *Perspectives on satipatthana*. Cambridge: Windhorse Publications.

Anderson, R. (2001). *Being upright: Zen meditation and the bodhisattva precepts*. Berkeley, CA: Rodmell Press.

Baer, R. (2003). Mindfulness training as a clinical intervention: A conceptual and empirical review. *Clinical Psychology: Science and Practice, 10*, 125–143.

Baer, R. (2015). Ethics, values, virtues, and character strengths in mindfulness-based interventions: A psychological science perspective. *Mindfulness, 6*(4), 956–969. https://doi.org/10.1007/s12671-015-0419-2

Barkham, M., & Mellor-Clark, J. (2003). Bridging evidence-based practice and practice-based evidence: Developing a rigorous and relevant knowledge for the psychological therapies. *Clinical Psychology and Psychotherapy, 10*, 319–327. https://doi.org/10.1002/cpp.379

Batchelor, S. (2017). *After Buddhism: Rethinking the dharma for a secular age*. New Haven, CT: Yale University Press.

Baumeister, R. F. (1999). The nature and structure of the self: An overview. In R. F. Baumeister (Ed.), *Self in social psychology: Key readings*. Philadelphia, PA: Psychology Press.

Baumeister, R. F. (2011). Self and identity: A brief overview of what they are, what they do, and how they work. *Annals of the New York Academy of Sciences, 1234*(1), 48–55. https://doi.org/10.1111/j.1749-6632.2011.06224.x

Beck, A. T., Rush, A. J., Shaw, B. F., & Emery, G. (1987). *Cognitive therapy of depresison*. New York: The Guilford Press.

Blum, L. A. (1993). Gilligan and Kohlberg: Implications for moral theory. In M. J. Larabee (Ed.), *An ethic of care*. New York: Routledge.

Bodhi, B. (2008). *The Noble Eightfold Path: The way to end suffering*. Onalaska, WA: BPS Pariyatti Editions.

Bodhi, B. (2011). What does mindfulness really mean? A canonical perspective. *Contemporary Buddhism, 12*(1), 19–39.

Bodhi, B. (2013). Nourishing the roots: Essays on Buddhist ethics. *Access to insight*. Retrieved from Access to Insight http://www.accesstoinsight.org/lib/bodhi/wheel259.html

Brown, K. W., Creswell, J. D., & Ryan, R. M. (Eds.). (2015). *Handbook of mindfulness: Theory, research, and practice*. New York: The Guilford Press.

Brown, K. W., & Ryan, R. M. (2003). The benefits of being present: Mindfulness and its role in psychological well-being. *Journal of Personality and Social Psychology, 84*, 822–848.

Brown, K. W., & Ryan, R. M. (2004). Peril and promise in defining and measuring mindfulness: Observations from experience. *Clinical Psychology: Science and Practice, 11*, 242–248.

Burns, J. P., Goodman, D. M., & Orman, A. J. (2013). Psychotherapy as moral encounter: A crisis of modern conscience. *Pastoral Psychology, 62*, 1–12.

Cayoun, B. A. (2011). *Mindfulness-integrated CBT: Principles and practice*. Chicester: Wiley-Blackwell.

Coffey, K. A., Hartman, M., & Fredrickson, B. L. (2010). Deconstructing mindfulness and constructing mental health: Understanding mindfulness and its mechanisms of action. *Mindfulness, 1*, 235–253.

Compson, J., & Monteiro, L. (2015). Still exploring the middle path: A response to commentaries. *Mindfulness, 7*(2), 548–564. https://doi.org/10.1007/s12671-015-0447-y

Crane, R. S. (2009). *Mindfulness-based cognitive therapy: Distinctive features*. New York: Routledge.

Crane, R. S., Kuyken, W., Hastings, R. P., Rothwell, N., & Williams, J. M. G. (2010). Training teachers to deliver mindfulness-based interventions: Learning from the UK experience. *Mindfulness, 1*(2), 74–86. https://doi.org/10.1007/s12671-010-0010-9

Crane, R. S., Kuyken, W., Williams, M. J. G., Hastings, R. P., Cooper, L., & Fennell, M. J. V. (2011). Competence in teaching mindfulness-based courses: Concepts, development and assessment. *Mindfulness*. https://doi.org/10.1007/s12671-011-0073-2

Cullen, M. (2011). Mindfulness-based interventions: An emerging phenomenon. *Mindfulness, 2*, 186–193.

Davis, J. H. (2015). Facing up to the question of ethics in mindfulness-based interventions. *Mindfulness, 6*(1), 46–48. https://doi.org/10.1007/s12671-014-0374-3

Derogatis, L. R. (1994). *Symptom Checklist-90-R: Administration, scoring, and procedure manual*. Minneapolis: National Computer Systems.

Dimidjian, S., & Segal, Z. V. (2015). Prospects for a clinical science of mindfulness-based intervention. *American Psychologist, 70*(7), 593–620. https://doi.org/10.1037/a0039589

Eberth, J., & Sedlmeier, P. (2012). The effects of mindfulness meditation: A meta-analysis. *Mindfulness, 3*, 174–189.

Eisenberg, N., & Eggum, N. D. (2008). Empathic responding: Sympathy and personal distress. In B. Sullivan, S. Snyder, & J. Sullivan (Eds.), *Cooperation: The political psychology of effective human interaction* (pp. 71–83). Malden, MA: Blackwell Publishing.

Ekman, P., & Davidson, R. J. (Eds.). (1994). *The nature of emotion: Fundamental questions*. New York: Oxford University Press.

Epstein, M. (2013). *Thoughts without a thinker: Psychotherapy from a Buddhist perspective* (Revised ed.). New York: Basic Books.

Epstein, M. (2014). *The trauma of everyday life*. New York: Penguin Books.

Evans, A., Crane, R. S., Cooper, L., Mardula, J., Wilks, J., Surawy, C., … Kuyken, W. (2014). A framework for supervision for mindfulness-based teachers: A space for embodied mutual inquiry. *Mindfulness, 6*(3), 572–581. https://doi.org/10.1007/s12671-014-0292-4

Fisher, B., & Tronto, J. C. (1990). Toward a feminist theory of caring. In E. Abel & M. Nelson (Eds.), *Circles of care*. Albany, NY: SUNY Press.

Fisher, J. W. (2010). Development and application of a spiritual well-being questionnaire called SHALOM. *Religions, 1*, 105–112.

Fisher, J. W. (2011). The four domains model: Connecting spirituality, health and well-being. *Religions, 2*, 17–28.

Fjorback, L. O., Arendt, M., Ornbol, E., Fink, P., & Walach, H. (2011). Mindfulness-based stress reduction and mindfulness-based cognitive therapy – A systematic review of randomized controlled trials. *Acta Psychiatrica Scandinavica, 124*, 102–119.

Flanagan, O. (1993). *Varieties of moral pesonality*. Cambridge, MA: Harvard University Press.

Geertz, C. (1973). *Thick description: Towards an interpretive theory of culture*. New York: Basic Books.

Germer, C. K. (2009). *The mindful path to self-compassion: Freeing yourself from destructive thoughts and emotions*. New York: The Guilford Press.

Gethin, R. (1998). *The foundations of Buddhism*. Oxford: Oxford University Press.

Giammarco, E. A. (2016). The measurement of individual differences inmorality. *Personality and Individual Differences, 88*, 26–34.

Gilbert, P., & Choden. (2014). *Mindful compassion*. Oakland, CA: New Harbinger.

Gilligan, C. (1993). *In a different voice: Psychological theory and women's development* (revised ed.). Cambridge, MA: Harvard University Press.

Gilligan, C. (2011). *Joining the resistance*. Cambridge: Ploity Press.

Gilligan, C. (2014). Moral injury and the ethic of care: Reframing the conversation about differences. *Journal of Social Philosophy, 45*(1), 89–106.

Gilligan, C., & Attanucci, J. (1988). Two moral orientations. In C. Gilligan, J. V. Ward, & J. Taylor (Eds.), *Mapping the moral domain*. Cambridge, MA: Harvard University Press.

Goldstein, J. (2013). *Mindfulness: A practical guide to awakening*. Louisville, CO: Sounds True.

Gombrich, R. (2009/2013). *What the Buddha thought*. Bristol, CT: Equinox Publishers.

Goyal, M., Singh, S., Sibinga, E. S., Gould, N. F., Rowland-Seymour, A., Sharma, R., … Haythornthwaite, J. A. (2014). Meditation programs for psychological stress and well-being: A systematic review and meta-analysis. *JAMA Internal Medicine, 174*(3), 357–368. https://doi.org/10.1001/jamainternmed.2013.13018

Grabovac, A., Lau, M., & Willett, B. (2011). Mechanisms of mindfulness: A Buddhist psychological model. *Mindfulness, 2*(3), 154–166. https://doi.org/10.1007/s12671-011-0054-5

Greenberg, M., & Mitra, J. (2015). From mindfulness to right mindfulness: the intersection of awareness and ethics. *Mindfulness, 6*(1), 74–78. https://doi.org/10.1007/s12671-014-0384-1

Grossman, G. (2009). *On killing: The psychological cost of learning to kill in war and society*. New York: Back Bay Books.

Grossman, P. (2015). Mindfulness: Awareness informed by an embodied ethic. *Mindfulness, 6*(1), 17–22. https://doi.org/10.1007/s12671-014-0372-5

Grossman, P., & Van Dam, N. (2011). Mindfulness, by any other name …: trials and tribulations of sati in western psychology and science. *Contemporary Buddhism, 12*(1), 219–239.

Gunaratana, B. (2001). *Eight mindful steps to happiness: Walking the Buddha's path*. Somerville, MA: Wisdom Press.

Gunaratana, B. (2012). *The four foundations of mindfulness in plain English*. Boston, MA: Wisdom Publishers.

Hamilton, R. (2013). The frustrations of virtue: The myth of moral neutrality in psychotherapy. *Journal of Evaluation in Clinical Practice, 19*, 485–492.

Hanh, T. N. (1998). *Interbeing: Fourteen guidelines for engaged Buddhism*. Berkeley, CA: Parallax Press.

Hanh, T. N. (1999). *The miracle of mindfulness: An introduction to the practice of meditation*. Boston: Beacon Press.

Hanh, T. N. (2006). *Transformation and healing: The sutra on the four foundations of mindfulness*. Berkeley CA: Parallax Press.

Hanh, T. N. (2007). *For a future to be possible: Buddhist ethics for everyday life*. Berkeley, CA: Parallax Press.

Hanh, T. N. (2009). *Breathe, You Are Alive! Sutra on the full awareness of breathing*. Berkeley, CA: Parallax Press.

Hanh, T. N. (2011). *Our appointment with life: Sutra on knowing the better way to live alone*. Berkley, CA: Parallax Press.

Hanley, A. W., Abell, N., Osborn, D. S., Roehrig, A. D., & Canto, A. I. (2016). Mind the Gaps: Are conclusions about mindfulness entirely conclusive? *Journal of Counseling & Development, 94*, 103–113. https://doi.org/10.1002/jcad.12066

Harrington, A., & Dunne, J. (2015). When mindfulness is therapy: Ethical qualms, historical perspectives. *American Psychologist, 70*(7), 621–631. https://doi.org/10.1037/a0039460

Harvey, P. (2000). *An introduction to Buddhist ethics*. Cambridge: Cambridge University Press.

Harvey, P. (2013). *An introduction to Buddhism: Teachings, history and practices* (2nd ed.). Cambridge: Cambridge University Press.

Hathaway, W. L. (2011). Ethical guidelines for using spiritually oriented interventions. In J. D. Aten, M. R. McMinn, & E. L. Worthington Jr. (Eds.), *Spiritually oriented interventions for counseling and psychotherapy* (pp. 65–81). Washington, DC: Ameerican Psychological Association.

Holmqvist, R., Philips, B., & Barkham, M. (2015). Developing practice-based evidence: Benefits, challenges, and tensions. *Psychotherapy Research, 25*, 20–31. https://doi.org/10.1080/10503307.2013.861093

Holzel, B. K., Lazar, S. W., Gard, T., Schuman-Olivier, Z., Vago, D. R., & Ott, U. (2011). How does mindfulness meditation work? Proposing mechanisms of action from a conceptual and neural perspective. *Perspectives on Psychological Science, 6*(6), 537–559.

Jackson, A. P., Hansen, J., & Cook-Ly, J. M. (2013). Value conflicts in psychotherapy. *Issues in Religion and Psychotherapy, 35*, 6–15.

Janoff-Bulman, R., Sheikh, S., & Hepp, S. (2009). Proscriptive versus prescriptive morality: Two faces of moral regulation. *Journal of Personality and Social Psychology, 96*(3), 521–537.

Kabat-Zinn, J. (2003). Mindfulness-based interventions in context: Past, present and future. *Clinical Psychology: Science and Practice, 10*, 144–156.

Kabat-Zinn, J. (2011). Some reflections on the origins of MBSR, skillful means, and the trouble with maps. *Contemporary Buddhism, 12*(1), 281–306.

Kabat-Zinn, J. (2013). *Full catastrophe living: Using the wisdom of your body and mind to face stress, pain, and illness*. New York, NY: Bantam.

Keltner, D. (2009). *Born to be good: The science of a meaningful life*. New York: W.W. Norton.

Keown, D. (2001). *The nature of Buddhist ethics*. New York: Palgrave.

Keown, D. (2005). *Buddhist ethics: A very short introduction*. Oxford: Oxford University Press.

Kernis, M. H., & Goldman, B. M. (2006). A multicomponent conceptualization of authenticity: Theory and research. *Advances in experimental social psychology, 38*, 283–357. https://doi.org/10.1016/S0065-2601(06)38006-9

Khoury, B., Lecomte, T., Fortin, G., Masse, M., Therien, P., Bouchard, V., … Hofmann, S. G. (2013). Mindfulness-based therapy: A comprehensive meta-analysis. *Clinical Psychology Review, 33*, 763–771.

Kohlberg, L. (Ed.). (1976). *Moral stages and moralization: The cognitive developmental approach*. New York: Holt, Rinehart, & Winston.

Kurchin, S. (2013). Thick concepts and thick descriptions. In S. Kurchin (Ed.), *Thick concepts* (pp. 60–77). Oxford: Oxford University Press.

Larabee, M. J. (Ed.). (1993). *An ethic of care*. New York: Routledge.

Lazarus, A. (1989). *The practice of multimodal therapy: Systematic, comprehensive and effective psychotherapy*. Baltimore, MD: Johns Hopkins University Press.

Lazarus, A. (2006). Multimodal therapy: A seven-point integration. In G. Stricker & J. Gold (Eds.), *A casebook of psychotherapy integration* (pp. 17–28). Washington, DC: American Psychological Association.

Lazarus, R. S., & Folkman, S. (1984). *Stress, appraisal, and coping*. New York: Springer.

Leiter, M. P., Jackson, N. J., & Shaughnessy, K. (2009). Contrasting burnout, turnover intention, control, value congruence and knowledge sharing between Baby Boomers and Generation X. *Journal of Nursing Management, 17*(1), 100–109. https://doi.org/10.1111/j.1365-2834.2008.00884.x

Levine, P. (1997). *Waking the Tiger*. Berkeley: North Atlantic Books.

Lindahl, J. (2015). Why right mindfulness might not be right for mindfulness. *Mindfulness, 6*(1), 57–62. https://doi.org/10.1007/s12671-014-0380-5

Machado, A. (2002). *Campos de Castilla y Soledades – Fields of Castille and Solitude*. London: Duckworth Publishers.

Maslach, C., Jackson, S. E., & Leiter, M. P. (1996). *Maslach burnout inventory manual* (3rd ed.). Palo Alto, CA: Consulting Psychologists Press.

Maslow, A. (2014). *Toward a psychology of being*. Floyd, VA: Sublime Books.

McCown, D. (2013). *The ethical space of mindfulness in clinical practice: An exploratory essay*. Philadelphia, PA: Jessica Kingsley Publishers.

McCown, D. (2014). *Mindfulness: Fulfilling the promise at last, with a relational view*. Paper presented at the Beyond the Therapeutic State: Collaborative Practices for Individual and Social Change, Drammen, Norway.

McCown, D. (2016). Being is relational: Considerations for using mindfulness in clinician-patient settings. In E. Shonin, W. van Gordon, & M. D. Griffiths (Eds.), *Mindfulness and Buddhist-derived approaches in mental health and addiction* (pp. 29–60). Switzerland: Springer.

McEwen, B. S. (2002). *The end of stress as we know it*. Washington, DC: Joseph Henry Press.

Mikulas, W. L. (2015). Ethics in Buddhist training. *Mindfulness, 6*(1), 14–16. https://doi.org/10.1007/s12671-014-0371-6

Monteiro, L. (2012). *Burnout and spiritual incongruence: An evidence-based counselling model for Buddhist chaplains*. Santa Fe, NM: Upaya Zen Institute.

Monteiro, L. (2015). Dharma and distress: Buddhist teachings that support psychological principles in a mindfulness program. In E. Shonin, W. Van Gordon, & N. N. Singh (Eds.), *Buddhist Foundations of Mindfulness* (pp. 181–215). New York: Springer.

Monteiro, L. (2016). Implicit ethics and mindfulness: Subtle assumptions that MBIs are values-neutral. *International Journal of Psychotherapy, 20*, 210–224.

Monteiro, L., & Musten, R. F. (2013). *Mindfulness starts here: An 8-week guide to skillful living*. Victoria, BC: Friesen Press.

Monteiro, L., Musten, R. F., & Compson, J. (2015). Traditional and contemporary mindfulness: Finding the middle path in the tangle of concerns. *Mindfulness, 6*(1), 1–13.

Monteiro, L., Nuttall, S., & Musten, R. F. (2010). Five skillful habits: An ethics-based mindfulness intervention. *Counselling and Spirituality, 29*(1), 91–103.

Musten, R. F., Monteiro, L., & Hollands, R. (2007). Self-administered psychosocial survey.

Narvaez, D. (2014). *Neurobiology and the development of human morality*. New York: W.W. Norton.

Neff, K. D. (2003). The development and validation of a scale to measure self-compassion. *Self and Identity, 2*(3), 223–250.

Neff, K. D. (2011). *Self-compassion: Stop beating yourself up and leave insecurity behind*. New York: William Morrow.

Nuttall, S. (2009). *Mindfulness-based symptom management: A naturalistic study of a new mindfulness-based intervention*. (B.A.), University of Ottawa.

Olendzki, A. (2008). The real practice of mindfulness. *Buddhadharma, 7*, 8.

Olendzki, A. (2011). The construction of mindfulness. *Contemporary Buddhism, 12*(1), 55–70.

Onken, L. S., Carroll, K. M., Shoham, V., Cuthbert, B. N., & Riddle, M. (2014). Reenvisioning clinical science: Unifying the discipline to improve the public health. *Clinical Psychological Science, 2*, 22–34. https://doi.org/10.1177/2167702613497932

Patterson, C. H. (1959). *Counseling and psychotherapy*. New York: Harper & Row.

Porges, S. (2007). The Polyvagal perspective. *Biological Psychology, 74*(2), 116–143.

Porges, S. (2011). *The Polyvagal theory: Neurophysiological foundations of emotions, attachment, communication, and self-regulation*. New York: W.W. Norton.

Purser, R. (2015). Clearing the muddles path of traditional and contemporary mindfulness: A response to Monteiro, Musten, and Compson. *Mindfulness, 6*(23–45).

Purser, R., & Loy, D. (2013). Beyond McMindfulness. *Huffington Post*. Retrieved from http://www.huffingtonpost.com/ron-purser/beyond-mcmindfulness_b_3519289.html website: http://www.huffingtonpost.com/

Riso, L. P., du Toit, P. L., Stein, D. J., & Young, J. E. (2007). *Cognitive schemas and core beliefs in psychological problems*. Washington, DC: American Psychological Association.

Roeser, R. W., Vago, D., Pinela, C., Morris, L. S., Taylor, C., & Harrison, J. (2014). Contemplative education: Cultivating ethical development through mindfulness training. In L. NUcci, D. Narvaez, & T. Krettenauer (Eds.), *Handbook of moral and character educaiton*. New York: Routledge, Taylor & Francis Group.

Rogers, C. (2003). *Client-centered therapy: Its current practice, implications and theory*. London: Constable Publisher.

Rogers, C., & Kramer, P. D. (1995). *On becoming a person: A therapist's view of psychotherapy* (2nd ed.). New York: Mariner Books.

Rosenbaum, R. M., & Magrid, B. (Eds.). (2016). *What's wrong with mindfulness (and what isn't)*. Somerville, MA: Wisdom Books.

Schachter, S., & Singer, J. (1962). Cognitive, social, and physiological determinants of emotional state. *Psychological Review, 69*, 379–399. https://doi.org/10.1037/h0046234

Segal, Z. V., Williams, J. M., & Teasdale, J. D. (2012). *Mindfulness based cognitive therapy for the prevention of depression relapse* (2nd ed.). New York: The Guilford Press.

Seligman, M. (2012). *Flourish: A visionary new understanding of happiness and well-being*. New York: Free Press.

Senauke, A. (2013). Wrong Mindfulness: An interview with Hozan Alan Senauke. Retrieved from http://www.tricycle.com/blog/wrong-mindfulness   website: http://www.tricycle.com/blog/wrong-mindfulness

Selye, H. (1974). *Stress without distress*. Toronto: HarperCollins.

Shapiro, S. L., & Carlson, L. E. (2009). *The art and science of mindfulness: Integrating mindfulness into psychology and the helping professions*. Washington, DC: American Psychological Association.

Shapiro, S. L., Carlson, L. E., Astin, J. A., & Freedman, B. (2009). Mechanisms of mindfulness. *Journal of Clinical Psychology, 62*(3), 373–386. https://doi.org/10.1002/jclp.20237

Shapiro, S. L., Jazaieri, H., & Goldin, P. R. (2012). Mindfulness-based stress reduction effects on moral reasoning and decision making. *The Journal of Positive Psychology, 7*(6), 504–515.

Shaw, C. (2012). *Mindfulness-based symptom management and the treatment of burnout* (M.A. Research, Carleton University, Ottawa, ON).

Smallenbroek, O., Zelenski, J. M., & Whelan, D. (2017). Authenticity as a eudaimonic construct: The relationships among authenticity, values, and valence. *The Journal of Positive Psychology, 12*(2), 197–209.

Stanley, S. (2013). 'Things said or done long ago are recalled and remembered': The ethics of mindfulness in early Buddhism, psychotherapy and clinical psychology. *European Journal of Psychotherapy and Counselling, 15*(2), 151–162.

Thanissaro, B. (1997a). Sallatha Sutta: The arrow. *Samyutta Nikaya*. Retrieved from http://www.accesstoinsight.org/tipitaka/sn/sn36/sn36.006.than.html

Thanissaro, B. (1997b). Simsapa Sutta: The Simsapa Leaves SN 56.31. *Samyutta Nikaya*. Retrieved from http://www.accesstoinsight.org/tipitaka/sn/sn56/sn56.031.than.html

Thanissaro, B. (1998). Cula-Malunkyovada Sutta: The shorter instructions to Malunkya. Retrieved from http://www.accesstoinsight.org/tipitaka/mn/mn.063.than.html

Thanissaro, B. (2004). Alagaddupama Sutta: The Water-Snake Simile. Retrieved from http://www.accesstoinsight.org/tipitaka/mn/mn.022.than.html

Thanissaro, B. (2012). *Right mindfulness: Memory and ardency on the Buddhist path.*

Tirch, D., Silberstein, L., & Kolts, R. (2016). *Buddhist psychology and cognitive-behavioral therapy: A clinician's guide*. New York: The Guilford Press.

Titmuss, C. (2013). The Buddha of mindfulness. The politics of mindfulness. http://christophertitmuss.org/blog/?p=1454. Retrieved from http://www.christophertitmuss.org/

Tjeltveit, A. C. (1999). *Ethics and values in psychotherapy*. London: Routledge.

Tronto, J. C. (1993). *Moral Boundaries: A political argument for an ethic of care*. New York: Routledge.

Tuske, J. (2013). The non-self theory and problems in philosophy of mind. In S. M. Emmanuel (Ed.), *A companion to Buddhist philosophy*. Chicehester, West Sussex: Wiley.

van Aalderen, J. R., Breukers, W. J., Reuzel, R. P. B., & Speckens, A. E. M. (2014). The role of the teacher in mindfulness-based approaches: A qualitative study. *Mindfulness, 5*, 170–178.

Van Gordon, W., Shonin, E., & Griffiths, M. (2015). Towards a second generation of mindfulness-based interventions. *Australian & New Zealand Joyrnal of Psychiatry, 49*(7), 591–592. https://doi.org/10.1177/0004867415577437

van Nistelrooij, I., Schaafsma, P., & Tronto, J. C. (2014). Ricoeur and the ethics of care. *Medical Health Care and Philosophy, 17*, 485–491.

Varela, F., Thompson, E., & Rosch, E. (2017). *The embodied mind: Cognitive science and human experience* (2nd ed.). Cambridge MA: MIT Press.

Walker, M. U. (2007). *Moral understandings: A feminist study in ethics*. New York: Oxford University Press.

Whitehill, J. (2000). Buddhism and the Virtues. In D. Keown (Ed.), *Contemporary Buddhist Ethics*. London: Routledge Curzon.

Williams, J. M., & Kabat-Zinn, J. (2013). *Mindfulness: Diverse perspectives on its meaning, origins and applications*. New York: Routledge.

Chapter 9
Promoting the Ethics of Care
in a Mindfulness-Based Program for Teachers

Patricia A. Jennings and Anthony A. DeMauro

A number of scholars (e.g., Monteiro, Musten, & Compson, 2015; Purser & Loy, 2013) have raised concerns about the absence of ethics in contemporary mindfulness-based interventions (MBIs). They fear that without including ethics as a component of mindfulness, MBIs might wrongly decontextualize and misappropriate many Buddhist values and traditions from which mindfulness originated and limit the scope of mindfulness to mere stress management. These scholars argue that such an approach may be problematic because MBIs may be misused to advance oppressive agendas—for example, corporations might exploit employees, but provide them with mindfulness training to help them tolerate being overworked. However, grounding MBIs in ethical frameworks may mitigate many of these threats by promoting ethical principles such as non-harm, alleviation of suffering, and moral virtue. Some MBIs draw upon the Buddhist ethical/moral frameworks that originally informed the mindfulness movement; although, many MBIs operate in settings where religious/spiritual references are prohibited, and as a result must solely rely on secular ethics. Monteiro et al. (2015) argue that MBIs do not need to ascribe to strictly religious ethical frameworks, and that non-faith-based ethics can guide MBIs if they are rooted in universal concepts of "moral responsibility, courage, expectations, and action" (p. 10).

Cultivating Awareness and Resilience in Education (CARE for Teachers) is one such MBI that is rooted in secular ethics, as it typically operates in US public schools (Jennings, 2016b). CARE for Teachers is a professional development program designed to build teachers' social and emotional competence and improve the quality of their learning environments (Jennings, 2016a). Combining emotion skills training, mindful awareness practices, and compassion/caring activities, CARE for

---

P.A. Jennings, PhD (✉) • A.A. DeMauro, PhD
CISE Department, Curry School of Education, University of Virginia,
PO Box 400273, 206D Bavaro Hall, Charlottesville, VA 22904, USA
e-mail: tishjennings@virginia.edu

© Springer International Publishing AG 2017   229
L.M. Monteiro et al. (eds.), *Practitioner's Guide to Ethics and Mindfulness-Based Interventions*, Mindfulness in Behavioral Health,
DOI 10.1007/978-3-319-64924-5_9

Teachers aims to foster the skills and dispositions K-12 teachers need to create supportive learning environments, while maintaining their well-being and love of teaching. CARE is an evidenced-based program shown to improve aspects of teachers' intrapersonal experiences such as mindfulness, efficacy, and emotion regulation, as well as interpersonal dimensions of their teaching practice, including their ability to create a positive classroom climate, be sensitive and responsive to students' needs, and sustain productive learning activities (Jennings, Frank, Snowberg, Coccia, & Greenberg, 2013; Jennings et al., 2017).

It is important to reiterate that CARE for Teachers is a strictly secular program, due to federal regulations regarding the separation of church and state and the restriction on promoting religious/spiritual teachings in public schools. Therefore, CARE for Teachers is rooted in various nonsectarian ethical traditions such as professional ethics for educators and Noddings' (2013) ethics of care. The ethics of care is particularly prominent in CARE for Teachers and will be discussed in more depth throughout the current chapter. The purpose of the chapter is to provide an example of how a strictly secular ethical framework, Noddings' ethics of care, can guide a MBI to promote ethical behavior in teachers. In the discussion of mindfulness and ethics, CARE for Teachers is a particularly illustrative case to examine because it operates in a highly ethics-laden and secular context.

The importance of ethics in teaching cannot be understated, as teaching is a highly interpersonal endeavor involving distinct power dynamics, where the outcomes of teaching have significant long-term consequences for many stakeholders (i.e., teachers, students, parents, administrators, the general public). In most cases, particularly for those working in public school settings, the ethics of teaching must be devoid of any religious/spiritual ethical dimensions. So, the ethics that explicitly guide the field are of a more universal nature and generally relate to responsibility to others and not causing harm. In the following chapter we will offer Noddings' ethics of care as a particularly useful framework for MBIs in the context of teaching and demonstrate how the ethics of care informs the CARE for Teachers program.

Professional Ethics in Education

Professional organizations like the National Education Association (NEA, 2016) and Association of American Educators (AAE, 2016) have published codes of ethics to outline basic principles, or the do's and don'ts, of ethical behavior for educators. Both NEA and AAE codes begin with a commitment to students—which includes taking responsibility for the learning and development of the student while not intentionally hindering students' learning, freedoms, or fulfillment of their potential. Both codes also contain principles related to maintaining the dignity of the teaching profession, which involves meeting professional qualifications and promoting national trust in educators. The AAE code additionally provides more specific principles regarding ethical treatment of colleagues, as well as parents and the communities that educators serve. There is a good deal of overlap between the two codes revolving around standards of responsibility and accountability for others and the profession as a whole.

In the scholarly literature on the ethics of teachers/educators, however, there is much less alignment. There is no one widely agreed upon code of ethics for teachers among researchers and educational scholars, and much of the work to date reflects diverse theoretical perspectives, each with its own underlying assumptions and principals. For example, in a review of the literature on ethics in education, Campbell (2008) distinguished between theories of virtue, responsibility and duty, caring, moral development, social justice, and applied practical ethics. Each approach is grounded in diverse philosophical orientations and thus holds varying rationales and ideals for ethical behavior. It is not in the purview of the current chapter to discuss each theory in depth, but to outline how one mindfulness-based program for teachers utilizes secular ethics. Noddings' (2013) theory of the ethics of care aligns particularly well with this chapter's mindfulness-based approach to teacher professional development and will thus be used as a theoretical framework for the discussion of CARE for Teachers.

Noddings' Ethics of Care

Noddings' (2013) ethics of care describes the characteristics and processes involved in healthy caring relationships. The theory draws upon a variety of caring dynamics including parent–child, friend–friend, teacher–student, etc., but highlights the underlying attitudes and behaviors that support ideal caring across all contexts. Being a relational process, caring requires at least two persons or entities (animals, plants, things, and ideas are also included in the theory), where Noddings labels the caregiver as "the one-caring" and the recipient of care to be "the cared-for."

The Relational Process From the perspective of the one-caring, caring involves both receptivity and motivation. Receptivity involves a state of attentiveness toward the cared-for and requires noticing that something is wrong or needs addressing (Noddings, 1996, 2012, 2013). Receptivity also involves "feel[ing] with the other," or what Noddings calls "engrossment" (2013, p. 30), but it is different from the western concept of empathy. Noddings states, "I do not 'put myself in the other's shoes,' so to speak, by analyzing his reality as objective data and then asking, 'How would I feel in such a situation?'" (p. 30). Rather, the one-caring truly feels the other's experience and shares it with them, as opposed to projecting one's own thoughts and feelings onto another's situation. Then, there is a motivational shift in the one-caring, or a call-to-action. The one-caring has a sense that, "I must do something" (p. 14) and directs her energy toward the cared-for to relieve pain, meet the needs of the cared-for, or foster progress toward a goal. The one-caring's energy moves in the direction of the other, which provides the cared-for a certain strength and hope.

The role of the cared-for is to show that the caring has been received by responding positively to the caring with a smile or nod, or to begin to take on the problem with a new energy. The cared-for's response completes the caring transaction. Without it, true caring has not occurred because caring is a strictly relational process. The cared-for's response also provides information to the one-caring in evaluating the impact of her efforts.

The Ethical Ideal There are many relations, such as mother–child, where caring occurs quite naturally and effortlessly, and would not be considered ethical nor moral behavior. However, the experience of natural caring is a key part of Noddings' (2013) ethics framework because repeated experiences of giving and receiving natural caring form memories of genuine care. These memories along with a desire to re-experience one's most caring moments create for each person a vision of goodness and the best picture of oneself—"the ethical ideal" (p. 49). One embodies the ethical ideal when one receives and accepts the "I must" feeling, and directs one's energy toward caring for the other. The call to care for another may at times conflict with one's own self-interests, and caring may require some effort; but in this effort one finds the *ethical* dimension of caring. "The source of ethical behavior is, then, in twin sentiments—one that feels directly for the other and one that feels for and with the best self…. It is our best picture of ourselves caring and being cared for" (p. 80). It is this remembering of one's most caring moments and the vision of the best self which ignites one's desire to care while guiding one's efforts to serve the other.

Constructing the ethical ideal also involves understanding humanity's need for relatedness and committing to openly receive others; although, the commitment to receive and care for others is not everlasting and must be nurtured. Noddings proposes the ethical ideal can be nurtured through listening, dialogue, and attributing others' behavior to their best possible motives. Ones-caring can also maintain the ethical ideal from within by celebrating everyday experiences of life, even such repetitive activities as cooking, eating, or gardening. Lastly, one's ethical ideal can be enhanced through experiences of joy. Each of these ways of constructing, nurturing, maintaining, and enhancing the ethical ideal will be discussed in more detail later in the chapter, along with a description of how CARE for Teachers contributes to each.

Teacher Stress and Ethics

There are a number of forces that can thwart the ethics of caring, and two that are particularly challenging for teachers are occupational stress and burnout. Teacher stress is currently a major concern in educational systems across the world (Aloe, Amo, & Shanahan, 2014; Greenberg, Brown, & Abenavoli, 2016; Kyriacou, 2001), and research indicates teaching to be among the most stressful occupations, with comparable levels of stress to nurses, physicians, police officers, and ambulance workers (Gallup, 2014; Johnson et al., 2005). Evidence suggests teacher stress is increasing, as ratings of stress and job satisfaction have dramatically changed over the last 30 years. In a nationally representative sample of K-12 teachers, 51% reported being under great stress several days per week, up from 36% in 1985 (Markow, Macia, & Lee, 2013). In the same survey, teachers' job satisfaction was at 39%, its lowest point in 25 years, and a drop of 23% points since 2008. Common sources of stress for teachers include lack of support in meeting the diverse needs of all students, having to take work home due to an overload of responsibilities, limited control in making school decisions, minimal time to relax during the day, trying to motivate difficult to reach students, and pressures of accountability (Richards, 2012).

Exposure to repeated stress over time leads to burnout (Bellingrath, Weigl, & Kudielka, 2009; Blasé, 1982; Fisher, 2011), which is conceptualized as involving three dimensions: emotional exhaustion, depersonalization, and lack of personal accomplishment (Maslach, 1976; Maslach, Schaufeli, & Leiter, 2001). According to Jennings and Greenberg (2009), teacher stress can trigger a "burnout cascade" (p. 492) whereby emotional exhaustion leads to depersonalization and finally a lack of personal accomplishment, when teachers often leave the profession. Emotional exhaustion is characterized by feelings of fatigue after repeatedly experiencing difficult emotions such as frustration and anger (Maslach, 1976). An emotionally exhausted person typically feels completely drained of physical and emotional resources at the end of the workday. Emotional exhaustion leads to depersonalization, or a certain detachment from those one works with. Depersonalization can include feelings of callousness, cynicism, and irritability toward others. In addition to losing a feeling of connection with others, one can also result in a feeling of lost connection to one's work and feelings of inadequacy and inefficacy (or a lack of personal accomplishment). This is the inability to find success in one's work or see one's efforts as meaningful contributions to a larger goal. Experiences of stress and burnout in teachers have been related to physical health risks (Bellingrath, Rohleder, & Kudiclka, 2010; Bellingrath et al., 2009; Katz, Greenberg, Jennings, & Klein, 2016) as well as teacher attrition (Chang, 2009; Fisher, 2011; Schaefer, Long, & Clandinin, 2012).

Noddings (2013) was keenly aware of the threat posed by experiences of stress and burnout to teachers' abilities to maintain their ethics of caring.

> It is certainly true that the "I must" can be rejected and, of course, it can grow quieter under the stress of living. I can talk myself out of the "I must," detach myself from feeling and try to think my way to an ethical life (p. 49).

The "I must" or the motivation to care for another can diminish under stressful circumstances, and experiences of emotional exhaustion and depersonalization can be particularly damaging to the caring relation between teachers and students. The caring relation depends on the teacher to "feel with" the student, in a way vicariously experiencing difficult emotions of the student. Emotional exhaustion, however, depletes one's emotional resources, to the point of feeling a certain emotional numbing (Maslach, 2003). This can prevent teachers from really feeling with their students' emotions. Not only does this distort teachers' perceptions of their students' needs by potentially misinterpreting experiences of suffering, but it can also suppress teachers' motivation to care. Feeling the student's difficult emotions triggers the "I must" feeling in the teacher, and as Noddings (2013) noted, the "I must" can grow quieter in stressful circumstances. The teacher might also "detach" from her students, avoiding, denying, or becoming numb to their emotions, and no longer be able to "feel with" her students. This process of depersonalization is a dysfunctional coping strategy: a means of protection for the teacher, an effort to halt the perceived drain of emotional resources. Although, it is antithetical to the process of "engrossment" required for caring. In depersonalization, the burned-out teacher begins to dehumanize her students, treating them as objects or cogs in a wheel so that she can invest fewer emotional resources into her relationships with them. It is important to stress that this process is simply a dysfunctional mechanism to cope with the repeated stress and emotional exhaustion. If the teacher avoids forming deep relationships with her students, she is less likely to feel with their suffering and avoids further depletion of her own emotional energy. Feeling with her students is the first step in the caring process, and true caring, by Noddings's definition, cannot occur in a teacher experiencing depersonalization.

There are a number of ways teacher stress and burnout can negatively impact students. Students with teachers experiencing burnout show disruptions in diurnal cortisol patterns, a physiological indicator of stress (Oberle & Schonert-Reichl, 2016), and students with teachers reporting greater levels of stress had higher internalizing and externalizing disorders (Milkie & Warner, 2011). Finally, teacher depression may be significantly related to deficits in classroom interaction quality (Jennings, 2015a). Thus, teacher stress and burnout is not a strictly intrapersonal problem, but can have negative impacts on students as well. Noddings (2013) repeatedly describes caring as a reciprocal process, and evidence is beginning to demonstrate the far-reaching consequences of teacher burnout. It is possible that a lack of caring, triggered by burnout, is involved in the deterioration of both teacher and student well-being.

To summarize, teacher burnout can hinder the ethics of caring and attainment of the ethical ideal when teachers no longer have the emotional resources to invest in caring for their students. However, this is not an inevitable reality of teaching. For one, not all teachers experience burnout. Additionally, even for teachers working in stressful settings at greater risk for burnout, there exist more adaptive coping mechanisms and ways of replenishing emotional resources to avoid emotional exhaustion and depersonalization. Noddings (2013) offers that protection from burnout can come through practice of self-care, support from others, and finding ways to reconnect with the source of caring—oneself.

> The one-caring must be maintained, for she is the immediate source of caring. The one-caring, then, properly pays heed to her own condition. She does not need to hatch out elaborate excuses to give herself rest, or to seek congenial companionship, or to find joy in personal work. Everything depends on the strength and beauty of her ideal, and it is an integral part of her. To go on sacrificing bitterly, grudgingly, is not to be one-caring and, when she finds this happening, she properly but considerately withdraws and repairs. When she is prevented by circumstances from doing this, she may still recognize what is occurring and make heroic efforts to sustain herself as one-caring. Some are stronger than others, but each has her breaking point. (Noddings, 2013, p. 105)

The one-caring cannot simply push through the feelings of burnout, as she will eventually reach a breaking point. Rather, she must intentionally make efforts to care for herself and replenish her resources. For Noddings, self-care is a critical piece in the caring relation, and ones-caring need no excuse for self-care. Connection with close others and finding joy in one's work are further ways the one-caring can care for herself. Practicing self-care is the foundational element of the CARE for Teachers program and is interwoven into all aspects of the training.

The following sections will introduce the intervention models underlying the CARE for Teachers theory of change. The CARE for Teachers components will be described and related to the cultivation of self-care and care for others in relation to Noddings' ethics of care.

Prosocial Classroom Model

Jennings and Greenberg (2009) articulated the prosocial classroom theoretical model proposing that certain social and emotional competencies are required to enable teachers to cope with the demands of teaching and to prevent burnout (see Fig. 9.1). These competencies include self-awareness of emotional states and cognitions and the ability to effectively regulate what are sometimes strong emotions while teaching. In this way, teachers can appropriately respond to students' needs while maintaining emotional energy and thereby preventing the emotional exhaustion associated with burnout. When teachers lack these social and emotional

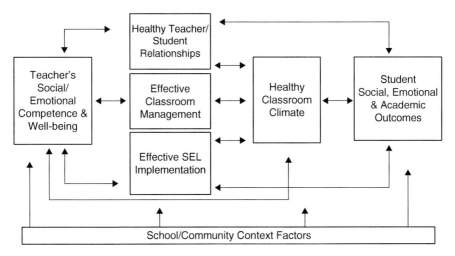

Fig. 9.1 A model of teacher well-being and social and emotional competence; and support and classroom and student outcomes. From: Jennings and Greenberg (2009). The Prosocial classroom: Teacher social and emotional competence in relation to student and classroom outcomes. *Review of Educational Research, 79*, 491–525. Reprinted with permission from SAGE Publications, Inc

competencies their well-being erodes, leading to a deterioration of the classroom climate and increase in teacher stress, triggering the "burnout cascade" (p. 492) mentioned above. In contrast, teachers with high levels of these social and emotional competencies can cope with the demands of the classroom, build and maintain a positive classroom climate, supportive relationships with their students, and consistent classroom interactions that promote student learning.

The CARE for Teachers Logic Model

Based upon the prosocial classroom model, CARE for Teachers is a comprehensive professional development program for teachers specifically designed to address teachers' social and emotional competencies as articulated in the CARE for Teachers logic model (Fig. 9.2). The CARE for Teachers program elements of emotion skills instruction, mindful awareness and stress reduction practices, and caring and listening practices are designed to promote reductions in psychological and physical distress, as well as improvements in adaptive emotion regulation, teaching efficacy, mindfulness, and classroom interactions that promote learning (e.g., emotional support and classroom organization). This model has been tested and refined in several studies (Jennings, Snowberg, Coccia, & Greenberg, 2011, Jennings et al., 2013, Jennings et al., 2017).

CARE for Teachers was developed in accordance with best practices in adult learning. Material is introduced sequentially, applying a blend of didactic, experiential, and interactive learning activities. While the CARE for Teachers program does

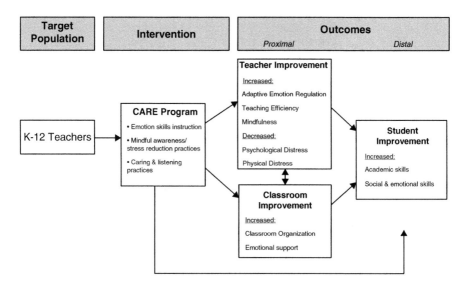

Fig. 9.2 The CARE for Teachers logic model

not explicitly advocate or teach the ethics of care, they are implied and embedded throughout the training in the form of various practices that assume that teachers bring to the program their deep commitment to caring for students based in values to promote learning, reduce suffering, and do no harm. The practices are intended to help teachers clarify the ethical basis of their profession for themselves and to provide opportunities for them to more consciously align their behavior with their ideals through the integration of mindful awareness practices (MAP) and emotion skills training. CARE for Teachers presents MAPs including breath awareness practice, mindful walking, listening and compassion practices, and didactic and experiential activities designed to promote emotion awareness and emotion regulation (see Jennings, 2016a for more extensive descriptions of the CARE for Teachers program model).

CARE for Teachers is typically delivered in 30 h over five in-person training days (6 h each) across the school year. The first two training days are offered consecutively and then two training days are offered over the course of several weeks. A booster session is offered 1 month later. The breaks in between sessions provide teachers with the opportunity to practice, reflect, and apply the material to their experience teaching and participants receive coaching by phone to support these processes. Participants receive a program workbook and an audio CD/MP3 of recorded mindful awareness practices for home practice.

Next, we describe program elements and activities in more detail and discuss how they support Noddings's ethics of care.

CARE for Teachers Program Components

Intention Setting or Renewing Commitment Noddings (2013) reminds us:

> I must make a commitment to act. The commitment to act in behalf of the cared-for, a continued interest in his reality throughout the appropriate time span, and the continual renewal of commitment over the span of time are the essential elements of caring from the inner view (p. 16).

A core component of CARE for Teachers is the intention-setting practice, which is a way to renew one's commitment to care on a regular basis. The intention-setting practice is intended to explicitly link teachers' own ethics and commitment to care in relation to their work by applying the program material to more consciously and consistently align their behavior with their ethics. To introduce the practice, participants are invited to reflect upon why they became a teacher and what values they hold that motivated them to choose this profession. Participants are invited to share their reflections in small group discussions. Typically, participants share the love they have for children and how they wanted to make a difference in their students' lives. They also share how they felt like their jobs had meaning for them, that they have the opportunity to make a valuable contribution to society. The next step in the process is to invite the participants to cultivate a vision for the world and for their schools and classrooms more specifically, e.g., "what does their classroom look like when they are their best?" Intention setting is described as a tool for aligning one's actions with this vision of one's "best self," what Noddings refers to as the ethical ideal. An intention is different than a goal in that it is an ongoing process rather than an end point. An intention does not have the tension or edge one feels when setting a goal; if she fails to reach the goal, she may feel like a failure. When she sets an intention, she clarifies her orientation toward becoming her best self and can use her intention as a guide, like a personal GPS, to keep herself on track. Then participants are invited to consider an intention for one particular day. Silently they are invited to use imagination or words to set their intention. They can direct their attention to imagining themselves behaving in alignment with this intention, or focus on words that describe the intention for a few minutes. Once the intention setting is completed, participants are invited to share their intentions with one another and/or to find an "intention buddy" to provide support to one another. They are encouraged to check in from time to time to see whether or not they are "on course" and to realign their behavior, or modify their intention accordingly. The intention-setting practice is introduced on the first day of training and is practiced at the beginning of each training segment, after a simple practice of mindfully taking three, deep diaphragmatic breaths to bring their attention to the present.

In this way, CARE for Teachers supports teachers' ability to hold the vision of their best caring self, their ethical ideals, as Noddings (2013) describes:

> As my receiving the other enables the "I must" to arise with respect to the other, so receiving the vision of what I might be enables the "I must" to arise with respect to the ethical self. I see what I might be, and I see also that *this* vision of what I might be is the genuine product of caring. I shall require that the ethical ideal be—in a way I must describe—realistic, attainable (p. 50).

As intentions are constantly revisited throughout the program, participants' visions of their ethical ideals frame all of their learning experiences. Teachers are also given recommendations for how to set intentions once they return to the classroom so that their best visions of themselves can constantly inform their teaching practice.

Self-care The CARE for Teachers program is based upon the understanding that to be an effective "carer" one must care for oneself. As Noddings (2013) noted, "The one-caring must be maintained, for she is the immediate source of caring (p. 105)." One of the first activities in the CARE for Teachers program involves participants completing a self-assessment of their daily activities, examining how much time they spend doing something primarily for self or other(s), how much they enjoy each activity, and how the activity might nurture their physical, emotional, psychological, or spiritual growth and development. Participants are encouraged to consider gaps in their current self-care and to think about ways to provide themselves with a more balanced set of self-care activities or practices in a way that works best for each individual. Part of the program involves creating a plan for self-care that may incorporate the MAPs and other activities such as reflective writing into their daily regimen. CARE for Teachers also emphasizes that teachers should not feel guilty in taking the time for self-care because without caring for themselves, they may not have the resources to care for others. This also aligns with Noddings' argument that ones-caring need no excuse for self-care, as it is essential to maintaining the ethical ideal.

Basic MAPs The CARE for Teachers program presents opportunities for instruction and practice of a variety of basic, secular MAPs. Mindfulness is introduced as a state of awareness, a trait, and a practice. The intention is to build the understanding that the aim of the practices is to be more mindful each moment of their day and that they can build this capacity with both formal and informal practices. They learn basic breath awareness practice, involving focusing one's attention on the sensation of the breath, noticing when they become distracted and their mind wanders, and then bringing the attention back to the breath. Depending upon the experience level of the participants, practices can range from 10–15 min at first and up to 20 min later in the program. Participants are encouraged to notice while they are practicing what thoughts or feelings have captured their attention before they return their attention back to the breath. The intention is to become more aware of habits of mind and emotion and to promote what have called *decentering*, the recognition that "I am not my thoughts and feelings" (Fresco, Segal, Buis, & Kennedy, 2007).

Several MAPs are introduced to promote awareness of the body and to support sense of being grounded in the body. Body awareness can help one recognize emotional reactivity, even when it's subtle. For example, some people clench their jaws when they are starting to become frustrated and the more awareness they have of this tendency when it is occurring, the more likely they are to be able to manage their emotional reactivity before it becomes so intense that it's more difficult to manage. A practice called *centering* is introduced early in the program. This practice involves standing with the feet parallel and focusing attention on the weight of the body on the floor through the soles of the feet and also on the anatomical center of gravity of the body, located in the lower abdomen and imagining that this center is connected to the center of the earth. Participants learn mindful walking where they are instructed to focus their attention on the sensation of the weight on their feet and it shifts from the heel, to the ball, and to the toe of the foot. Again, when they find their mind wandering, they are instructed to bring their attention back to the sensation of the weight on their feet. CARE for Teachers also introduces a version of the body scan. Participants are invited to practice either sitting or lying down. They are guided through a practice of focusing their attention on each part of their body, noticing sensations. Participants also learn a number of informal mindful awareness practices, such as mindful eating, as a way of cultivating mindful awareness during everyday experiences.

While Noddings (2013) never explicitly discusses mindfulness or mindful awareness practices, her work often echoes many related themes such as present moment awareness and beginners' mind. In describing how ones-caring nurtures the ethical ideal, she describes celebrating everyday experiences: "The one-caring chooses to celebrate the ordinary, human-animal life that is the source of her ethicality and joy… Thus repetition is not mere repetition, leading to boredom and disgust, but it represents opportunities to learn, to share, and to celebrate" (p. 125). She explains how ones-caring can find great pleasure in activities like walking, cooking, or gardening as a way to nurture oneself. Throughout CARE for Teachers, participants are encouraged to engage in informal mindfulness practices such as noticing how they feel when talking or listening, when enacting a role play, and when eating. They are encouraged to build informal practices into their self-care plans in order to find moments of joy and rejuvenation throughout their everyday lives.

Compassion Practices Similar with Noddings's conception of care as involving a process of receptivity, motivation, and action, the CARE for Teachers program defines compassion as the capacity to attend to the experience of others, to feel concern for them, to sense into what will really serve, and then to be in service, the best one is able (Halifax, 2014). According to this definition, compassion requires attunement, similar to Noddings's (2013) concept of *engrossment*:

> When my caring is directed to living things, I must consider their natures, ways of life, needs, and desires. And, although I can never accomplish it entirely, I try to apprehend the reality of the other. This is the fundamental aspect of caring from the inside. When I look at and think about how I am when I care, I realize that there is invariably this displacement of interest from my own reality to the reality of the other…I must see the other's reality as a possibility for my own (p. 14).

The definition also aligns with Noddings's motive to act:

> We also have aroused in us a feeling, "I must do something." When we see the other's reality as a possibility for us, we must act to eliminate the intolerable, to reduce the pain, to fill the need, to actualize the dream (Noddings, 2013, p. 14)

The CARE for Teachers program introduces a series of practices designed to promote care and compassion for self and others. The first of the series invites participants to remember a time when they felt loved or cared for and to imagine themselves at that time. While they do this, they are encouraged to explore the sensations in their body that they feel when they are feeling loved and cared for. The next practice is a secular adaptation of the traditional loving-kindness (or *metta*) practice that is called *caring practice*. This practice involves offering feelings and well-wishes of well-being, happiness, and peace to oneself, to a dear loved one, to a neutral person, and to a person for whom one has difficult feelings. The facilitator guides the practitioner through each of these steps suggesting either holding the person (or self) in the mind's eye and silently repeating the phrase, "May you enjoy well-being, happiness, and peace." Or alternatively, imagining the person (or oneself) being well, happy, and peaceful. Later in the program, participants explore positive or "pleasant" emotions such as happiness and gratitude through guided practices of accessing memory in order to build the capacity to recognize and re-experience these emotions when they need them to build resilience and to strengthen their emotional capacity, a means to prevent emotional exhaustion and burnout (Cohn, Brown, Fredrickson, Milkels, & Conway, 2009).

Listening and Dialogue

> Listening is the oldest and perhaps the most powerful tool of healing. It is often through the quality of our listening and not the wisdom of our words that we are able to effect the most profound changes in the people around us. When we listen, we offer with our attention an opportunity for wholeness. Our listening creates sanctuary for the homeless parts within the other person. (Remen, 2006, p. 219)

According to Noddings (2013), listening plays a critical role in receiving the cared-for. Often teachers are trained to be *active listeners* whereby they demonstrate that they understand what the other is saying by nodding and making confirmational statements. However, this approach to listening can interfere with the listening process because the active listener spends a great deal of energy trying to express understanding, that they may not be fully present for the listening experience. During the program, CARE for Teachers participants often make comment such as, "I realized how much time I spend preparing for what I'm going to say, rather than actually listening."

Mindful listening is an integral part of CARE for Teachers. The intention of the practice is to bring one's full openhearted and accepting presence to the act of simple listening, which can include noticing thoughts and feelings that may be triggered in the process. The program includes a sequence of listening activities intended to cultivate the ability to listen mindfully, but to also attend to one's experience while speaking, noticing one's comfort or discomfort, thoughts and feelings associated with telling a mindful listener something. This practice often begins with participants choosing a poem they like from an offered selection. They find a partner and the instructions are to begin by gathering their attention by taking several mindful breaths, then the reader reads the poem to the listener. It is recommended that the reader and listener do not look at one another so that the facial expressions do not interfere with the simple act of speaking and listening. The listener is invited to hold an openhearted and accepting space for the speaker. The speaker is invited to offer themselves the same acceptance and notice thoughts and feelings as they read their poem. After the reader has read the poem once, the pair sits quietly for a moment, noticing how they feel. Then the reader reads the poem a second time following the same instructions. After the second reading is completed, the pair is invited to take a moment to notice how they feel again and then answer some reflection questions in their workbooks. Once they are finished reflecting, they trade places and complete the process. After the second session is completed and they have finished their private reflections, they are invited to discuss the experience with their partner. Often participants share that listening this way can feel uncomfortable at first because they are not engaging in their normal active listening. With practice, many realize how often they are not really listening, even when they think they are. The listeners often notice a heightened sensation of the other's emotional tone. Speakers often share that it feels comforting to speak without worrying about the social niceties of social conversation, and how deeply they felt heard. Others also feel that the exercise is somewhat uncomfortable because they do not get feedback. In either case, participants learn to bring more awareness to their speaking and listening which can help them attune to others, which can support their ability to care.

The beginning listening practice sets a standard of listening and discussion practiced throughout the rest of the program. Participants are encouraged to give one another space when talking by allowing for pauses and silences between thoughts. After this beginning practice, the program offers a series of listening practices involving noticing thoughts and feelings of both speakers and listeners, while one is talking about situations that are challenging and elicit difficult emotions. Participants learn to recognize the subtleties of emotional patterns that they may have developed to cope with the emotional demands of teaching. In this process, as they begin to recognize these patterns, they can shift their behavior toward engaging in more effective and healthful coping processes.

Later in the program, the listening and compassion practices merge into role play practices where participants are invited to enact a challenging experience from the past to begin to better understand their reaction to that experience and to apply CARE for Teachers skills to developing a more effective and compassionate response to similar situations in the future. This small group activity involves inviting a participant to think about a classroom situation that was emotionally challenging and to coach her group members to play the roles of the other people in the scenario, which can be students, colleagues, or parents. Once everyone understands their role, the role play is performed twice. The first time it is enacted as it unfolded in the past. After the first run, all the participants reflect in writing on how they felt and what they experienced. Then the group discusses this and the protagonist (teacher) decides what CARE for Teachers skills she will use to respond to the situation, rather than reacting automatically. Then the role play is performed a second time with the teacher using the CARE for Teachers skills. The group again reflects in writing and then discusses how they felt this time. Often there is a dramatic change in the way the teacher and the other cast members feel and experience the situation. Participants often recognize emotional patterns or "scripts" about the situation that triggered the emotional reaction and how the CARE for Teachers skills helped them recognize the script and set it aside so they could be more supportive to the needs of the other.

Noddings (2013) urges, "Listening, that supremely important form of receiving, is essential" (p. 121). Listening allows the one-caring to truly understand the cared-for's dilemma, feelings, and needs, and through a sequence of mindful listening exercises, CARE for Teachers participants learn how to listen more receptively to others.

Emotion Skills Instruction CARE for Teachers introduces a series of mini-lectures and experiential exercises focused on helping participants understand the nature of emotional experience and how it affects teaching and learning. Participants learn about the fight-flight-freeze response including the role of the brain and body in the process. They learn about the role of the prefrontal cortex in higher-order executive processes and self-regulation and how strong emotional reactivity can interfere with these brain processes, which are critical to learning. They learn about emotional triggers and scripts and how to recognize the bodily signals or physical sensations that arise at the beginning of emotional arousal. Most importantly, they learn that all emotions, even so-called "negative" emotions, are necessary and useful. In CARE for Teachers, we explain that when describing positive emotions, such as joy, gratitude, and enthusiasm, we like to use the words "comfortable" or "pleasant" rather than "positive" and for negative emotions such as anger, fear, and sadness, we like to use the words "uncomfortable" or "unpleasant." We make this distinction because the negative and positive terms imply that negative emotions are bad and positive emotions are good. It is our intention to clarify that all emotional experience results from natural, biological processes that evolved to help us adapt to situations of threat. In this way, we want to honor all emotional experience and learn from it, rather than to judge, suppress, or dismiss it.

Teachers learn that uncomfortable or unpleasant emotions are adaptive biological functions that arise under predictable situations. For example, anger typically arises when we feel that our goals are thwarted, when we feel attacked, or when we feel that an ethical norm has been broken. The physical reaction associated with anger prepares us to fight. Teachers learn the common physical sensations associated with the rise of anger, such as tension in the jaw, shoulders, and fists. This tension signals the body's preparation to fight. Cognitive processes are also affected. Attention is narrowed to center on the perceived threat and often higher-order cognitive processes are impaired. This reaction arises whether we are actually physically threatened or only psychologically threatened. While the reaction is adaptive when we are physically threatened, it is not adaptive under situations of psychological threat because the impaired cognitive functioning interferes with thoughtful consideration, planning, and good decision-making. Participants learn that they can apply mindful awareness to recognizing the early signals of emotional reactivity and to use deep mindful breathing to calm themselves so they can respond thoughtfully rather than react unconsciously.

Noddings (2013) explains why self-awareness and emotional awareness more specifically are critical to the caring process:

> When we honestly accept our loves, our innate ferocity, our capacity to hate, we may use all this information in building the safeguards and alarms that must be part of the ideal. We know better what we must work toward, what we must prevent, and the conditions under which we are lost as ones-caring. Instead of hiding from our natural impulses and pretending that we can achieve goodness through lofty abstractions, we accept what is there—all of it—and use what we have already assessed as good to control that which is not. (p. 100)

Similar to CARE for Teachers, Noddings does not reject the uncomfortable emotions like ferocity and hate, but underscores the need to have deep familiarity with them so that they do not subdue the ethical ideal. The uncomfortable emotions are merely innate reactions humans have to threatening situations, and by respecting and recognizing the full range of emotional experiences, participants are better equipped to regulate them. When teachers begin to understand their emotional experience, patterns, and scripts, they begin to better understand their emotional reactivity that sometimes interferes with their ability to provide care for their students and that may eventually result in emotional exhaustion and burnout.

For example, one teacher in a CARE for Teachers program was having a difficult time with a second-grade student who was coming to class late every day. When she would arrive, often 30–60 min late, the teacher immediately felt anger and the student would respond by giggling. The teacher tried punishing her with time-out but the girl would continue to disrupt the class. During the training, this teacher realized that she had a script about being late that she learned from her childhood. As a child, she was punished severely for being late so she learned that being late is very bad and disrespectful. When this student turned up late every day, it automatically triggered this script and the associated anger. She then realized that she had never asked this child why she was late, so one day she did. She learned that this second grader had to get herself to school without any adult support because her single mother worked at night and was asleep in the morning. You can imagine how this information changed this teacher's perception and feelings toward this child. From then on, when she arrived, she welcomed her to class with a big smile. The girl's giggling, caused by deep embarrassment and shame, stopped and the student became more engaged. Over time, the student was able to come to school earlier and her classroom climate dramatically improved (from Jennings, 2015b). This is an excellent example of how the CARE for Teacher program is designed to support teachers' ability to behave according to their ethics of care. When they have greater self-awareness, and can regulate their emotions better, they can be their "best selves." Their classroom environments improve and their students flourish. This aligns with Noddings's (2013) understanding of the importance of perspective-taking: "The one caring receives the child and views his world through both sets of eyes… The one-caring assumes a dual perspective and can see things from both her own pole and that of the cared for" (p. 63). Noddings also poses that the ethical ideal is maintained when the one-caring sees the best possible motives as the source of the cared-for's actions. When teachers are better able to see events from the viewpoints of their students, they may be more likely to see that challenging behaviors, like the event of the student coming late to class, are a result of the students' own challenging experiences and not personal attacks on the teacher. Then they may be more likely to maintain the caring relationship and ethical ideal.

The CARE for Teachers program also introduces the adaptive functions of comfortable or pleasant emotions. Based upon Fredrickson's (2004) "broaden and build" theory, participants learn that "positive" emotions broaden our perspective, helping us recognize context and build relationships with individuals and groups by creating a sense of belongingness and connection. When teachers understand the power of comfortable emotions, they can skillfully use these emotions to enhance their classroom social and emotional climate. The participants are introduced to activities that provide opportunities for teachers to re-experience comfortable emotions, such as joy or happiness. Once the participant is feeling the emotion, they are encouraged to apply mindful awareness to deeply feel the physical sensations associated with this experience and to savor them. According to Fredrickson (2004), savoring emotions can build resilience to stress.

Noddings (2013), too, poses that the experience of joy can be a way of enhancing the ethical ideal. In addition to cultivating the ideal by finding joy in the everyday experiences of life, as described above, joy is also essential to the caring process because it can be experienced in relation to others. This certain form of receptive joy, what Noddings calls "joy-feeling," creates connectedness and harmony and is unique to the caring relation.

> Now I do not control this receptive joy. It comes to me. I cannot say, with any reasonable expectation of success, "I shall go sit on the front steps and be filled with joy," but I can increase the likelihood that joy will come to me. I can quit thinking and manipulating. I can be quiet, emptying consciousness of its thought-objects and, then, a receptive mood may take over… In "joy-feeling," we are receptive, spoken to, supplied with intention. (p. 140)

This final quote by Noddings again contains allusions of mindful awareness by setting aside the thinking and manipulating mind and opening to the experience of joy. CARE for Teachers includes specific exercises aimed at cultivating and savoring the experience of joy. These mindful awareness practices are valuable both as an end in themselves and to enhance teachers' ethical ideals by cultivating the joy-feeling with colleagues, as well as with their students once they return to the classroom.

In the following section of the chapter, we review the evidence that the CARE for Teachers program supports teachers' ethics of caring.

Efficacy of CARE for Teachers

Since 2009, the first author and her colleagues have been conducting a series of both quantitative and qualitative studies based upon the CARE for Teachers logic model to examine the efficacy of the CARE for Teachers program for promoting teachers' social and emotional competencies and their capacity to create and maintain a supportive learning environment for their students.

Quantitative Evidence Building upon a series of pilot studies that demonstrated the promise of CARE for Teachers to improve teachers' social and emotional competencies (Jennings et al., 2011, 2013), the most recent and most rigorous study to date suggests that CARE for Teachers may promote teachers' care ethic and enable them to provide better care to their students. Jennings et al., (2017) recruited 224 teachers from 36 elementary schools located in high-poverty regions of New York City. Teachers were randomly assigned within schools to receive the CARE for Teachers program or be in a waitlist control group. Teachers completed self-report questionnaires at baseline in the fall, before randomization, and then again in the spring, after the treatment group had received the CARE for Teachers program. Measures assessed teachers' adaptive emotion regulation, teaching efficacy, mindfulness, psychological distress, and time urgency (see Jennings et al., 2017, for more details regarding measurement model). At the same time points, teachers' classrooms were observed by a trained researcher blind to the teachers' assignment and the study aims. The researchers coded the classrooms using the *Classroom Assessment Scoring System* (CLASS; Pianta, La Paro, & Hamre, 2008), a well-validated and commonly used observational measure of classroom interaction quality that assesses emotional support, classroom organization, and instructional support. Results showed that compared to controls, teachers who participated in the CARE for Teachers program showed increases in self-reported adaptive emotion regulation and mindfulness and decreases in self-reported psychological distress and time urgency. There were no significant direct impacts on efficacy; however, at baseline teachers' efficacy scores were quite high, suggesting ceiling effects may have interfered with the measurement of efficacy. The interactions in the classrooms of the teachers who received the CARE for Teachers program were significantly more emotionally supportive. This was reflected by improvements in teacher sensitivity and positive emotional climate (two dimensions of the emotional support domain of the CLASS). The classrooms were also marginally improved on classroom organization reflected by significant improvements in productivity (one dimension of the classroom organization domain of the CLASS). These results demonstrate that the CARE for Teachers program improved the social and emotional competencies teachers require to cope with the demands of the classroom. This may have supported their ability to maintain their "ethical ideals" in the caring relationship allowing them to create and maintain a classroom environment that was more emotionally supportive and there was more productive use of time for learning. The results of this study are particularly notable because they are the first to show that a mindfulness-based intervention can have significant observable impacts on a social context.

Qualitative Evidence Two qualitative studies on the CARE for Teachers program have begun to shed light on the mechanisms of change involved in the quantitative outcomes. Schussler, Jennings, Sharp, and Frank (2016) conducted a series of focus groups with a total of 50 CARE for Teachers participants to investigate their experiences with the program and changes they saw in their teaching since completing the program. Participants felt CARE for Teachers helped them gain greater self-awareness in relation to both physical and emotional responses to stress. They noticed how they held stress in their bodies and learned strategies to alleviate physical tension. They also gained familiarity with emotional triggers and became less reactive to challenging situations in the classroom. Lastly, teachers reported gaining a greater appreciation for self-care and felt less guilty about taking the time to do it. Sharp and Jennings (2016) had similar findings in conducting in-depth interviews with eight CARE for Teachers participants. Teachers in this study also described an enhanced emotional awareness and less emotional reactivity as a result of the program. Participants also described being able to reappraise situations in the classroom, or shift their perspective to see a situation differently. This allowed them to consider multiple viewpoints or see the situation in a broader context to not react so emotionally to it. Some teachers gained a greater understanding for their students' own emotional experiences, which led to more compassionate responses to their difficult behaviors.

The qualitative findings suggest CARE for Teachers helped participants cultivate the ethical ideal through emotional awareness and self-care to prevent emotional exhaustion, along with the ability to see events from multiple perspectives, which develops the compassion and understanding necessary to maintain the relational process of caring for their students. Reappraising difficult situations also allows teachers to shift their perspective from students' challenging behaviors being a personal attack on the teacher to an understanding that students' own difficult emotions trigger behaviors. This reappraisal process creates the opportunity for teachers to ascribe the best possible motives for their students' behaviors, which Noddings (2013) holds to be a necessary part of the ethical ideal.

Next Steps: Verifying Assumptions

The research described above suggests that CARE for Teachers promotes teachers' ethics of care. However, more research is required to more clearly link participation in the program to specific outcomes associated with the ethics of care. For example, future studies should include measures that specifically tap teachers' impressions of their ethics of care to see whether these change in response to the CARE for Teachers program. However, this poses an interesting measurement issue as, to date, there are no such measures that were designed to assess teachers' ethics of care. Therefore, the first step would be the development and validation of such a measure and then use in a randomized controlled trial to examine the measure's sensitivity to change. However, a shortcoming of asking individuals about their assessment of their ethics of care is likely subject to social desirability biases and may not reflect teachers' behavior. It's likely that teachers may not be aware that their behavior does not always align with their ethics of care. For this reason, rather than developing additional self-report measures, observational measures may need to be refined to better articulate specific changes in teachers' caring behavior that reflect ethics of care. Yet, observational measures alone may be insufficient to assess individuals' ethics of caring as an observer cannot accurately determine the receptivity and motivation of another's actions simply by viewing their outward behavior. Noddings (2013) identifies this as a significant challenge: "When we consider the action component of caring in depth, we shall have to look beyond observable action to acts of commitment, those acts that are seen only by the individual subject performing them." These internal "acts of commitment" can only be understood through in-depth dialogue with the one-caring. Additionally, caring is not simply an outcome, but a *process*, and purely quantitative work is not always best suited to study processes.

Therefore, qualitative or mixed methods research using both observations and interviews may be the best way to capture the complexity and nuance of the ethics of care. Interviews would allow CARE for Teachers participants to describe how the program influenced aspects of their ethics of care including receptivity, engrossment, ethical ideal, etc., and observations provide the opportunity to see these processes in the classroom. The interviews and observations would also have to be iterative and reflexive to allow the researcher to ask questions about what was observed in the classroom in order to uncover the more internal acts of commitment behind the external behaviors.

A further challenge of researching the ethics of care is Noddings' constant framing of care as a relational process. Thus, only studying teachers might be insufficient to fully capture the caring relation if the cared-for's experiences and contributions to the relation may be overlooked. Interviewing students would strengthen the trustworthiness of the study by providing insight into how students feel cared for by their teacher. Although, classroom observations may provide a more parsimonious, yet still rigorous method for capturing the relational processes between teacher and student. Noddings holds that the cared-for completes caring interactions with some response such as a thank you or a newly gained energy in solving their problem, and these responses can certainly be observed by a researcher and inferred to be related to the teachers' caring behavior.

Thus, both interviews and observations are likely needed to accurately represent the ethics of care. Conducting reflexive interviews and classroom observations of CARE participants requires significant time and resources; yet, a study of similar size ($n = 224$) to the latest CARE for Teachers trial by Jennings et al., (2017) may not be needed to verify some of the links between CARE for Teachers and the ethics of care. A smaller scale qualitative or mixed methods study of program participants designed using Noddings' ethics of care as a theoretical framework could provide sound evidence regarding the relationship between participants' experiences with CARE for Teachers influencing their ethics of care in the classroom. If teachers were to describe how program elements influenced their ability to care for students, and these changes manifested in observable interactions with students, there would be sufficiently rigorous evidence to link CARE for Teachers and the ethics of care.

Conclusion

Concerns have been raised that the absence of ethics in contemporary MBIs might wrongly decontextualize and misappropriate the Buddhist values from which mindful awareness practices originated and limit the scope of mindfulness to mere stress management (Monteiro et al., 2015; Purser & Loy, 2013). While these concerns have merit, some MBIs were designed to support individuals working in secular settings where religious or spiritual references are inappropriate. However, values and ethical standards need not be linked to a spiritual or religious tradition and many secular settings have well-established ethical standards. Furthermore, individuals drawn to the helping professions, such as teachers, typically hold personal values and ethical standards that motivate them to do good that can be drawn upon in developing MBIs for these populations.

This chapter articulated an example of Monteiro et al.' (2015) proposition that MBIs can ascribe to secular ethical frameworks, and that such ethics can guide MBIs if they are rooted in universal concepts of "moral responsibility, courage, expectations, and action" (p. 10). The CARE for Teachers program provides participants the opportunity to explore the values and ethics they hold that motivated them to choose the teaching profession. Through the practice of intention setting, they learn to envision their "best self" rooted in their ethical idea and to better align their behavior with this vision. This practice is introduced at the beginning of every session, to remind teachers of the overall intention of the program: to apply mindful awareness to developing the self-awareness and self-management they need to cope with the stressors and demands of teaching. In this way, the program aims to break the cycle of the "burnout cascade" that can seriously impact the quality of our schools and children's learning. When teachers lack the social and emotional competencies to manage the demands of teaching, they may lose touch with their ethical ideals and find it difficult, if not impossible to consistently bring their "best selves" into their classrooms day after day. In contrast, when teachers have these skills and they are linked to their ethical ideal, they are more able to enact the values they hold in their day-to-day interactions with their students.

References

Aloe, A. M., Amo, L. C., & Shanahan, M. E. (2014). Classroom management self-efficacy and burnout: A multivariate meta-analysis. *Educational Psychology Review, 26*, 101–126.

Association of American Educators. (2016). *Code of ethics for educators*. Retrieved from https://www.aaeteachers.org/index.php/about-us/aae-code-of-ethics

Bellingrath, S., Rohleder, N., & Kudielka, B. M. (2010). Healthy working school teachers with high effort–reward-imbalance and overcommitment show increased pro-inflammatory immune activity and a dampened innate immune defence. *Brain, Behavior, and Immunity, 24*, 1332–1339.

Bellingrath, S., Weigl, T., & Kudielka, B. M. (2009). Chronic work stress and exhaustion is associated with higher allostastic load in female school teachers: Original research report. *Stress, 12*, 37–48.

Blasé, J. J. (1982). A social–psychological grounded theory of teacher stress and burnout. *Educational Administration Quarterly, 18*, 93–113.

Campbell, E. (2008). The ethics of teaching as a moral profession. *Curriculum Inquiry, 38*, 357–385.

Chang, M. L. (2009). An appraisal perspective of teacher burnout: Examining the emotional work of teachers. *Educational Psychology Review, 21*, 193–218.

Cohn, M. A., Brown, S. L., Fredrickson, B. L., Milkels, J. A., & Conway, A. M. (2009). Happiness unpacked: Positive emotions increase life satisfaction by building resilience. *Emotion, 9*(3), 361–368.

Fisher, M. H. (2011). Factors influencing stress, burnout, and retention of secondary teachers. *Current Issues in Education, 14*. Retrieved from http://cie.asu.edu/

Fredrickson, B. L. (2004). The broaden-and-build theory of positive emotions. *Philosophical Transactions of the Royal Society B Biological Sciences, 359*, 1367–1378. https://doi.org/10.1098/rstb.2004.1512

Fresco, D. M., Segal, Z. V., Buis, T., & Kennedy, S. (2007). Relationship of posttreatment decentering and cognitive reactivity to relapse in major depression. *Journal of Consulting and Clinical Psychology, 75*(3), 447–455.

Gallup. (2014). *State of American schools report: The path to winning again in education*. Retrieved from http://www.gallup.com/services/178709/state-america-schools-report.aspx

Greenberg, M. T., Brown J. L., & Abenavoli, R. M. (2016). *Teacher stress and health: Effects on teachers, students, and schools*. Edna Bennett Pierce Prevention Research Center, Pennsylvania State University.

Halifax, J. (2014). G.R.A.C.E. for nurses: Cultivating compassion in nurse/patient interactions. *Journal of Nursing Education and Practice, 4*, 121–128.

Jennings, P. A. (2015a). Early childhood teachers' well-being, mindfulness and self-compassion in relation to classroom quality and attitudes towards challenging students. *Mindfulness, 6*, 732–743. https://doi.org/10.1007/s12671-014-0312-4

Jennings, P. A. (2015b). *Mindfulness for teachers: Simple skills for peace and productivity in the classroom*. New York: W. W. Norton.

Jennings, P. A. (2016a). CARE for teachers: A mindfulness-based approach to promoting teachers' well-being and improving performance. In K. Schonert-Reichl & R. Roeser (Eds.), *The handbook of mindfulness in education: Emerging theory, research, and programs* (pp. 133–148). New York: Springer.

Jennings, P. A. (2016b). Mindfulness-based programs and the American public school system: Recommendations for best practices to ensure secularity. *Mindfulness, 7*, 176–178. https://doi.org/10.1007/s12671-015-0477-5

Jennings, P. A., Brown, J. L., Frank, J. L., Doyle, S., Oh, Y., Tanler, R., …, Greenberg, M. T. (2017). Impacts of the CARE for teachers program on teachers' social and emotional competence and classroom interactions. *Journal of Educational Psychology*. Advance online publication. http://dx.doi.org/10.1037/edu0000187

Jennings, P. A., Frank, J. L., Snowberg, K. E., Coccia, M. A., & Greenberg, M. T. (2013). Improving classroom learning environments by cultivating awareness and resilience in education (CARE): Results of a randomized controlled trial. *School Psychology Quarterly, 28*, 374–390. https://doi.org/10.1037/spq0000035

Jennings, P. A., & Greenberg, M. T. (2009). The prosocial classroom: Teacher social and emotional competence in relation to student and classroom outcomes. *Review of Educational Research, 79*, 491–525. https://doi.org/10.3102/0034654308325693

Jennings, P. A., Snowberg, K. E., Coccia, M. A., & Greenberg, M. T. (2011). Improving classroom learning environments by cultivating awareness and resilience in education (CARE): Results of two pilot studies. *Journal of Classroom Interactions, 46*, 27–48.

Johnson, S., Cooper, C., Cartwright, S., Donald, I., Taylor, P., & Millet, C. (2005). The experience of work-related stress across occupations. *Journal of Managerial Psychology, 20*, 178–187.

Katz, D. A., Greenberg, M. T., Jennings, P. A., & Klein, L. C. (2016). Associations between the awakening responses of salivary α-amylase and cortisol with self-report indicators of health and wellbeing among educators. *Teaching and Teacher Education, 54*, 98–106.

Kyriacou, C. (2001). Teacher stress: Directions for future research. *Educational Review, 53*, 27–35.

Markow, D., Macia, L., & Lee, H. (2013). *The MetLife survey of the American teacher: Challenges for school leadership*. New York: Metropolitan Life Insurance Company.

Maslach, C. (1976). Burned-out. *Human Behavior, 5*, 16–22.

Maslach, C. (2003). *Burnout: The cost of caring*. Los Altos, CA: ISHK.

Maslach, C., Schaufeli, W. B., & Leiter, M. P. (2001). Job burnout. *Annual Review of Psychology, 52*, 397–422.

Milkie, M. A., & Warner, C. H. (2011). How does the classroom learning environment affect children's mental health? *Journal of Health and Social Behavior, 52*, 3–21.

Monteiro, L. M., Musten, R. F., & Compson, J. (2015). Traditional and contemporary mindfulness: Finding the middle path in the tangle of concerns. *Mindfulness, 6*, 1–13.

National Education Association. (2016). *Code of ethics*. Retrieved from http://www.nea.org/home/30442.htm

Noddings, N. (1996). The caring professional. In S. Gordon, P. Benner, & N. Noddings (Eds.), *Readings in knowledge, practice, ethics, and politics*. Philadelphia: University of Pennsylvania Press.

Noddings, N. (2012). The caring relation in teaching. *Oxford Review of Education, 38*, 771–781.

Noddings, N. (2013). *Caring: A relational approach to ethics and moral education*. Oakland, CA: Univ of California Press.

Oberle, E., & Schonert-Reichl, K. A. (2016). Stress contagion in the classroom? The link between classroom teacher burnout and morning cortisol in elementary school students. *Social Science and Medicine, 159*, 30–37.

Purser, R., & Loy, D. (2013). Beyond McMindfulness. *Huffington post*. Retrieved from http://www.huffingtonpost.com/ron-purser/beyondmcmindfulness_b_3519289.html

Remen, R. N. (2006). *Kitchen table wisdom: Stories that heal, 10th anniversary edition*. New York: Riverhead Books.

Richards, J. (2012). Teacher stress and coping strategies: A national snapshot. *The Educational Forum, 76*, 299–316.

Schaefer, L., Long, J. S., & Clandinin, D. J. (2012). Questioning the research on early career teacher attrition and retention. *Alberta Journal of Educational Research, 58*(1), 106–121.

Schussler, D. L., Jennings, P. A., Sharp, J. E., & Frank, J. L. (2016). Improving teacher awareness and well-being through CARE: A qualitative analysis of the underlying mechanisms. *Mindfulness, 7*, 130–142. https://doi.org/10.1007/s12671-015-0422-7

Sharp, J. E., & Jennings, P. A. (2016). Strengthening teacher presence through mindfulness: What educators say about the Cultivating Awareness and Resilience in Education (CARE) program. *Mindfulness, 7*, 209–218. https://doi.org/10.1007/s12671-015-0474-8

Chapter 10
Compassion as the Highest Ethic

James N. Kirby, Stanley R. Steindl, and James R. Doty

Compassion as the Highest Ethic

Ethics are moral principles that guide a person's behavior, and ethics have been at the heart of philosophical, religious, and spiritual discussions for thousands of years. One source for the word "ethic" can be derived from the Ancient Greek word *êthikos*, which means "*relating to one's character.*" Ethical principles provide a framework for people to help make decisions about how best to live their life and what actions are right or wrong in a particular situation. Definitions of ethics typically emphasize the importance of what is the best way for people to live or what is the science of the "*ideal*" human character (Kidder, 2003). Consequently, ethical codes have been developed and applied in a number of modern-day professions, such as medicine, politics, psychology, law, education, and business. As technology advances, ethics are also becoming of great interest in the development and programming of artificial intelligence (AI). Indeed, current ethical issues inherent in AI developments can inform our understanding of how ethics and compassion are related. By way of example, consider driverless cars. In a scenario where either the driverless car needs to avoid crashing and harming a group of people or avoiding

J.N. Kirby, PhD
The University of Queensland, St Lucia, QLD, Australia

The Center for Compassion and Altruism Research and Education, Stanford University, Stanford, CA, USA

S.R. Steindl, PhD
The University of Queensland, St Lucia, QLD, Australia

J.R. Doty, MD (✉)
The Center for Compassion and Altruism Research and Education, Stanford University, Stanford, CA, USA
e-mail: jrdoty@stanford.edu

© Springer International Publishing AG 2017   253
L.M. Monteiro et al. (eds.), *Practitioner's Guide to Ethics and Mindfulness-Based Interventions*, Mindfulness in Behavioral Health,
DOI 10.1007/978-3-319-64924-5_10

and harming the individual in the car—what is the ethical choice, what is the driverless car programmed to do? These are difficult decisions to contemplate, as whose life or lives are more important. In the driverless car scenario, one would often argue from a principle of greater good, thus protecting the group of people and sacrificing the driver. However, would this response change if we were informed that the group of people were criminals guilty of murder and the driver was a parent of two young children? AI developers might argue that the program design would avoid such dilemmas altogether, but how certain can we be? One of the main principles of compassion is to avoid doing harm (Dalai Lama, 1995), and this is where compassion as an ethical guide can be most useful. The focus of this chapter is to suggest that compassion may be our highest ethic, which can help provide the guiding motivation to address life difficulties. Therefore, there are five key parts to this chapter: (1) defining compassion; (2) understanding compassion in terms of evolutionary processes and physiology; (3) examining the benefits of compassion; (4) linking compassion with ethics; and (5) examining how compassion-based interventions are aiming to help aid individuals in making ethically wise decisions.

Defining Compassion

Compassion is a growing area of interest within different fields of research, particularly psychotherapy (Gilbert, 2014; Kirby, 2016). For example, according to Google Scholar, in 2016 the term "compassion" was referred to in a staggering 38,800 publications. Many researchers around the world are responsible for the rise of compassion as an area of scientific enquiry (Ekman & Ekman, 2013; Germer, 2009; Gilbert & Choden, 2013; Keltner, Marsh, & Smith, 2010; Neff, 2003; Ricard, 2015; Singer & Bolz, 2013). As a result, compassion research is being conducted from the differing perspectives of evolutionary science, psychological science, and neuroscience, often in collaboration with spiritual teachers, to enhance our understanding of compassion and its associated impacts.

Compassion has been defined in various ways (Gilbert, 2014; Goetz et al., 2010; Jinpa, 2010; Strauss et al., 2016). Most theorists focus on the preparedness and wish to sensitively attend to suffering and the needs of others, and also the preparedness to do something to help reduce that suffering. Many researchers focus on describing certain qualities and attributes that comprise compassion (Strauss et al., 2016). These qualities include elements such as recognizing and having a sensitivity to suffering, being non-judgmental, recognizing the common humanity of suffering, having empathy, distress tolerance, equanimity, patience and a motivation to act to do something to alleviate and to prevent suffering (Feldman & Kuyken, 2011; Gilbert, 2014; Goetz et al., 2010; Neff, 2003; Strauss et al., 2016). Goetz et al. (2010) specifically define compassion "as the feeling that arises in witnessing another's suffering and that motivates a subsequent desire to help" (p. 351). Geshe Thupten Jinpa, who developed the Stanford Compassion Cultivation Training program, defines compassion as a complex multidimensional construct that is comprised of four components: (1) an awareness of suffering (cognitive component),

(2) sympathetic concern related to being emotionally moved by suffering (affective component), (3) a wish to see the relief of that suffering (intentional component), and (4) a responsiveness or readiness to help relieve that suffering (motivational component; Jazaieri et al., 2013). The notion of self-compassion has received increasing attention with the work of Kristen Neff, who defined self-compassion based on her interpretations of Buddhist teachings as having three components: (1) being mindful, rather than over-identifying with problems; (2) connecting with others, rather than isolating oneself; and (3) adopting an attitude of self-kindness, rather than being judgmental (Neff, 2003).

When reviewing the definition of compassion, it becomes clear how many researchers tend to develop lists of qualities and attributes that are identified as being part of compassion. Some definitions stress the motivational nature of compassion, exploring its goal and focus and the various competencies necessary for that motive to operate successfully. Compassion as motivation is central to many of the contemplative traditions (Armstrong, 2010; Dalia Lama, 1995; Junpa 2015). This is captured in such definitions as having *a sensitivity to suffering in self and others, with a commitment to alleviate and prevent it* (for a review Gilbert, 2014). Importantly, compassion includes three directions: giving compassion to others (e.g., friend, family member), being open and responding to receiving compassion from others, and self-compassion (Gilbert, 2014; Gilbert, McEwan, Matos, & Rivis, 2010; Jazaieri et al., 2014; Neff & Germer, 2013). Viewing compassion as a motive requires an increased understanding of evolution and physiological processes and brain functioning, which provide insights as to why compassion could be regarded as our highest ethic.

Compassion: Evolutionary Insights

One way to help understand compassion is via evolutionary insights into its origins and functioning situated within its neurophysiological architecture (Brown & Brown, 2015; Gilbert, 2014; Kirby, 2016). Theorists suggest that compassion is rooted in the evolved mammalian caring motivational system (Gilbert, 2014; Mayseless, 2016), and motives are a key cause of behavior (Neel et al., 2016). Derived from the Latin word motivus, meaning "*moving*" or "*to move*," motives are linked to desires, wishes, and wants; they give rise to specific incentives and concerns, but differ from values and emotions (Klinger, 1977). Emotional arousal or attention evolved as mechanisms to "*move*" or motivate an animal toward biosocial goals such as to support reproduction or survival (Dunbar & Barnett, 2007). Along with compassion, there are many human motives including self-protection (harm-avoidance), sexual (finding a mate and reproducing), and caring-based motives (Bernard, Mills, Swenson, & Walsh, 2005; Gilbert, 2014; Huang & Bargh, 2014). All motives have two basic processes, which when applied to compassion include, (1) having a motive-appropriate signal detection (input) to suffering (i.e., sensitivity and awareness of distress), and (2) having a behavior output repertoire that allows appropriate responsiveness to suffering (i.e., taking action to alleviate and prevent suffering).

Parental investment in evolutionary biology and psychology is a concept that refers to, "any parental expenditure that benefits one offspring at a cost to parent's ability to invest in other components of fitness" (Clutton-Brock, 1991). Animals vary greatly in the amount of parental investment they provide. For example, sea turtles (reptiles) provide no parental investment to their young hatchlings after they are born on sandy beaches, while in contrast humans (mammals) provide the most significant amount, with children needing over a decade of parental investment to ensure their safety and healthy development (Gilbert, 2014). The caring system of humans, and indeed mammals, is a critical motive to enable offspring survival. The caring system motive or compassionate motive (Gilbert, 2014) requires parents to be sensitive to the distress signal of their offspring—for example, noticing a newborn infant that could be crying (first process), and then having the capacity to move toward that crying infant (suffering) so that the infant can be cared for through some kind of soothing affiliative behavior, for example, touch or voice tone (second process). This interaction between care-giver (parent) and care-seeker (infant) then helps facilitate the attachment system between parent and child (see Swain & Ho, 2016), and also demonstrates how affection and affiliative behaviors are fundamental in the affect regulation of mammals.

Many species such as fish, turtles, and other egg laying reptiles produce large numbers of young who need to disperse rapidly afterbirth to avoid predation, including, at times, from their own parents (MacLean, 1985). Thus, fish and reptilian young are born to be mobile, be able to seek their own protection, and be self-sustaining. This is sometimes referred to as r selection. The evolution of warm-bloodedness, live birth, small numbers of young, and post birth parental/caring investment, sometimes referred to as k selection, required substantial changes to the physiology of threat avoidance and approach behavior, allowing for close interpersonal contact and connection. To facilitate these interactional sequences, k selected regulation processors operate through a sequence of adaptations. One of these major adaptations was the evolution of part of the myelinated parasympathetic system—the dorsolateral vagal nerve that links a range of internal organs to central control systems. Indeed, the vagus is connected to a range of organs including the heart and gut, and with the brain through its link to inhibitory prefrontal-subcortical circuits. One of the key functions of parental investment is sensitivity to distress and preparedness to act appropriately to relieve that distress. This is also the basic sentiment and core of compassion (Gilbert, 2014), and compassion utilizes the same evolved physiological pathways as basic caring behavior.

Compassion: Physiological Processes

It is now well-recognized that a key process that assists with affect regulation is through caring affiliative and affectionate behaviors. Polyvagal theory, outlined by Porges (2007), details how the activation of the myelinated parasympathetic nervous system helps in the regulation of fight/flight (autonomic sympathetic nervous system), thus enabling calmness and soothing to be achieved through having close proximity to others, giving/receiving affiliative, caring, and prosocial behavior (Davidson, 2012; Depue & Morrone-Strupinsky, 2005; Gilbert, 2014). This is reflected in the dynamic balancing of the sympathetic and parasympathetic nervous systems that give rise to the variability in heart rate (Porges, 2007). Hence, feeling safe is linked to heart rate variability (HRV), and higher HRV is linked to a greater ability to self-soothe when stressed (Porges, 2007). Specific strategies such as breathing practices, friendly voice tones, and facial and body expressions can activate the parasympathetic system, aiming to calm and soothe the individual, which improves heart rate variability (Krygier et al., 2013). Moreover, when the sympathetic system is activated under threat this decreases the ability for higher order cognitive capacities such as mentalizing to occur (e.g., theory of mind, empathizing, perspective taking), whereas activating the parasympathetic system helps provide a feeling of safeness, which increases the ability to activate the prefrontal cortex and enable mentalization (Liotti & Gilbert, 2011; Klimecki et al., 2014; Thayer & Lane, 2000). It is important to distinguish between feelings of safety and safeness. The former is related to being removed from elements that bring the possibility of threat or harm, such as a distressing situation, thought, or feeling. The latter refers to a greater freedom to explore the distress despite the possibility of harm (Gilbert, 2014). Compassion is not about the avoidance of threatening stimuli, rather it involves developing the courage to engage with what we need to do (Gilbert, 2014). Thus, the focus on activating affiliative processing systems (e.g., parasympathetic system) assists in the regulation of affect, and helps calm individuals when distressed.

Compassion: Brain Functioning and Affect Regulation

The human brain is a product of evolution and can be understood in terms of Darwinian "selection for function", and so can many mental health problems. Social processing and early social contexts influence brain development and are central to understanding mental health problems. Relationships based on affection and caring show many physiological and psychological beneficial effects, even on genetic expression (Cozolino, 2007, 2008, 2013; Siegel, 2009). We recognize that as an evolved species many of our basic motives, emotions, and their genetic polymorphisms are products from the challenges of survival and reproduction (Conway & Slavich, 2017). This understanding of how humans evolved as biological, gene-built systems that (phenotypically) adapt to their environments and operate a range of evolved motivation and emotion processing systems has important implications not only for our understanding of mental health difficulties but their prevention and alleviation.

The view that the human brain can be considered as an evolved organ shaped by contextual factors to help with survival and reproduction also warns us that assumptions like "*all is well until something goes wrong*" are unhelpful, misleading, and basically often wrong (Brune et al., 2012; Nesse & Williams, 1995). Therefore, our brains although capable of wonderful capacities such as imagination, creativity, and being able to forecast the future and reflect on the past, also comes at a cost, as it permits rumination, worry, and self-criticism, that can underpin so many mental health difficulties (Gilbert, 2014; Kirby & Gilbert, 2016). Moreover, our evolved brain has a number of inbuilt biases, for example, having kin preferences (nepotism), in-group preferences (tribalism), a negativity bias (better safe than sorry), and biased learning (e.g., fear of snakes but not electricity). These biases indicate that our evolved minds, although with many advantages, also have a number of problematic evolutionary trade-offs and glitches. This view is in contrast to the Western medical model of mental health, where the idea is conveyed that there is nothing fundamentally wrong with our mind (i.e., nothing inherently bad or tricky about its evolved construction) and it is only "*when things go wrong*" that we have mental "*disorder,*" requiring therapies "*to correct*" and "*fix*" (Brune et al., 2012).

In contrast, the Buddha highlighted that our *normal unenlightened* states were problematic—that the mind is, in a way, inherently crazy, especially if it lacks compassion (Dalai Lama, 1995). Thus, when presented with ethical dilemmas it can be difficult to make judgments and decisions, due to our "*tricky mind,*" and mistakes are made. Importantly, from this perspective one can view our "craziness" as not being our fault, but as a consequence of the evolved human mind, for which we need to take responsibility.

One of the aims of compassion is to help individuals take responsibility for their "tricky mind" by providing psychoeducation on the human mind, specifically regarding how the brain regulates emotions, which can cloud our judgment and decision making. One way to consider emotions, other than individually, is to group them in terms of evolutionary function. For example, we can identify a whole set of emotions whose primary functions are self-protective and defensive, and are triggered in the context of threats but not in the context of being safe or content. Another set of emotions is associated with rewards and acquiring resources and achievements. These functions help to direct and energize individuals to things conducive to their well-being and need to be acquired (e.g., food, shelter). Once acquired however, and without threats, emotions will be conducive to calmness, peacefulness, and "rest and digest." Importantly, the three types of emotional systems need not be mutually exclusive, rather it is referring to the degree to which these blend. This simple three-function heuristic approach to emotions has been suggested by Gilbert (2009, 2014) and is depicted in Fig. 10.1. This model is informed by affective neuroscience research into the evolutionary functions of emotion (Depue & Morrone-Strupinsky, 2005.

These three emotion regulation systems interact and include: (a) the threat/self-protect system, (b) the drive-reward system, and (c) the affiliative/soothing system. Gilbert (2014) and others (Kirby, 2016; Tirch, Schoendroff, & Silberstein, 2014) have emphasized how people (children and adults) often find themselves trapped between the threat and reward systems because of the family environments and the Western culture in which we live—a culture that increasingly

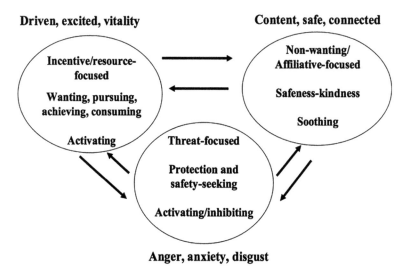

Fig. 10.1 The interaction between the three major emotion-regulation systems

focuses on individualistic values that promote achievement and independence (Kasser, 2011; Park, Twenge, & Greenfield, 2014). This model of emotion regulation can help when dealing with ethical dilemmas and decision making. For example, if asked to lie to protect somebody, we could feel heightened anxiety and fear about the potential of being "caught" or making a "wrong" decision, and as such would be operating from a threat-base. When operating from this threat-system we are more likely to be focused on self-protection, making it more difficult to think broadly and abstractly about the problem, and rather we might be angry about being put in this position, thus narrowing our perspective. In contrast, lying to protect somebody might lead to significant gain, for example financially, and this can result in a short-term feeling of excitement and this activation of the drive system also narrows perspective, as we focus on pursuing what we want. However, the long-term continued anxiety and fear of being caught may also linger. Therefore, being able to recognize our emotional systems, and how they can influence what we attend to, how we think and behave is important when considering ethical dilemmas and decision making.

One of the problems of being caught between the threat and reward systems is that this then can become the only way of regulating emotions for individuals, and the soothing/affiliative system becomes underdeveloped (Kirby & Gilbert, 2016). The trap of being caught between the drive and threat system in Western cultures is evidenced in the current education system. Despite the increasing evidence highlighting the importance of skills such as understanding emotions, compassion, and emotion regulation, these skills are often not taught explicitly in schools. Rather, the focus of schools is on teaching skills to enhance academic knowledge and achievement resulting in a heavy focus on comparative, competitive, and achievement-based goals. This is evidenced by Western countries solely emphasizing and valuing student performance as measured by outcomes on standardized testing. Moreover, a problem of an educational approach based on competition and achievements is that students' ethical integrity becomes compromised in the search for better outcomes, as evidenced in the Making Caring Common Project (MCCP) at Harvard University.

The MCCP project authors surveyed 10,000 adolescents across the United States and found that 80% said that *"achievement or happiness"* (personal success) is their top priority compared to 20% saying *"caring for others"* is their top priority (Making Caring Common, Harvard, 2014). The study also found youths were three times more likely to agree than disagree with the statement: *"my parents are prouder if I get good grades than if I'm a caring community member."* Approximately 80% of youths also reported perceiving teachers as prioritizing students' achievements over their caring. Youths also ranked "hard work" above fairness. Importantly, previous research has found that valuing personal success and achievement comes at a price, with half of high school students admitting to cheating on a test and nearly 75% admitting to copying someone else's homework (Josephson Institute, 2012). These findings underscore the significant influence competitive based pressures can have on youth, and how it can impact their ethical decision making. Importantly though, there are now educators, psychologists, parents, and policymakers eager to address childhood social, emotional, and behavioral learning as equally important as academic knowledge, but how to achieve this remains unclear. One potential option to help children and adolescents is to introduce compassion-based programs in the school context (which is already beginning to happen and one we support), given the many benefits associated with compassion and mental health (Kirby, 2016).

Benefits of Compassion

There is now considerable evidence that being the giver and recipient of caring behaviors, particularly compassion, has a range of health benefits (Cozolino, 2007; Mayseless, 2016) and can affect genetic expression (Fredrickson et al., 2013). Compassion training improves general well-being and social relationships (e.g., Jazaieri, et al., 2014; Seppala, Rossomando, & Doty, 2012), with increasing evidence of its effectiveness as a psychotherapy (Leaviss & Uttley, 2015; Kirby, 2016; Kirby & Gilbert, in press). Practicing compassion has an impact on neurophysiology due to neuroplasticity (e.g., Klimecki, Leiberg, Ricard, & Singer, 2014), with a recent study showing that it has significant impacts on heart rate variability (Matos et al., 2016).

With the rise of an awareness of the power of prosocial, compassionate interactions for well-being, and how their opposite (criticism and neglect) is linked to mental distress, there has been a growth of different approaches to help people cultivate compassion for themselves and others. These approaches include Mindful Self-Compassion (MSC; Neff & Germer, 2013), Compassion Cultivation Training (CCT; Jazaieri et al., 2013), Cognitively-Based Compassion Training (CBCT; Pace et al., 2009), Cultivating Emotional Balance (CEB). Compassion and Loving-Kindness Meditations (e.g., CM & LKM; Hoffmann, Grossman, & Hinton, 2011), and Compassion-Focused Therapy (CFT, Gilbert, 2014; Kirby, 2016). Hybrids are also constantly appearing such as the mindful compassionate living course that combines CFT with more intense mindfulness training or the integration of CFT with therapies such as Acceptance and Commitment Therapy.

To date, there has only been one meta-analysis conducted on compassion-based interventions (Kirby, Tellegen, & Steindl, 2016), which included 23 randomized controlled trials (RCTs) over the last 10 years. Results found significant short-term moderate effect sizes for compassion ($d = 0.559$), self-compassion ($d = 0.691$), and mindfulness ($d = 0.525$). Significant moderate effects were also found for reducing suffering-based outcomes of depression ($d = 0.656$), anxiety ($d = 0.547$), and small to moderate effects for psychological distress ($d = 0.374$). Significant moderate effects were also found for well-being ($d = 0.540$). These results indicate the promising nature of compassion-based approaches in helping with a range of difficulties. The question remains though, do individuals who participate in compassionate-based interventions experience an emerging of ethical importance in their daily life.

Compassion and Ethics

The Dalai Lama has frequently said, "Buddhist ethics can be summed up in two statements: If you are able to help others, then help. If you are not able to help, at least do not harm." (Dalai Lama, 1995). These statements from the Dalai Lama are in alignment with the motivation of compassion, which is to both alleviate and prevent suffering (Gilbert, 2014), and it is arguable that compassion might be the highest ethical principle that guides our behaviors in all domains of life. To support this premise, we would like to emphasize two important points. First, the evolution of mammalian caregiving, which involves hormones such as oxytocin, vasopressin, and the myelinated vagal nerve as part of the ventral parasympathetic system, enables humans to come together, co-regulate each other's emotions and create prosociality. Second, the dynamic balancing of the sympathetic and parasympathetic nervous systems gives rise to variability in heart rate (Heart Rate Variability (HRV); Kirby, Doty, Petrocchi, & Gilbert, 2017). In fact, the autonomic nervous system enables emotion-related action tendencies, which, in the case of compassion, are approach and caregiving. The inhibition of heart rate through the activity of the parasympathetic nervous system has shown to be linked to the orienting response and sustained outward attention, which constitute a core action tendency of compassion (Suess, Porges, Plude, 1994). Consistently, compassion-evoking stimuli (videos of other's suffering) have shown to generate vagally mediated heart rate deceleration in children (Eisenberg et al., 1998) and in adults, whose self-reports of sympathy and compassion were positively related to heart rate deceleration (Eisenberg et al., 1991). Moreover, children with higher heart rate deceleration during evocative films showed increased subsequent compassionate behavior (Eisenberg et al., 1989). Interestingly, children with higher baseline HRV were rated by teachers and parents as more helpful and more able to regulate their emotions than those with lower HRV (Eisenberg et al., 1996) and showed increased self-reports of sympathy, both dispositionally and in response to distress-inducing films (Fabes, Eisenberg, & Eisenbud, 1993). This suggests that tonic HRV might represent the physiological signature of a trait-like compassionate responding, indicating that perhaps in some way we are "*hard-wired*" for the compassionate motive to be our in-built ethical compass.

When considering compassion as a guiding ethic, it is important to note the *motive* component. For example, the action of not speeding when driving might be due to an underlying motive of wanting to avoid harm to self by not getting a speeding ticket—put simply, avoiding punishment/harm to self. Harvey (2000) would suggest that this kind of action is done for prudential reasons, "*I do not want a fine or go to jail*," and thus is not really done from a compassionate ethical perspective or motive. From an evolutionary perspective, this action can be considered as stemming from the threat-system, which is focused on self-protection, and has a different physiological pattern compared to caring/compassionate motives (Gilbert, 2014). In contrast, if the motive was one of compassion, not speeding when driving is part of being a good citizen on the road and attempting to prevent harm due to caring for others well-being.

Buddhist Ethics and Compassion Ethics are an important component in Buddhist teaching and the foundation of the Buddha's Eightfold Path is ethics or a wholesome lifestyle. The Eightfold Path has specific steps suggested for the alleviation of suffering for ourselves and others. Traditionally, the eight practices are presented in the following order: (1) right view, (2) right resolve, (3) right speech, (4) right action, (5) right livelihood, (6) right effort, (7) right mindfulness, and (8) right concentration (Bodhi, 2000). The Eightfold Path is characterized by a sense of ethical direction, determined by the cultivation of the wholesome and helpful, and relinquishment of the unwholesome and unhelpful (Bodhi, 2000). Ricard (2015) describes it this way: "In Buddhism, an act is essentially unethical if its aim is to cause suffering and ethical if it is meant to bring genuine well-being to others." (p. 239). The Eightfold Path is sometimes considered in three categories of (1) moral virtue (right speech, right action, right livelihood); (2) meditation (right effort, right mindfulness, right concentration); and (3) insight or wisdom (right view, right resolve). It offers an ethical framework in which to live and interact with others and the world, aimed at promoting a reduction in suffering and an increase in well-being, but also at a deeper level it may lead to liberation, Nirvana, or complete release from *dukkha*. Compassion is the heart of the Eightfold Path and provides the guidance toward ethical action, or more accurately, an ethical way of being.

Whereas the ethical intention of Buddhist practice is to cultivate a way of being, that is, a life that feels good or consistent with one's values, Aristotle takes a different view. For Aristotle, the primary purpose for ethics is to help guide human beings toward living a good life. This is, of course, distinct from living a life that *feels* good. Rather, the good life, according to Aristotle, is one in which the activities of living are performed not simply for some sort of specific outcome, such as wealth or power, but rather the activity is performed because of the inherent worth, value or quality of the activity itself (1999). We choose to be a good friend, not because the friendship will benefit us with some sort of payoff, but because the activities of friendship are worthwhile in and of themselves. Aristotelian ethics also promotes the view of teleology, which attempts to describe things in terms of apparent purpose, principle, or goal (Fowers, 2015a). This can be further divided into *extrinsic* purpose—a purpose imposed by humans, and *intrinsic* purpose which are irrespective of human use or opinion. For example, Aristotle claimed that an acorn's intrinsic telos is to become a fully grown oak tree (Fowers, 2015a).

Aristotle also argued that there is a hierarchy of activities and goods. For example, he considered activities that were a means to an end, and the end was possessed or experienced by an individual only (for example, money or possessions), as lower-order activities than those activities that were of value in and of themselves, and that value is shared (for example, friendship or teamwork). These ethical views proposed by Aristotle reflect an eudemonic way of being, which Plato and Socrates also wrote. An eudemonic view equates happiness with the human ability to pursue complex goals, which are meaningful to society. This contrasts with a hedonic view, which equates happiness with pleasure, comfort, and enjoyment (Delle Fave, Massimini, & Bassi, 2010). Often it seems in today's modern world that the pursuit of a hedonic lifestyle has become the imperative, and this is reflected in Western cultures desire to pursue drive-based goals based on individualistic achievements (Kasser, 2011).

Young people in Western cultures are increasingly endorsing individualistic values (Park, Twenge, & Greenfield, 2014). Although the increase in individualism may be the necessary result of a competitive market economy, this focus may diminish collectivistic and community values. For example, researchers have found that recent generations are lower in empathy for others (Konrath, O'Brien, & Hsing, 2011) and concern for others (Twenge, Campbell, & Freeman, 2012), which may negatively impact societal ties and mental health (Park et al., 2014). Moreover, other correlational studies have found that a strong focus on goals like money and status (compared to community feeling) is associated with being less warm and more controlling toward one's children (Kasser, Ryan, Zax, & Sameroff, 1995). These results suggest the more an individual cares about self-interested and materialistic goals, the less likely the person is to prioritize the values that help facilitate the well-being of current and future children (Kasser, 2011).

In a large study by Kasser (2011) that examined cultural values and future well-being, data were collected from 20 wealthy nations (e.g., the United States, Australia, the United Kingdom, Germany) on the indices of childhood well-being, the amount of maternity leave available, and country CO_2 emissions (data collected from archival data and multiple sources). Specifically, Kasser (2011) was interested in whether countries would perform better if they prioritized egalitarian-based values (i.e., that promote cooperation and a sense that everyone is equal and should be cared for (i.e., eudemonic)) over hierarchy-based values (i.e., that validate the unequal distribution of power and resources often found in cultures) and harmony values (i.e., that promote an acceptance and appreciation of the world as it is) over mastery values (i.e., hedonic or those that attempt to actively change the world to fit one's own self-interests). What he found was the more a nation prioritized egalitarianism and harmony-based values over hierarchy and mastery values, the higher children's well-being was in the nation, the more generous the national laws were regarding maternal leave, and the less CO_2 the nation emitted (Kasser, 2011).

Contemporary philosopher Thomas Metzinger suggests that we need to consider an ethics of consciousness (2009). This becomes even more important with the advancement of artificial intelligence. He postulated there are three desirable states of consciousness: (1) it should minimize the suffering in humans and all other beings capable of suffering; (2) it should ideally possess an epistemic potential (that is, it should have a component of insight and expanding knowledge); and (3) it should have behavioral consequences that increase the probability of the occurrence of future valuable types of experience (2009). Metzinger concedes that how to achieve this is unclear, however, some possibilities include meditation in high school, and familiarizing people with the brain–body connection. Metzinger (2009) emphasizes that the brain is part of the body, and dualistic philosophy has had negative impacts, as disconnecting the brain from our bodies creates unrealistic and potentially dangerous ideologies. Rather, Metzinger (2009) suggests teaching people from an early age about how our nervous systems work will help people to take responsibility for how their own body–brain works, which will enable them to show empathy and compassion toward others as they mature. These sentiments of Metzinger's (2009) are shared by Compassion Focused Therapy (Gilbert, 2014; Kirby & Gilbert, 2016) where the aim is to teach about the evolved functions of our brains and body so we can better relate to ourselves and to others.

Compassion and Ethical Conflict

Importantly, despite the advantages of holding compassion as a guiding ethic it does not resolve and provide answers to all ethical dilemmas. Ekman (2014) postulates that we should be more precise when referring to the target of compassion, and whether it is a familial (e.g., family member, offspring, sibling), a familiar (e.g., friend, neighbor, colleague), a stranger (e.g., somebody you do not know)—which could also be further assessed in terms of in- and out-group variations (e.g., gender, race, ethnicity), or any sentient being (e.g., any living being, pet, animal). Indeed, research has found it is easier to be compassionate to those whom we like and are part of our group than those who are not (Gilbert, 2014). For example, take the notion of heroic compassion, or as Paul Ekman refers to it, non-referential compassion (Ekman & Ekman, 2013). In this form of compassion, the idea is that you extend compassion to all despite potential consequences to oneself.

Franco, Blau, and Zimbardo (2011) define heroism as:

> A social activity: (a) in service to others in need—be it a person, group, or community, or in defense of socially sanctioned ideals, or new social standard; (b) engaged in voluntarily (even in military contexts, heroism remains an act that goes beyond actions required by military duty); (c) with recognition of possible risks/costs, (i.e., not entered into blindly or blithely, recalling the 1913 Webster's definition that stated, 'not from ignorance or inconsiderate levity'); (d) in which the actor is willing to accept anticipated sacrifice; and (e) without external gain anticipated at the time of the act. (2011, p. 101)

A common example that comes to mind when considering heroic compassion is that of the families who took Jews into their homes during World War II. Kristin Monroe (1996) published a book on heroic compassion, which was made up of individual interviews with people who had risked their own life to save others including many Germans who took in Jews during the Nazi régime. What was poignant and most powerful about this book was that the only unifying aspect of all her interviewees was a feeling that they simply had to do what they did, it was not a choice. This suggests that for these people, risking their life was a necessary response to the perceived threat toward others. It sounds as though these people did not experience "out group" biases and in fact had almost familial compassion toward those people they rescued, often with great risk to their own livelihood. Perceiving the target of compassion to be like us, irrespective of external differences, has been called a universal orientation, one that is likely to precede a globally compassionate approach.

Although the example of German families taking Jewish people into their homes to protect them during World War II is unquestionably brave, one must also consider all members in this situation: (1) the Jewish family; (2) the German parents who took the Jewish family in; and (3) the children of the German parents. If we direct compassion to the Jewish family, one could consider this as heroic compassion. However, if we direct our compassion to the children of the German parents would it still be compassion? Could a potentially inadvertent consequence of the actions of the German parents to let the Jewish people into their homes potentially lead to a devastating outcome for these children? If German parents did not let Jewish people into their homes because of the risk of harm to their own children would that be considered a more "selfish" action? Or would it still constitute compassionate action for their children? When one considers all members in this very difficult ethical dilemma it becomes clear that although compassion can help guide us in our ethical choices, it does not lead to easy, simple, correct/incorrect answers or ways of being (see Jennings & DeMauro and Monteiro & Musten in this book).

What is important, however, is that compassion can help ground us, and it can help direct our attention from being caught up in threat, where we have an increased likelihood of acting out of fear and anger. And it can help activate the physiological systems within our body that help provide calmness and permits empathic perspective taking, empathy, and mentalizing to occur. In doing so, compassion interventions perhaps offer hope to help ethics emerge.

Compassion-Based Interventions

Over the last 10 years, there has been an increase in the number of compassion-based interventions with many options available for individuals. A review by Kirby (2016) on compassion-based interventions found at least six current empirically supported interventions that focus on the cultivation of compassion: Compassion-Focused Therapy (CFT; Gilbert, 2014), Mindful Self-Compassion (Neff & Germer, 2013), Compassion Cultivation Training (Jazaieri et al., 2013), Cognitively Based Compassion Training (Pace et al., 2009), Cultivating Emotional Balance, and Compassion and Loving-Kindness Meditations (e.g., Hoffmann, Grossman, & Hinton, 2011). To date, all six forms of intervention have been subject to the "gold standard" evaluations of randomized controlled trials (RCTs); however, only CFT and Compassion and Loving-Kindness Meditations have been evaluated in a systematic review (Hoffmann et al., 2011; Leaviss & Uttley, 2015). Kirby and Gilbert (2016), in an effort to understand the current state of compassion-based interventions, created a table that provides a brief description of some of the elements that are similar and different across some of these compassion-based approaches, which can be seen in Table 10.1.

Importantly, when viewing the elements in each of the compassion-based interventions it becomes clear that many compassion-training programs include teachings and instruction on ethics, specifically concerning the ethic of compassion. Although the psychoeducation, strategies, and exercises across the interventions are presented within a primarily secular framework, many of the key concepts and core practices are drawn from Buddhist traditions, and all programs were developed with consultation or advice from Buddhist teachers or scholars. This inclusion of ethical views, specifically the ethical view of compassion, in compassion-based interventions is an important distinction compared to mindfulness-based interventions. In the literature (e.g., Monteiro, Musten, & Compson, 2015), it has been discussed that the inclusion of overt reference to ethics in mindfulness training is often considered as if it is imposing Buddhist values. A key feature of scientifically driven contemporary psychology is for its practices and strategies to be value-free (Monteiro, 2016). In addition, many contemporary mindfulness-based programs do not overtly address the importance of ethics within their participants' mindfulness practice. Many therapists and program leaders feel that to discuss the ethics of their patients or program participants' behaviors would somehow be an imposition of values (Monteiro, 2016). Thus, current mindfulness-based interventions have been criticized as being

Table 10.1 Common and specific features of compassion-based training and therapy (Kirby & Gilbert, 2016)

Common features

- Designed to be secular in approach, utilizing western psychology science and therapies but also informed, to greater or lesser degrees by contemplative traditions.
- Define what compassion is, with each intervention having a different definition.
- Attention and mindfulness-based training components.
- Compassion-focused visualizations and meditation practices.
- Some form of psychoeducation where rationale provided for intervention.
- Active experiential components.
- Focus on intention or values.
- Homework exercises and regular practice.

Specific features

CFT	MSC	CBCT	CCT	CEB
• Compassion definition includes two psychologies: (1) engagement and (2), alleviation and prevention, each with 6 trainable competencies. • Psychoeducation of evolved "tricky mind" due to old and new brain interactions. • Evolved function of emotions of threat/protection drive/acquisition, and soothing /contentment and the links to (neuro)physiological processes and emotional balance. • The concept of multiple (phenotypic) versions of self arising from gene and social context.	• Based primarily on Neff's conceptualization of self-compassion using bipolar constructs of: (1) Kindness vs self-judgment; (2) common humanity vs isolation; (3) mindfulness vs over-identifying. • Informed by various approaches including self-experiences of life difficulties. Insight Meditation, CFT, and other mindfulness-based interventions such as MSBR.	• Based primarily on Buddhist *lojong* tradition. • Examines compassion as aspirational and active. • Focus on four immeasurables, equanimity, loving-kindness, appreciative joy, and compassion. • Teaches active contemplation of loving-kindness, empathy and compassion towards loved ones, strangers, and enemies.	• Based on definition of compassion by Jinpa involving four constructs cognitive, affective, intentional, and motivation. • Begin and end each session with a meditation practice, which includes breath focus meditation. • Inclusion of *tong-len.* • Primary focus is on meditative practices to cultivate compassion and loving-kindness towards self and others.	• Compassion more focused on others as a prosociality. • Concentration and directive practice meditations. • Recognizing emotions. • Understanding emotional patterns. • Recognizing emotions in others (face, verbal) to promote empathy. • Yoga and movement practices. • Knowledge of functions, sensations, triggers, appraisals, and cognitions associated with affective states.

(continued)

Table 10.1 (continued)

| | | Specific features | | |
CFT	MSC	CBCT	CCT	CEB
• Cultivating a compassionate Mind as an inner organizing motivation and self-identity process made up from cultivating the combined "flows" of compassion: Compassion for others, open to compassion from others, self-compassion. • Developing compassionate imagery and sense of self using acting techniques of becoming and then "acting from" constructed self-role. • Developing and using the compassionate mind to address difficulties such as shame self-criticism and relational conflicts. • Addressing fears block and resistances to positive affect and compassion. • Letter-writing exercises. • Breath, postural training, with "thinking emotional tones." • Expecting and addressing fears blocks and resistances to positive and affiliative emotions and the three orientations of compassion. • Administered both individually and in groups.	• Inclusion of the self-compassion break exercise, based on self-compassion definition. • Breaks meditations into core, other, and informal practices. • Focus on savoring and positive psychology. • Includes letter-writing. • Working with backdraft problems with compassion blocks.	• Integrates cognitive interventions		

Therapy Approach:	Follows eight-steps:	Training Program Components:	Follows six-steps:	Training Program Components:
1. Individualized and group interventions based on client's presentation and case conceptualization 2. Compassionate Mind Training an 8-week intervention is also available	1. Developing attention and stability of Mind 2. The nature of mental experience 3. Developing self-compassion 4. Developing equanimity for others 5. Developing appreciation and gratitude for others 6. Developing affection and empathy 7. Realizing, wishing and aspirational compassion 8. Realizing Active Compassion for others	1. Introduction and review of self-compassion 2. Mindfulness training 3. Application of self-compassion to daily life 4. Developing a compassionate inner voice 5. Living in accordance with values 6. Dealing with difficult emotions 7. Dealing with challenging interpersonal relationships 8. Relating to positive aspects of oneself and one's life with appreciation 9. A mid-program 4-h retreat often included	1. Settling and focusing the mind 1. Loving-kindness and compassion for a loved one 3a. Compassion for self 3b. Loving-kindness for oneself 4. Embracing shared common humanity and developing appreciate of others 5. Cultivating compassion for others 6. Active compassion practice (tong-len) and integrated daily compassion cultivation practice	1. Concentration training 2. Mindfulness training 3. Promotion of empathy and compassion 4. Yoga and other movement practices 5. Conceptual discussion including a focus on values, life meaning 6. Knowledge of functions, sensations, triggers, automatic appraisals, and cognitions associated with specific affective states (e.g., anger, fear, sadness) 7. Recognizing one's own emotions 8. Understanding one's own emotional patterns 9. Recognizing emotion in others (face, verbal) to promote empathy
Initial Development: • Complex clinical problems of high shame and self-criticism.	**Initial Development:** • University students and adolescents at risk to develop emotional resilience.	**Initial Development:** • The general population who struggle with self-criticism.	**Initial Development:** • The general population to help with emotion regulation and cultivate compassion.	**Initial Development:** • The general population to reduce destructive enactment of emotions and enhance prosocial responses.
Source: • Gilbert (2014)	**Source:** • Ozawa-de Silva, B & Dodson-Lavelle, B (2011)	**Source:** • Neff and Germer (2013)	**Source:** • Jazaieri et al. (2014)	**Source:** • Kemeny, M. et al. (2012)

more of a bare attention training (Farias & Wikholm, 2015). Monteiro et al. (2015) pointed out the differences between the contemporary and traditional approaches to mindfulness, and highlighted the concerns expressed in Buddhist communities. The main concerns expressed were: (1) the practice of mindfulness has been de-contextualized from the Eightfold Path; (2) the scientific reductionist approach to defining mindfulness may have devolved to it being, for the most part, just bare attention and does not contain all the elements of what Buddhists call right mindful-ness; and (3) that mindfulness as it is taught in contemporary settings is most often devoid of any explicit reference to ethics though implicit transmission of ethics is presumed.

Although compassion-based interventions focus on the ethic of compassion in their intervention approaches, and these interventions have been found to be effec-tive in a meta-analysis (Kirby, Tellegen, & Steindl, 2016), there is presently no data from compassion-based interventions that have directly examined the emergence of ethics as an outcome variable. Rather, evaluation studies of compassion-based inter-ventions are currently focused on the alleviation of suffering-based outcomes, such as depression and anxiety, most commonly through using self-report measures. Despite this, some interventions have tried to assess the impact of compassion train-ing on helping behavior. For example, Leiberg et al. (2011) examined the impact of a 6-h workshop based on a compassion meditation. The major focus of this study was to determine whether compassion training increased prosocial behavior toward strangers, based on responses in a computerized game called the "Zurich Prosocial Game." Results found that compassion training significantly increased helping behavior toward strangers—to date the only study to directly assess behavior as an outcome.

In contrast to this finding, a recent RCT of compassion training on charitable donation giving found that compassion meditation did not significantly increase donations (Ashar et al., 2016). The study randomized 58 participants to either a smartphone-based compassion meditation program, or to a placebo oxytocin condi-tion, or a Familiarity intervention (to control for expectancy effects and demand characteristics). In the compassion meditation condition, participants were instructed to listen to a 20-min guided meditation daily. Overall, participants donated an average of $21.57 per donation trial, out of $100 maximum. In the compassion meditation and oxytocin conditions, participants' donations did not change over the course of the intervention, however the Familiarity participants' donations decreased. The authors provided some possible reasons for this outcome, including, participants may tend to donate less over time to the same recipients, or possibly that compassion meditation directly targets thoughts and feelings and not overt behavior (Ashar et al., 2016). It could also be that the sample size did not have adequate power to detect a small effect.

Overall, what these findings indicate is current evaluations of compassion-based interventions are focused on alleviation of suffering, and some are also moving toward examining the impact on prosociality. To better assess the emergence of ethics as an outcome from compassion training, a different study design may poten-tially be useful. For example, the use of diary entries or group discussions pertain-ing to ethical dilemmas could begin to shed light on whether compassion interventions increase ethical thinking and behavior. In addition, researchers are now developing questionnaires that aim to assess whether individuals have not only experienced an increased motivation to be compassionate, but also whether they have engaged in behavioral acts (Steindl et al., 2016). Given the theoretical notion that compassion is the foundation for morality and ethics (e.g., Halifax, 2012), future research may benefit from examining the relationship between moral reasoning or ethical decision making and compassion training. Importantly, evaluation work in mindfulness is beginning to examine this relationship, with Shapiro, Jazaieri, and Goldin (2012) finding that the Mindfulness-Based Stress Reduction (MSBR) program led to improvement in moral reasons and ethical decision making 2 months post-intervention.

Future of Compassion and Ethics Research

In terms of future research, examining physiological markers such as Heart Rate Variability may be one of the key elements in understanding the emergence of ethical thinking and behavior. For example, an innovative study by Leon, Hernandez, Rodriguez, and Vila (2008) found that HRV modulates perception of other-blame, reducing anger. Specifically, 84 college participants were asked to read a story that was constructed in such a way to be emotionally meaningful and involve a negative consequence for the reader. The story involved the reader being dismissed from his/her part-time job due to the actions of a colleague. Participants were randomized to the story either having an intentional or non-intentional ending, where a colleague is deliberately or not-deliberately responsible for the job loss. Participants are measured on a range of variables including the primary measure of HRV. Researchers found that in the situations of intentionality, individuals with higher HRV made less extreme evaluation of the offender's blame, versus those with lower HRV, thus leading to a reduction in anger reaction. These results suggest that HRV is a direct index of cognitive rather than emotional regulation. These results provide some preliminary evidence indicating how the physiological measure of HRV can influence how we feel and think about a situation, which can directly impact our decision making in ethical dilemmas.

Kirby, Doty, Perocchi, and Gilbert (2016) have recently suggested that HRV is the key primary outcome that needs to be measured in compassion training as it is a direct measure of physiology. Moving beyond the use of self-report, which is of limited reliability, or the more complex and expensive fMRI, HRV is relatively easy to measure and offers windows to a number of important physiological systems, including the frontal cortex and people's relative state of psychological flexibility. The value of using HRV both as a process/state and outcome measure in compassion research is linked to three major domains. First, that psychopathology (depression, anxiety, paranoia) and underlying processes such as self-criticism, negative rumination, shame, and worry are linked to lower levels of HRV (Beevers et al., 2011; Brosschot et al., 2007; Rockliff, Gilbert, McEwan, Lightman, & Glover, 2008). Second, that compassion is correlated with HRV

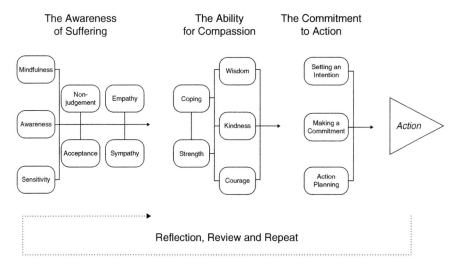

Fig. 10.2 The motivational flow from mindfulness to compassionate action

(Svendsen et al., 2016). Third, compassion-based practices can directly increase HRV and potentially other biological, physiological, and neurophysiological measures such as cortisol and blood inflammation (Rockliff et al., 2008; Kok et al., 2013; Petrocchi, Ottaviani, & Couyoumdjian, 2016). These results perhaps highlight how the precursors of compassion are, in a way, "hard-wired" into our physiology, and if we can impact our physiology we increase our ability to be more compassionate and therefore more likely to act ethically. Thus, future research needs to measure individuals' levels of HRV in compassion-based interventions, as well as how this impacts the emergence of ethics, potentially through how they respond to ethical dilemmas. This would shed further light on the interconnection between compassion, ethics, and physiology.

A final potential way to promote the ethic of compassion in training is to have a pragmatic flow diagram on how the flow of mindfulness to compassionate action may look. We have proposed such a model in Fig. 10.2, outlining how the awareness of suffering can lead to the ability for compassion, which can impact on committed action. This model is just a preliminary conceptualization that requires testing to determine whether a pragmatic flow would be helpful theoretically, for researchers, and for individuals engaging in compassion training to help improve ethical thinking and behavior.

Conclusion

The focus of this chapter was to suggest that compassion may be our highest ethic. We discussed how compassion can be a guiding motivation to address life difficulties, and how compassion is understood in terms of evolutionary processes and physiology. Based on the recent research conducted in compassion science, we put forward the view that compassion holds potential as being our "*hard-wired*" ethical compass. However, our modern-day Western cultural values diminish its impact. Compassion-based interventions hold promise to help increase compassion, and potentially, influence our physiology, so we can begin to become more ethical beings.

References

Armstrong, K. (2010). *Twelve steps to a compassionate life*. New York: Random House.

Ashar, Y. K., Andrews-Hanna, J. R., Yarkoni, T., Sills, J., Halifax, J., Dimidjian, S., & Wager, T. D. (2016). Effects of compassion meditation on a psychological model of charitable donation. *Emotion, 16*, 691–705. https://doi.org/10.1037/emo0000119

Beevers, C. G., Ellis, A. J., & Reid, R. M. (2011). Heart rate variability predicts cognitive reactivity to a sad mood provocation. *Cognitive Therapy and Research, 35*, 395–403. https://doi.org/10.1007/s10608-010-9324-0

Bernard, C., Mills, M., Swenson, L., & Walsh, R. P. (2005). An evolutionary theory of human motivation. *Genetic, Social, and General Psychology Monographs, 131*, 129–184.

Bodhi, B. (2000). *The noble eightfold way: Way to the end of suffering*. Onalaska, WA: BPS Pariyatti Editions.

Brosschot, J. F., Van Dijk, E., & Thayer, J. F. (2007). Daily worry is related to low heart rate variability during waking and the subsequent nocturnal sleep period. *International Journal of Psychophysiology, 63*, 39–47. https://doi.org/10.1016/j.ijpsycho.2006.07.016

Brown, S. L., & Brown, R. M. (2015). Connecting prosocial behavior to improved physical health: Contributions from the neurobiology of parenting. *Neuroscience and Biobehavioral Reviews, 55*, 1–17.

Brune, M., Belsky, J., Fabrega, H., Feierman, J. R., Gilbert, P., Glantz, K., … Wilson, D. R. (2012). The crisis of psychiatry – Insights and prospects from evolutionary theory. *World Psychiatry, 11*, 55–57.

Clutton-Brock, T. H. (1991). *The evolution of parental care*. Princeton, NJ: Princeton University Press.

Conway, C., & Slavich, G. M. (2017). Behavior genetics of prosocial behavior. In P. Gilbert (Ed.), *Compassion: Concepts, research and applications* (pp. 151–170). New York: Routledge.

Cozolino, L. (2007). *The neuroscience of human relationships: Attachment and the developing brain*. New York: W. W. Norton.

Dalai Lama. (1995). *The power of compassion*. India: Harper Collins.

Davidson, R. J. (2012). The biology of compassion. In C. Germer & D. Siegel (Eds.), *Wisdom and compassion in psychotherapy: Deepening mindfulness in clinical practice* (pp. 111–110: 111–118). New York: Guilford Press.

Delle Fave, A., Massimini, F., & Bassie, M. (2010). Hedonism and eudaimonism in positive psychology. In A. Delle Fave, F. Massimini, & M. Bassie (Eds.), *Psychological selection and optimal experience across cultures* (pp. 3–18). Springer: New York.

Depue, R. A., & Morrone-Strupinsky, J. V. (2005). A neurobehavioral model of affiliative bonding. *Behavioral and Brain Sciences, 28*, 313–395. https://doi.org/10.1017/S0140525X05000063

Dunbar, R. I. M., & Barrett, L. (2007). *The Oxford handbook of evolutionary psychology*. Oxford: Oxford University Press.

Eisenberg, N., Fabes, R. A., Bustamante, D., Mathy, R. M., Miller, P. A., & Lindholm, E. (1998). Differentiation of vicariously induced emotional reactions in children. *Developmental Psychology, 24*, 237–246. https://doi.org/10.1037/0012-1649.24.2.237

Eisenberg, N., Fabes, R. A., Miller, P. A., Fultz, J., Shell, R., & Mathy, R. M. (1989). Relation of sympathy and personal distress to prosocial behavior: A multimethod study. *Journal of Personality and Social Psychology, 57*, 55–66. https://doi.org/10.1037/0022-3514.57.1.55

Eisenberg, N., Fabes, R. A., Murphy, B., Karbon, M., Smith, M., & Maszk, P. (1996). The relations of children's dispositional empathy-related responding to their emotionality, regulation, and social functioning. *Developmental Psychology, 32*, 195–209. https://doi.org/10.1037/0012-1649.32.2.195

Eisenberg, N., Fabes, R. A., Schaller, M., Miller, P., Gustavo, C., & Poulin, R. (1991). Personality and socialization correlates of vicarious emotional responding. *Journal of Personality and Social Psychology, 61*, 459–470. https://doi.org/10.1037/0022-3514.61.3.459

Ekman, P. (2014). *Moving toward global compassion.* Lexington, KY: Paul Ekman Group.

Ekman, E., & Ekman, P. (2013). Cultivating emotional balance: Structure, research, and implementation. In T. Singer & M. Bolz (Eds.), *Compassion: Bridging practice and science* (pp. 398–414). Munich: Max Planck Society.

Fabes, R. A., Eisenberg, N., & Eisenbud, L. (1993). Behavioral and physiological correlates of children's reactions to others in distress. *Developmental Psychology, 29*, 655–663. https://doi.org/10.1016/S0065-2601(08)60412-8

Farias, M., & Wikholm, C. (2015). *The Buddha Pill: Can meditation change you?* London: Watkins Publishing.

Feldman, C., & Kuyken, W. (2011). Compassion in the landscape of suffering. *Contemporary Buddhism, 12*, 143–155.

Fowers, B. J. (2015a). *The evolution of ethics: Human sociality and the emergence of ethical mindedness.* London: Palgrave/McMillan.

Franco, Z., Blau, K., & Zimbardo, P. G. (2011). Heroism: A conceptual analysis and differentiation between heroic action and altruism. *Review of General Psychology, 15*, 99.

Fredrickson, B. L., Grewen, K. M., Coffey, K. A., Algoe, S. B., Firestine, A. M., Arevalo, J. M. G., … Cole, S. W. (2013). A functional genomic perspective on human well-being. *Proceedings of the National Academy of Sciences, 110*, 13684–13689. https://doi.org/10.1073/pnas.1305419110

Germer, C. K. (2009). *The mindful path to self-compassion: Freeing yourself from destructive thoughts and emotions.* New York: Guilford Press.

Gilbert, P. (2009). *The compassionate mind: A new approach to life's challenges.* Oakland, CA: New Harbinger Publications.

Gilbert, P. (2014). The origins and nature of compassion focused therapy. *British Journal of Clinical Psychology, 53*, 6–41. https://doi.org/10.1111/bjc.12043

Gilbert, P., & Choden. (2013). *Mindful compassion.* London: Constable-Robinson.

Gilbert, P., McEwan, K., Matos, M., & Rivis, A. (2010). Fears of compassion: Development of three self-report measures. *Psychology and Psychotherapy: Theory, Research and Practice, 84*, 239–255. https://doi.org/10.1348/147608310X526511

Goetz, J. L., Keltner, D., & Simon-Thomas, E. (2010). Compassion: An evolutionary analysis and empirical review. *Psychological Bulletin, 136*, 351–374. https://doi.org/10.1037/a0018807

Halifax, J. (2012). A heuristic model of enactive compassion. *Current Opinion in Supportive and Palliative Care, 6*, 228–235. https://doi.org/10.1097/SPC.0b013e3283530fbe

Harvey, P. (2000). *An introduction to Buddhist ethics.* Cambridge: Cambridge University Press.

Hoffmann, S. G., Grossman, P., & Hinton, D. E. (2011). Loving-kindness and compassion meditation: Potential for psychological intervention. *Clinical Psychology Review, 13*, 1126–1132. https://doi.org/10.1016/j.cpr.2011.07.003

Huang, J. Y., & Bargh, J. A. (2014). The selfish goal: Autonomously operating motivational structures as the proximate cause of human judgement and behavior. *Behavioral and Brain Sciences, 37*, 121–135.

Jazaieri, H., Jinpa, T., McGonigal, K., Rosenberg, E. L., Finkelstein, J., Simon-Thomas, E., … Goldin, P. R. (2013). Enhancing compassion: A randomized controlled trial of a compassion cultivation training program. *Journal of Happiness Studies, 14*, 1113–1126.

Jazaieri, H., McGonigal, K., Jinpa, T., Doty, J. R., Gross, J. J., & Goldin, P. R. (2014). A randomized controlled trial of compassion cultivation training: Effects on mindfulness, affect, and emotion regulation. *Motivation and Emotion, 38*, 23–35. https://doi.org/10.1007/s11031-013-9368-z

Jinpa, G. T. (2010). *Compassion cultivation training (CCT): Instructor's manual.* Unpublished.

Junpa, G. T. (2015). *Fearless heart.* New York: Avery Publishing Group.

Kasser, T. (2011). Cultural values and the well-being of future generations: A cross-national study. *Journal of Cross-Cultural Psychology, 42,* 206–215. https://doi.org/10.1177/0022022110396865

Kasser, T., Ryan, R. M., Zax, M., & Sameroff, A. J. (1995). The relations of maternal and social environments to late adolescents' materialistic and prosocial values. *Developmental Psychology, 31,* 907–914. https://doi.org/10.1037/0012-1649.31.6.907

Keltner, D., Marsh, J., & Smith, J. A. (2010). *The compassionate instinct.* New York: Norton & Company.

Kidder, R. (2003). *How good people make tough choices: Resolving the dilemmas of ethical living.* New York: Harper Collins.

Kirby, J. N. (2016). Compassion interventions: The programs, the evidence, and implications for research and practice. *Psychology and Psychotherapy: Theory, Research and Practice.* Advanced online publication. doi:https://doi.org/10.1111/papt.

Kirby, J. N., Doty, J. R., Petrocchi, N., & Gilbert, P. (2017). The current and future role of heart rate variability for assessing and training compassion. *Frontiers in Public Health.* https://doi.org/10.3389/fpubh.2017.00040

Kirby, J. N., & Gilbert, P. (2016). The emergence of compassion focused therapies. In P. Gilbert (Ed.), *Compassion: Concepts, research and application.* London: Routledge.

Kirby, J. N., Tellegen, C. L., & Steindl, S. R. (2016). Cultivating compassion: A systematic review and meta-analysis of compassion-based interventions. Manuscript under review.

Klimecki, O. M., Leiberg, S., Ricard, M., & Singer, T. (2014). Differential pattern of functional brain plasticity after compassion and empathy training. *Social Cognitive & Affective Neuroscience, 7*(9), 873–879. https://doi.org/10.1093/scan/nst060

Klinger, E. (1977). *Meaning and void.* Minneapolis, MN: University of Minnesota Press.

Kok, B. E., Coffey, K. A., Cohn, M. A., Catalino, L. I., Vacharkulksemsuk, T., Algoe, S. B., & Fredrickson, B. L. (2013). How positive emotions build physical health: Perceived positive social connections account for the upward spiral between positive emotions and vagal tone. *Psychological Science, 24,* 1123–1132. https://doi.org/10.1177/0956797612470827

Konrath, S. H., O'Brien, E. H., & Hsing, C. (2011). Change in dispositional empathy in American college students over time: A meta-analysis. *Personality and Social Psychology Review, 15,* 180–198. https://doi.org/10.1177/1088868310377395

Krygier, J. R., Heathers, J. A., Shahrestani, S., Abbott, M., Gross, J. J., & Kemp, A. H. (2013). Mindfulness meditation, well-being, and heart rate variability: A preliminary investigation into the impact of intensive Vipassana meditation. *International Journal of Psychophysiology, 89,* 305–313. https://doi.org/10.1016/j.ijpsycho.2013.06.017

Leaviss, J., & Uttley, L. (2015). Psychotherapeutic benefits of compassion-focused therapy: An early systematic review. *Psychological Medicine, 45,* 927–945. https://doi.org/10.1017/S0033291714002141

Leiberg, S., Klimecki, O., & Singer, T. (2011). Short-term compassion training increases prosocial behavior in a newly developed prosocial game. *PLoS One, 6,* e17798. https://doi.org/10.1371/journal.pone.0017798

Leon, I., Hernandez, J. A., Rodriguez, S., & Vila, J. (2008). When head is tempered by heart: Heart rate variability modulates perception of other-blame reducing anger. *Motivation & Emotion, 33,* 1–9. https://doi.org/10.1007/s11031-008-9112-2

Liotti, G., & Gilbert, P. (2011). Mentalizing, motivation, and social mentalities: Theoretical considerations and implications for psychotherapy. *Psychology and Psychotherapy: Theory, Research and Practice, 84,* 9–25. https://doi.org/10.1348/147608310X520094

Making Caring Common Project, Harvard. (2014). *MCCP Report: The Children We Mean to Raise.* Retrieved from: http://mcc.gse.harvard.edu/files/gse-mcc/files/mcc-research-report.pdf?m=1448057487

MacLean, P. (1985). Brain evolution relating to family, play and the separation call. *Archives of General Psychiatry, 42,* 405–417.

Matos, M., Duarte, C., Duarte, J., Pinto-Gouveia, J., Petroscchi, N., Basran, J, & Gilbert, P. (2016). Psychological and physiological effects of compassionate mind training: A randomised controlled trial. Under Review.

Mayseless, O. (2016). *The caring motivation: An integrated theory*. New York: Oxford University Press.

Metzinger, T. (2009). *The ego tunnel – the science of the mind and the myth of the self*. New York: Basic Books.

Monroe, K. R. (1996). *The heart of altruism: Perceptions of a common humanity*. Princeton, NJ: Princeton University Press.

Monteiro, L. (2016). Implicit ethics and mindfulness: Subtle assumptions that MBIs are values-neutral. *International Journal of Psychotherapy, 20*, 210–224.

Monteiro, L. M., Musten, R. F., & Compson, J. (2015). Traditional and contemporary mindfulness: Finding the middle path in the tangle of concerns. *Mindfulness, 6*, 1–13.

Neel, R., Kenrick, D. T., White, A. E., & Neuberg, S. L. (2016). Individual differences in fundamental social motives. *Personality and Individual Differences, 110*, 887–907.

Neff, K. (2003). The development and validation of a scale to measure self-compassion. *Self and Identity, 2*, 223–250. https://doi.org/10.1080/15298860390209035

Neff, K. D., & Germer, C. K. (2013). A pilot study and randomized controlled trial of the mindful self-compassion program. *Journal of Clinical Psychology, 69*, 28–44. https://doi.org/10.1002/jclp.21923

Nesse, R. M., & Williams, G. C. (1995). *Evolution & healing*. London: Weidenfeld & Nicolson.

Pace, T. W., Negi, L. T., Adame, D. D., Cole, S. P., Sivilli, T. I., Brown, T. D., … Raison, C. L. (2009). Effect of compassion meditation on neuroendocrine, innate immune and behavioral responses to psychosocial stress. *Psychoneuroendocrinology, 34*, 87–98. https://doi.org/10.1016/j.psyneuen.2008.08.011

Park, H., Twenge, J. M., & Greenfield, P. M. (2014). The great recession: Implications for adolescent values and behavior. *Social Psychological and Personality Science, 5*, 310–318. https://doi.org/10.1177/1948550613495419

Petrocchi, N., Ottaviani, C., & Couyoumdjian, A. (2016). Compassion at the mirror: Exposure to a mirror increases the efficacy of a self-compassion manipulation in enhancing soothing positive affect and heart rate variability. *The Journal of Positive Psychology*. https://doi.org/10.1080/17439760.2016.1209544

Porges, S. W. (2007). The polyvagal perspective. *Biological Psychology, 74*, 116–143. https://doi.org/10.1016/j.biopsycho.2006.06.009

Rockliff, H., Gilbert, P., McEwan, K., Lightman, S., & Glover, D. (2008). A pilot exploration of heart rate variability and salivary cortisol responses to compassion-focused imagery. *Journal of Clinical Neuropsychiatry, 5*, 132–139.

Ricard, M. (2015). *Altruism*. London: Atlantic Books.

Seppala, E., Rossomando, T., & Doty, J. R. (2012). Social connection and compassion: Important predictors of health and well-being. *Social Research, 80*, 411–430. https://doi.org/10.1353/sor.2013.0027

Shapiro, S. L., Jazaieri, H., & Goldin, P. R. (2012). Mindfulness-based stress reduction effects on moral reasoning and decision making. *Journal of Positive Psychology*. [Epub ahead of print]. doi:https://doi.org/10.1080/17439760.2012.723732.

Siegel, D. J. (2009). *Mindsight: Change your brain and your life*. Melbourne: Scribe.

Singer, T., & Bolz, M. (2013). *Compassion. Bridging practice and science*. Munich: Max Planck Society.

Strauss, C., Taylor, B. L., Gu, J., Kuyken, W., Baer, R., Jones, F., & Cavanagh, K. (2016). What is compassion and how can we measure it? A review of definitions and measures. *Clinical Psychology Review, 47*, 15–27. https://doi.org/10.1016/j.cpr.2016.05.004

Suess, P. A., Porges, S. W., & Plude, D. J. (1994). Cardiac vagal tone and sustained attention in school-age children. *Psychophysiology, 31*, 17–22. https://doi.org/10.1111/j.1469-8986

Svendsen, J. L., Osnes, B., Binder, P. E., Dundas, I., Visted, E., Nordy, H., … Sorensen, L. (2016). Trait self-compassion reflects emotional flexibility through an association with high vagally mediated heart rate variability. *Mindfulness*, *7*, 1103–1113. https://doi.org/10.1007/s12671-016-0549-1

Swain, J.E., & Ho, S.S. (2016). Parental brain – The crucible of compassion. In J. Doty and E. Seppala (Eds.) *Oxford handbook on compassion science*. Oxford: USA.

Tirch, D., Schoendorff, B., & Silberstein, L. R. (2014). *The ACT practitioner's guide to the science of compassion*. New York: New Harbinger.

Thayer, J. F., & Lane, R. D. (2000). A model of neurovisceral integration in emotion regulation and dysregulation. *Journal of Affective Disorder*, *61*, 201–216. https://doi.org/10.1016/S0165-0327(00)00338-4

Twenge, J. M., Campbell, W. K., & Freeman, E. C. (2012). Generational differences in young adults' life goals, concern for others, and civic orientation, 1966–2009. *Journal of Personality and Social Psychology*, *102*, 1045–1062. https://doi.org/10.1037/a0027408

Chapter 11
Core Values in Mindful Self-Compassion

Pittman McGehee, Christopher Germer, and Kristin Neff

There's a thread you follow. It goes among things that change. But it doesn't change.

William Stafford

Compassion may be understood as "a sensitivity to suffering in self and others with a commitment to try to alleviate and prevent it" (Gilbert, 1989/2016). *Self-compassion* is simply compassion directed inward. It is a humble enterprise—remembering to include ourselves in the circle of compassion.

The construct of self-compassion was operationally defined and introduced to the scientific community over a decade ago by Kristin Neff (2003). She proposed self-compassion as a type of self-to-self relating that consists of three components: (1) *self-kindness* versus *self-judgment*, (2) *common humanity* versus *isolation*, and (3) *mindfulness* versus *over-identification*. These components combine and mutually interact to create a self-compassionate frame of mind. *Self-kindness* entails being gentle, supportive, and understanding toward oneself. Rather than harshly judging oneself for personal shortcomings, we offer ourselves warmth and unconditional acceptance. *Common humanity* involves recognizing the shared human experience, understanding that all humans fail and make mistakes, and that all people lead imperfect lives. Rather than feeling isolated by one's imperfection—egocentrically feeling as if "I" am the only one who has failed or suffers—the self-compassionate

P. McGehee, PhD
University of Texas, 508 Deep Eddy, Austin, TX 78703, USA
e-mail: pittman@mcgeheephd.com

C. Germer, PhD (✉)
20 Meacham Road, Cambridge, MA 02140, USA
e-mail: ckgermer@gmail.com

K. Neff, PhD
University of Texas, 1 University Station D5800, Austin, TX 78712, USA
e-mail: kneff@austin.utexas.edu

© Springer International Publishing AG 2017
L.M. Monteiro et al. (eds.), *Practitioner's Guide to Ethics and Mindfulness-Based Interventions*, Mindfulness in Behavioral Health,
DOI 10.1007/978-3-319-64924-5_11

person takes a broader and more connected perspective with regard to personal shortcomings and individual difficulties. *Mindfulness* involves being aware of one's present moment experience of suffering with clarity and balance, without being swept away by a storyline about one's negative aspects or life experience—a process that is termed "over-identification." Taken together, the three components of self-compassion comprise a state of "loving, connected presence."

The research on self-compassion has increased exponentially over the past decade, with over 1000 journal articles, chapters, and dissertations currently available on the topic (based on a Google Scholar search of entries containing "self-compassion" in the title). Most research on self-compassion has been correlational, using the Self-Compassion Scale (SCS; Neff, 2003) that measures the three components described above. Increasingly, however, researchers are using additional methods to explore self-compassion such as experimentally inducing a self-compassionate state of mind or evaluating the impact of short- and long-term interventions on psychological, physiological, and behavioral measures of well-being. Research findings tend to converge regardless of the methodology used.

In general, the scientific literature provides clear support for the link between self-compassion and well-being. Self-compassion has been associated with greater levels of happiness, optimism, life satisfaction, body appreciation, and motivation (Albertson et al., 2014; Breines and Chen, 2013; Hollis-Walker & Colosimo, 2011; Neff, Kirkpatrick, & Rude, 2007) as well as lower levels of depression, anxiety, stress, rumination, body shame, and fear of failure (Webb, Fiery, & Jafari, 2016; Finlay-Jones, Rees, & Kane, 2015; Neff, Hseih, & Dejitthirat, 2005; Odou & Brinker, 2014; Raes, 2010). Self-compassion is also predictive of healthier physiological responses to stress (Arch et al., 2014; Breines et al., 2015; Breines, Thoma et al., 2014).

Ethical Values and the three Components of Self-Compassion

Self-Kindness Versus Self-Judgment Contrary to what might be expected, research suggests that most people are more compassionate toward others than themselves (Neff, 2003). To illustrate this point, one of the first exercises in the MSC program invites participants to imagine a close friend who is suffering and reflect upon how they might respond to their friend, especially noting their words, tone, gestures, or attitudes. Then participants are asked, "How do you respond to *yourself* when you find yourself struggling in some way?" Typically, MSC participants discover that they are markedly less kind and more judgmental toward themselves than others. With this realization, participants begin to explore what they themselves may need in a tough moment, such as attention, validation, warmth, and patience, which launches participants on the path to self-compassion.

Most everyone seems to have an instinct for compassion (Keltner, Marsh, & Smith, 2010). Compassion is also a basic value in all the world's religions that "reflects something essential to the structure of our humanity" (Armstrong, 2010). For example, Confucius wrote, "Never do to others what you would not like them to do to you" and Jesus said, "Love your neighbor as yourself" (Mark 12:31).

However, ancient definitions of compassion were usually prescriptions for how people should relate to *others,* and they assume that we naturally love ourselves. This is no longer the case, however. We are more often our own worst enemy. In MSC, our instinct to be kind to others (sometimes just a select few) becomes a vehicle for learning self-kindness. We learn to tuck ourselves into the circle of our compassion. In this manner, the training of self-compassion is based on the basic human value of compassion for others.

Common Humanity Versus Isolation Unfortunately, when we struggle, we are more likely than ever to feel separate and alone. This is because our field of perception narrows when we feel under threat and it is hard to see beyond ourselves. We may further isolate ourselves in embarrassment or shame, as if we were solely responsible for our misfortune. However, when we are self-compassionate, we actually feel *more* connected to others in our awareness of shared human suffering and imperfection—we ourselves as a thread in a very large cloth.

Furthermore, we are likely to have a sense that our misfortune is the product of a universe of interacting causes and conditions rather than entirely due to personal error. This less egocentric view is known as the wisdom of interdependence. Insight into interdependence, or common humanity, opens the door to compassion because it engenders a sense of humility and mutuality. In this way, the ethical values of wisdom, compassion, interconnection, and selflessness are contained in the common humanity component of self-compassion.

Mindfulness Versus Over-Identification Mindfulness is commonly defined as "the awareness that emerges through paying attention, on purpose, in the present moment, and non-judgmentally to the unfolding of experience moment by moment" (Kabat-Zinn, 2003, p. 145). It is "knowing what you are experiencing *while* you are experiencing it." The opposite of mindfulness is losing perspective and becoming overly identified with our experience. Our tendency to ruminate can become particularly troublesome when we are absorbed in negative thoughts and feelings about ourselves. Mindfulness allows us to see our thoughts and feelings as just that— thoughts and feelings—rather than becoming swept up in them and reacting in regrettable ways.

Mindfulness is the foundation of self-compassion insofar as we can only respond self-compassionately when we know we are struggling. Ironically, we may be the last to know it when we suffer. A mindful moment could simply be the recognition that, "*This* is a moment of suffering!" rather than being lost in rumination, such as "I can't believe she said that," and "why did I do it?" The space created by mindful awareness opens the possibility of compassion. Mindfulness is also important in self-compassion training as a means for anchoring awareness in the present moment (e.g., the breath, soles of the feet) when we feel emotionally distressed. Finally, mindfulness helps to generate equanimity, or balanced awareness, which ripens into wisdom. Wisdom refers to understanding the complexity of a situation and the ability to see our way through. When we disentangle for our experience with mindfulness, we are more likely to see the larger picture, the options available to us, and to behave accordingly. In short, mindfulness creates the conditions for wise and compassionate action.

Needs and Core Values

The starting point of self-compassion training is the question, "What do I need?" When we know what we truly need, we are more likely to give it to ourselves. However, finding an answer to the question, "What do I need?" can be a challenge. Understanding our core values may help us discover our deepest needs.

Needs are universal and shared by everyone, albeit to different degrees by different individuals. Examples of needs are safety, belonging, health, and happiness. Needs are deeper than wants. Needs tend to come from the neck down—associated with physical and emotional survival—whereas wants arise from the neck up. Wants can be infinite in number, such as wanting a big house, a fancy car, a beautiful partner, and amazing children.

Sigmund Freud (1923) believed that needs are rooted in primal instincts and drives. Carl Jung (1961) expanded Freud's model of human needs to include the search for meaning, reflected in his theory of individuation. Maslow (1943) put needs into a hierarchy beginning with physical needs such as food and shelter that must be satisfied before graduating to higher needs associated with individuation, connection, and love. Glasser (1998) described humans as having five basic needs: survival, love, belonging, power, freedom, and fun. Recent theorists suggest that our drive for care and connection might subsume all other human needs (Cacioppo & Patrick, 2008; Gilbert & Choden, 2014). Ryan and Deci (2000) consider psychological health and well-being as linked to three basic human needs: autonomy, competence, and psychological relatedness.

Core values are the principles that determine the choices we make in life. Core values are discovered rather than determined by social desirability. They are a thread that runs through our lives. Examples of core values are compassion, generosity, honesty, friendship, loyalty, courage, tranquility, and curiosity. Thomas Merton (1969) wrote:

> If you want to identify me, ask me not where I live, or what I like to eat, or how I comb my hair, but ask me what I am living for, in detail, and ask me what I think is keeping me from living fully for the things I want to live for. (p. 160–161).

There is also a difference between core values and goals. Goals can be achieved whereas core values guide us after achieving our goals. Goals are destinations; core values are directions. Goals are something we do; core values are something we are. A good eulogy reflects a deceased person's core values, the *axis mundi* of his or her life.

Ruth Baer (2015) highlights Ryan and Deci's (2000) need for autonomy as a central link between our biological needs and our core values. In her discussion of values, Baer also makes reference to Peterson and Seligman's (2004) virtues (e.g., wisdom, courage, humanity, justice, temperance, and transcendence) and their associated character strengths (e.g., creativity, bravery, love, loyalty, humility, and appreciation). Peterson and Seligman consider human virtues to be biologically adaptive and essential for promoting the well-being of individuals and their communities. In that context, Baer suggests that the human need for autonomy is especially important as a basis for looking into our core values and thereby contribute to human flourishing.

Knowing our core values can help us orient us to our deepest needs. For example, if "friendship" is a core value for a particular individual, it points toward the basic need for love and connection described by Cacioppo et al. (2008). If "honesty" is a core value, it may point to a person's need for emotional safety, and if "curiosity" is a value, the underlying need may be for growth and freedom.

Both needs and values seem to reflect something essential in human nature. Needs are more commonly associated with physical and emotional survival, such as the need for health and safety, whereas values tend to have an element of choice, such as the choice to focus on friendship or autonomy. *Knowing* our needs and values supports our ability to respond with compassion in challenging times regardless whether we are struggling for survival or searching for happiness.

Mindful Self-Compassion (MSC) Training

MSC was the first training program created for the general public that was specifically designed to enhance a person's self-compassion. Mindfulness-based training programs such as mindfulness-based stress reduction (MBSR; Kabat-Zinn, 1991) and mindfulness-based cognitive therapy (MBCT; Segal et al., 2002) also increase self-compassion (Kuyken et al., 2010), but they do so implicitly, as a welcome byproduct. The developers of MSC, Chris Germer and Kristin Neff, wondered, "What would happen if self-compassion skills were *explicitly* taught as the primary focus of the training?"

MSC is loosely modeled on the MBSR program especially by the focus on experiential learning inquiry-based teaching and 8 weekly sessions of two or more hours each. Some key practices in MBSR have been adapted for MSC by highlighting the *quality* of awareness—warmth kindness—in those practices. Most MSC practices are explicitly designed to cultivate compassion for self and others.

MSC can be accurately described as *mindfulness-based self-compassion training*. It is a hybrid mix of mindfulness and compassion with an emphasis on self-compassion. MSC was designed for the general public yet it also blends personal development training and psychotherapy. The focus of MSC is on building the resources of mindfulness and self-compassion. In contrast, therapy tends to focus on healing old wounds. The therapeutic aspect of MSC is typically a byproduct of developing inner strengths. A corrective emotional experience occurs when relational injury is uncovered through awareness and compassion training and participants learn to hold themselves and their pain in a new way—with greater kindness and understanding.

There are currently three other structured time-limited empirically supported *compassion* training programs: Compassion Cultivation Training (CCT; Jazairi et al., 2014), Cognitively-Based Compassion Training (CBCT; Pace et al., 2009), and Mindfulness-Based Compassionate Living (MBCL; Bartels-Velthuis et al.,

2016; van den Brink & Koster, 2015). Each of these programs has a different origin and emphasis and may vary in format and target audience but they all share the common goal of cultivating compassion toward self and others. In addition, Compassion Focused Therapy (CFT; Gilbert, 2010) is a model of psychotherapy with a well-articulated theoretical base and an abundance of practical exercises. Compassion-Focused Therapy does not follow the 6- to 8-week group training structure of the other compassion training programs although a structured program for the general public is currently under development with promising early evidence of effectiveness.

The MSC curriculum has been carefully scaffolded so that the content of each session builds upon the previous session:

- Session 1 is a welcome session, introducing the participants to the course and to one another. Session 1 also provides a conceptual introduction to self-compassion with informal practices that can be practiced during the week.
- Session 2 anchors the program in mindfulness. Formal and informal mindfulness practices are taught to participants as well as the rationale for mindfulness in MSC. Participants learn about "backdraft"—when self-compassion activates difficult emotions—and how to manage backdraft with mindfulness practice. Sessions 1 and 2 include more didactic material than subsequent sessions to establish a conceptual foundation for practice.
- Session 3 introduces loving-kindness and the intentional practice of warming up awareness. Loving-kindness is cultivated before compassion because it is less challenging. Participants get a chance to discover their own loving-kindness and compassion phrases for use in meditation. An interpersonal exercise helps develop safety and trust in the group.
- Session 4 broadens loving-kindness meditation into a compassionate conversation with ourselves, especially how to motivate ourselves with kindness rather than self-criticism. By session 4, many participants discover that self-compassion is more challenging than expected so we explore what "progress" means and encourage participants to practice compassion when they stumble or feel like a failure during the course.
- Session 5 focuses on core values and the skill of compassionate listening. These topics and practices are less emotionally challenging than others, and are introduced in the middle of the program to give participants an emotional break while still deepening the practice of self-compassion.
- The retreat comes after Session 5. It is a chance for students to immerse themselves in the practices already learned and apply them to whatever arises in the mind during 4 h of silence. Some new practices that require more activity are also introduced during the retreat—walking, stretching out on the floor, and going outside.
- Session 6 gives students an opportunity to test and refine their skills by applying them to difficult emotions. Students also learn a new informal practice—soften-soothe-allow—that specifically addresses difficult emotions. The emotion of shame is described and demystified in this session because shame is so often

associated with self-criticism and is entangled with sticky emotions such as guilt and anger.

- Session 7 addresses challenging relationships. Relationships are the source of most of our emotional pain. This is the most emotionally activating session in the course, but most students are ready for it after practicing mindfulness and self-compassion for 6–7 weeks. Themes of Session 7 are anger in relationships, caregiver fatigue, and forgiveness. Rather than trying to repair old relationships, students learn to meet and hold their emotional needs, and *themselves*, in a new way.

- Session 8 brings the course to a close with positive psychology and the practices of savoring, gratitude, and self-appreciation—three ways to embrace the good in our lives. To sustain self-compassion practice, we need to recognize and enjoy positive experiences as well. At the end of the course, students are invited to review what they have learned, what they would like to remember, and what they would like to practice after the course has ended.

Neff and Germer (2013) conducted a randomized controlled study of the MSC program in which MSC participants demonstrated significantly greater increases in self-compassion, mindfulness, compassion for others, and life satisfaction, as well as greater decreases in depression, anxiety, stress, and emotional avoidance compared to wait-listed controls. Moreover, all gains in self-compassion were maintained 6 months and 1 year later. A second randomized controlled trial of MSC was conducted by Friis, Johnson, Cutfield, and Consedine (2016) with people suffering from type 1 and type 2 diabetes. MSC participants demonstrated a significantly greater increase in self-compassion and decrease in depression and diabetes distress compared to controls, and a statistically meaningful decrease in HbA1c between baseline and 3-month follow-up. Other empirically supported adaptations of MSC have been developed, such as for MSC for adolescents (Bluth, Gaylord, Campo, Mullarkey, & Hobbs, 2016) or shorter training without meditation (Smeets, Neff, Alberts, & Peters, 2014).

Core Values in the MSC Curriculum

The necessity of self-compassion became evident to the developers of MSC as they struggled with personal difficulties in their lives. For Kristin Neff, it was the stress of parenting a child with autism and for Chris Germer it was intense public speaking anxiety. Both had been practicing mindfulness for many years. Mindfulness is typically associated with spacious awareness of moment-to-moment *experience* whereas compassion emphasizes loving awareness of the *experiencer*. Chris and Kristin realized that when we are caught in intense and disturbing emotions like shame, grief, or despair, we need to hold *ourselves* in loving awareness before we can hold our moment-to-moment experience with mindfulness. Furthermore, although mindfulness is suffused with love and compassion when mindfulness is in full bloom, those qualities are likely to slip away when we encounter intense emotions. That is when we need to intentionally warm up our awareness. Loving-kindness and compassion cannot be expected to arise spontaneously when we need them the most.

In traditional Buddhist psychology, there are four virtues (*brahmaviharas*) that confer peace and happiness upon the practitioner. These are loving-kindness, compassion, appreciative joy, and equanimity (Hahn, 2002). They are traditionally taught in sequence and build upon one another. For example, loving-kindness is taught before compassion because it is easier to be kind when we are not caught in the pain of suffering. However, when loving-kindness meets suffering and stays loving, that is compassion. Similarly, our loving-kindness and compassion may be challenged when others are more fortunate than we are, so our love and compassion need to be strong before we can experience "appreciative joy"—delight over the success of others. Finally, equanimity—the ability to experience pain and pleasure, success and failure, or happiness and sorrow with balanced awareness—is an advanced skill that can only arise when we are already established in the other three virtues.

Although the MSC program is not built around the four virtues, they are nonetheless embedded in the curriculum. For example, we give participants a direct experience of loving-kindness in Session 3 before activating emotional distress and showing how to meet it with kindness in Session 4. In Session 7, when discussing empathic distress and caregiver fatigue, we teach phrases that cultivate equanimity. The equanimity phrases help caregivers get perspective and disentangle from the needs of others so they can access self-compassion and compassion for others. Finally, we teach savoring, gratitude, and self-appreciation at the closing session of the program. (Self-appreciation is taught in the context of gratitude for those who helped us develop our personal strengths.) All of these virtues also represent core values of MSC, and are necessary to help participants maintain a positive attitude as they do the work of learning self-compassion. Self-compassion cannot be taught in isolation of these values.

When we begin to give ourselves loving-kindness, we inevitably discover difficult emotions or unlovely parts of ourselves that make it difficult to remain in a loving state of mind. That is when we need self-compassion. Compassion is a positive emotion (Singer & Klimecki, 2014) that transforms the experience of suffering without denying or sugar-coating our difficulties.

As an illustration, consider the case of Karen, a working mom, and her 14-year-old daughter, Samantha. They have a heated argument about Samantha's homework that makes Samantha storm off and slam her bedroom door. Karen then finds herself sitting in the living room until late at night ruminating about the encounter. The usual thoughts intrude, such as "I'm not a good parent. I work too much and don't focus on my children. I've already messed up my child." Her despair might also turn to anger: "Samantha is a spoiled brat and deserves my anger." Karen has a strong impulse to get a glass of wine and binge on her favorite TV series. Instead, Karen takes a Self-Compassion Break (Neff, 2011).

While sitting alone in her darkened living room, Karen began to notice, "OK, this hurts. I feel tension in my neck. There's a voice in me that says, 'I'm not a good

Self-Compassion Break

When you notice that you're feeling stress or emotional discomfort, see if you can find the discomfort in your body. Where do you feel it the most? Make contact with the discomfort that you feel in your body. Then say to yourself, slowly and kindly:

- *"This is a moment of suffering"*

  That is mindfulness. Other options include:

- *This hurts.*
- *Ouch!*
- *This is stressful.*

- *"Suffering is a part of life"*

  That is common humanity. Other options include:

- *I'm not alone. Others are just like me.*
- *We all struggle in our lives*
- *This is how it feels when a person struggles in this way*

- *"May I be kind to myself"*

  That is self-kindness. Other options might be:

- *May I give myself what I need.*
- *May I accept myself as I am*
- *May I live in love*

- If you're having difficulty finding the right words, imagine that a dear friend or loved one is having the same problem as you. What would you say to this person, heart-to-heart? If your friend were to hold just a few of your words in their mind, what would you like them to be? What message would you like to deliver? Now, can you offer the same message to yourself.

parent.' This is all very painful." Then Karen reminded herself, "Literally NO ONE ever said parenting was easy, especially with teenagers. I know I'm not alone in my struggles with Samantha." Finally, Karen put a hand over her heart and breathed in deeply for herself and out for her daughter as an expression of her maternal interest and care. The tone of her inner dialogue slowly began to change and she heard herself saying, "I know I'm not a perfect mom, but I'm a good-enough mom. Sometimes I don't know what to do or say, but I really want my children to be happy and succeed in life. Perhaps next time I can stay calmer and it will go better." Karen's self-talk corresponds to the three components of self-compassion in the Self-Compassion Break: mindfulness, common humanity, and self-kindness.

Karen's response to her parenting distress illustrates how core values and self-compassion practice naturally overlap. For starters, Karen would not have been disturbed by the interaction if she had not had the core value of being a "good parent." When she recognized that she was feeling miserable, especially in her body, she tenderly reminded herself that she was not alone. Karen also began to reassure herself in the same manner as she might speak with a friend who was raising children of the same age. Finally, naming her core value of being a good parent helped Karen feel better about herself despite the challenging encounter she had with her daughter.

Participants in MSC are encouraged to recognize and hold difficult parts of themselves in a compassionate embrace—all parts are welcome. For example, most of us have a critical part that is struggling to make us improve, albeit in harsh, counterproductive ways. In MSC, we turn toward such difficult parts, explore their motivation, and then make room for a more compassionate voice or part of ourselves to guide us onward. Parts psychology, such as Internal Family Systems (IFS) by Richard Schwartz (1995), is inherently a compassionate theory of personality because it reduces the tendency toward overgeneralized negative attributions and shame ("I'm unworthy" versus "A part of me feels unworthy"). An interesting difference between IFS and MSC is that IFS assumes that our innate self-compassion naturally emerges as parts are relieved of their burdens whereas MSC intentionally strengthens our capacity to meet our parts with compassion.

A unique aspect of MSC is that we actively cultivate compassion for others as a precursor to activating compassion for ourselves. There are seven MSC practices and exercises that develop compassion for others, and research has shown that activating care of others can increase state self-compassion (Brienes & Chen, 2013). One explanation is that compassion for others helps us to experience common humanity, which makes it safer to accept our own suffering and shortcomings. Research has also shown that increases in self-compassion lead to enhanced compassion for others (Neff & Germer, 2013). In other words, there seems to be a reciprocal relationship between self-compassion and compassion for others.

Since MSC can be emotionally challenging, participants are encouraged to relate to the training program itself in a compassionate manner. In other words, participants are invited to ask themselves, "What do I need?" before engaging in an exercise or practice. If they determine that they are emotionally closing (less receptive, perhaps fatigued, or overwhelmed), they are encouraged to skip the exercise or allow their attention to wander during the instructions. If they are emotionally opening (receptive, alert, curious), then they can allow themselves to fully experience what the practice has to offer.

If self-compassion training feels like a struggle or is harmful in any way, we are not learning self-compassion. The goal and the process should be the same. Self-compassion is about subtraction—letting go of the unnecessary stress that we impose on ourselves through self-criticism, self-isolation, and rumination. Emotional safety is a prerequisite for experiencing compassion, so practicing non-harm and cultivating safety in the classroom is intrinsic to self-compassion training.

Safety is also a basic human need, and non-harm is a core value at the heart of most ethical systems.

Core values are directly addressed in Session 5 of the MSC program. This part of the program was inspired by Acceptance and Commitment Therapy (Hayes, Strosahl, & Wilson, 2011). Core values give meaning to our lives and frame our difficulties. For example, if we value novelty and learning, losing a job may be a blessing; if we want to provide for our families, losing a job would probably be a catastrophe. Furthermore, when we become confused, core values can serve as a compass or GPS to guide us home. In Session 5, participants do an exercise in which they discover their core values and identify inner and outer obstacles to living in accord with their values. Importantly, the exercise helps participants learn how to have self-compassion for that fact that we cannot always live in accord with our core values, and explore how self-compassion help us nourish and sustain our values even when they are difficult to manifest in our lives.

Discovering Our Core Values
- This is a written reflection exercise so please take out a pen and paper.
- Now, place your hand over your heart or elsewhere, feeling the warmth of your touch.

Looking Back

- Imagine that you are near the end of your life, looking back on the years *between now and then*. What gives you deep satisfaction, joy and contentment? What values did you embody that gave your life meaning and satisfaction? In other words, what core values were expressed in your life? Please write them down.

Not Living in Accord with Values?

- Now, please write down any ways you feel you are *not living in accord with your core values,* or ways in which your life feels out of balance with your values—especially personal ones. For example, perhaps you are too busy to spend much quiet time in nature, even though nature is your great love in life.
- If you have several values that feel out of balance, please choose one that is especially important for you to work with for the remainder of this exercise.

External Obstacles?

- Of course, there are often obstacles that prevent us from living in accord with our core values. Some of these may be *external obstacles*, like not having enough money or time, or having other obligations. If there are, please write down any external obstacles.

Internal Obstacles?

- There may also be some *internal obstacles* getting in the way of you living in accord with your core values. For instance, are you afraid of failure, do you doubt your abilities, or is your inner critic getting in the way? Please write down any internal obstacles.

Could Self-Compassion Help?

- Now consider if *self-kindness and self-compassion could help you live in accord with your true values.* For example, by helping you deal with internal obstacles like your inner critic. Or is there a way self-compassion could help you feel safe and confident enough to take new actions, or risk failure, or to let go of things that are not serving you?

Compassion for Insurmountable Obstacles?

- Finally, if there are *insurmountable obstacles* to living in accord with your values, can you give yourself compassion for that hardship? And what might enable you to keep your values alive in your heart in spite of the conditions? And if the insurmountable problem is that you are *imperfect*, as all human beings are, can you forgive yourself for that, too?

Teaching Self-Compassion as Ethics Training

The best way to teach self-compassion is to *be* compassionate. Students learn self-compassion by internalizing how their teachers embody compassion—loving, connected presence. There is no escape in the influence we have on others by our emotions and attitudes. The reason for this is that our brains are hardwired to resonate with the brains of others. If a teacher feels worried or irritated, their students will feel it. When the teacher is in an accepting, peaceful, and receptive frame of mind, that attitude will pervade the classroom. The phenomenon of "transmission" described in some meditation traditions (such as Zen) occurs when a teacher embodies a desirable state of mind that rubs off on the student.

There are a number of teaching prerequisites that select for personal embodiment of mindfulness and self-compassion. For example, all prospective MSC teachers are expected to have meditated for a few years before taking the intensive teacher training and to have participated in a silent meditation retreat. After teacher training, teacher trainees are expected to continue personal meditation practice and to participate in online consultation while teaching their first MSC course. Finally, teachers are asked to agree to MSC ethical guidelines that include embracing diversity, financial integrity, acknowledging the limitations of the program, respecting the integrity of other contemplative training programs and teachers, and engaging in continuing education.

In the teacher training, prospective teachers are taught to "teach from within" regardless whether they are guiding a meditation, leading a class exercise, delivering a mini-lecture, or reading a poem. Teachers are encouraged to present the curriculum in their own voice in a manner that reflects their passion and inspiration.

Class discussions are conducted using the inquiry method. Inquiry is a particular way of engaging in conversation with individual students about their experience of practice, usually immediately after the practice is completed. The purpose of inquiry is to strengthen the resources of mindfulness and self-compassion. Inquiry is a self-to-other dialogue that ideally mirrors the tone and quality of the self-to-self relationship that we are hoping to cultivate.

Inquiry has three R's: resonance, resources, and respect. The main task of a MSC teacher during inquiry is to emotionally resonate with their students. Resonance is embodied listening. Resonance occurs when students *feel felt* (Siegel, 2010, p. 136). The second task of teachers is to strengthen the resources of mindfulness and self-compassion by validating those qualities when they see them, or by drawing them out through collaborative exploration. The third "R" is respect—honoring the needs, boundaries, and vulnerabilities of our students. Since we know relatively little about our students' lives, we need to proceed with caution. Respect refers to safety, and protecting a student's safety is central to the inquiry process.

In summary, MSC is a mindfulness-based program designed primarily to cultivate the resource of self-compassion. Since compassion is an essential value in most ethical and religious systems, MSC is a fundamentally ethical enterprise. Self-compassion is taught in the context of compassion for others, and increases in self-compassion generally lead to increased compassion for others. Self-compassion training can also be emotionally challenging, so it is best taught in the context of other positive human values such as loving-kindness, gratitude, appreciation, wisdom, equanimity, and joy. The central question in self-compassion training is "What do I need?" and understanding of personal core values helps to connect with our basic human needs and respond to them in a compassionate manner. The MSC program is an experiential learning environment designed to give participants a direct experience of self-compassion as well as learn the principles and practices needed to evoke self-compassion in daily life. MSC has a unique pedagogy based on emotional resonance, resource building, and respect for the individuality and emotional safety of each participant. The best way to *teach* self-compassion is to *be* compassionate, and the best way to *learn* self-compassion is to treat the process of learning as the goal itself, tenderly nurturing, and encouraging ourselves every step of the way.

References

Albertson, E. R., Neff, K. D., & Dill-Shackleford, K. E. (2014). Self-Compassion and Body Dissatisfaction in Women: A Randomized Controlled Trial of a Brief Meditation Intervention. *Mindfulness*, 1–11.

Arch, J. J., Brown, K. W., Dean, D. J., Landy, L. N., Brown, K. D., & Laudenslager, M. L. (2014). Self-compassion training modulates alpha-amylase, heart rate variability, and subjective responses to social evaluative threat in women. *Psychoneuroendocrinology, 42*, 49–58.

Armstrong, K. (2010). *Twelve steps to a compassionate life*. New York: Knopf.

Baer, R. (2015). Ethics, values, virtues, and character strengths in mindfulness-based interventions: A psychological science perspective. *Mindfulness, 6*, 956–969.

Bartels-Velthuis, A. A., Schroevers, M. J., van der Ploeg, K., Koster, F., Fleer, J., & van den Brink, E. (2016). A mindfulness-based compassionate living training in a heterogeneous sample of psychiatric outpatients: A feasibility study. *Mindfulness, 7*(4), 809–818.

Bluth, K., Gaylord, S. A., Campo, R. A., Mullarkey, M. C., & Hobbs, L. (2016). Making friends with yourself: A mixed methods pilot study of a mindful self-compassion program for adolescents. *Mindfulness, 7*(2), 479–492.

Breines, J. G., & Chen, S. (2013). Activating the inner caregiver: The role of support-giving schemas in increasing state self-compassion. *Journal of Experimental Social Psychology, 49*(1), 58–64.

Breines, J. G., McInnis, C. M., Kuras, Y. I., Thoma, M. V., Gianferante, D., Hanlin, L., ... & Rohleder, N. (2015). Self-compassionate young adults show lower salivary alpha-amylase responses to repeated psychosocial stress. *Self and Identity, (ahead-of-print)*, 1–13.

Cacioppo, J. T., & Patrick, W. (2008). *Loneliness: Human nature and the need for social connection*. New York: Norton.

Finlay-Jones, A. L., Rees, C. S., & Kane, R. T. (2015). Self-Compassion, Emotion Regulation and Stress among Australian Psychologists: Testing an Emotion Regulation Model of Self-Compassion Using Structural Equation Modeling. *PloS one, 10*(7), e0133481.

Freud, S. (1923). The ego and the id.

Friis, A. M., Johnson, M. H., Cutfield, R. G., & Consedine, N. S. (2016). Kindness matters: A randomized controlled trial of a mindful self-compassion intervention improves depression, distress, and HbA1c among patients with diabetes. *Diabetes Care*, dc160416

Gilbert, R. (1989/2016). *Human nature and suffering*. London: Routledge.

Gilbert, P. (2010). *The compassionate mind: A new approach to life's challenges*. Oakland: New Harbinger Publications.

Gilbert, P., & Choden. (2014). *Mindful compassion: How the science of compassion can help you understand your emotions, live in the present, and connect deeply with others*. Oakland, CA: New Harbinger Publications.

Glasser, W. (1998). *Choice theory: A new psychology of personal freedom*. New York: Harper.

Hayes, S. C., Strosahl, K. D., & Wilson, K. G. (2011). *Acceptance and commitment therapy, second edition: The process and practice of mindful change*. New York: Guilford Press.

Hollis-Walker, L., & Colosimo, K. (2011). Mindfulness, self-compassion, and happiness in non-meditators: A theoretical and empirical examination. *Personality and Individual Differences, 50*, 222–227.

Jazaieri, H., McGonigal, K., Jinpa, T., Doty, J. R., Gross, J. J., & Goldin, P. R. (2014). A randomized controlled trial of compassion cultivation training: Effects on mindfulness, affect, and emotion regulation. *Motivation and Emotion, 38*(1), 23–35.

Jung, C. G. (1961). *Memories, dreams, reflections*. New York: Random House.

Kabat-Zinn, J. (1991). *Full catastrophe living: Using the wisdom of your body and mind to face stress, pain, and illness*. New York: Dell.

Kabat-Zinn, J. (2003) Mindfulness-Based Interventions in Context: Past, Present, and Future. *Clinical Psychology: Science and Practice, 10*, 144–156.

Keltner, D., Marsh, J., & Smith, J. A. (2010). Introduction to part three. In D. Keltner, J. Marsh, & J. A. Smith (Eds.), *The compassionate instinct: The science of human goodness* (pp. 177–178). New York: W. W. Norton.

Kuyken, W., Watkins, E., Holden, E., White, K., Taylor, R., et al. (2010). How does mindfulness-based cognitive therapy work? *Behaviour Research and Therapy, 48*, 1105–1112.

Maslow, A. H. (1943). A theory of human motivation. *Psychological Review, 50*(4), 370–396.

Merton, T. (1969). *My argument with the gestapo: A macaronic journal*. New York: New Directions Books.

Neff, K. D. (2003). Development and validation of a scale to measure self-compassion. *Self and Identity, 2*, 223–250.

Neff, K. D. (2011). *Self-compassion: The proven power of being kind to yourself.* New York: William Morrow.

Neff, K. D., & Germer, C. (2013). A pilot study and randomized controlled trial of the mindful self-compassion program. *Journal of Clinical Psychology, 69*(1), 28–44.

Neff, K. D., Hseih, Y., & Dejitthirat, K. (2005). Self-compassion, achievement goals, and coping with academic failure. *Self and Identity, 4*, 263–287.

Neff, K. D., Kirkpatrick, K. L., & Rude, S. S. (2007). Self-compassion and adaptive psychological functioning. *Journal of Research in Personality, 41*, 139–154.

Odou, N., & Brinker, J. (2014). Exploring the Relationship between Rumination, Self-compassion, and Mood. *Self and Identity, 13*(4), 449–459.

Pace, T. W., Negi, L. T., Adame, D. D., Cole, S. P., Sivilli, T. I., Brown, T. D., … Raison, C. L. (2009). Effect of compassion meditation on neuroendocrine, innate immune and behavioral responses to psychosocial stress. *Psychoneuroendocrinology, 34*(1), 87–98.

Peterson, C., & Seligman, M. E. P. (2004). *Character strengths and virtues: A handbook and classification.* New York: Oxford University Press.

Raes, F. (2010). Rumination and worry as mediators of the relationship between self-compassion and depression and anxiety. *Personality and Individual Differences, 48*, 757–761.

Ryan, R. M., & Deci, E. L. (2000). Self-determination theory and the facilitation of intrinsic motivation, social development, and well-being. *American Psychologist, 555*, 68–78.

Schwartz, R. C. (1995). *Internal family systems.* London: Guilford Press.

Segal, Z. V., Williams, M. G., & Teasdale, J. D. (2002). *Mindfulness-based cognitive therapy for depression.* New York: The Guilford Press.

Siegel, D. J. (2010). *The mindful therapist.* New York: Norton.

Singer, T., & Klimecki, O. M. (2014). Empathy and compassion. *Current Biology, 24*(18), R875–R878.

Smeets, E., Neff, K. D., Alberts, H., & Peters, M. (2014). Meeting suffering with kindness: Effects of a brief self-compassion intervention for female college students. *Journal of Clinical Psychology, 70*(9), 794–807.

van den Brink, E., & Koster, F. (2015). *Mindfulness-based compassionate living: A new training programme to deepen mindfulness with heartfulness.* London: Routledge.

Webb, J. B., Fiery, M. F., & Jafari, N. (2016). You better not leave me shaming!: Conditional indirect effect analyses of anti-fat attitudes, body shame, and fat talk as a function of self-compassion in college women. *Body Image, 18*, 5–13.

Chapter 12
Mindfulness, Compassion, and the Foundations of Global Health Ethics

David G. Addiss

Introduction

Mindfulness is generally considered a characteristic or quality of individual persons. Its focus is primarily inward, directed toward one's thoughts, emotions, and bodily sensations, as well as toward one's immediate environment. Yet the accelerating pace of globalization compels us to consider mindfulness in a broader context. What is the role of mindfulness for the increasing number of people who work at the global level, who actively seek to improve health and quality of life for entire populations, for people they will never meet, from whom they are separated by great geographic, cultural, and economic distances? How can mindfulness help to guide them through the ethical minefields inherent in such a complex undertaking? Indeed, what *kind* of mindfulness is required? How does globalization affect our fundamental understanding of what mindfulness is and what determines ethical action?

I approach these questions not as a trained ethicist or expert in mindfulness-based interventions, but as one who has worked in the field of global health for almost 30 years. At times during this period, a lack of mindfulness limited the effectiveness of my work. I lacked equanimity, was emotionally reactive, and was unaware of much that was happening—not only within myself, but also among my international colleagues and within the agencies for which we worked. I did not understand the huge gaps in power, opportunity, and privilege that separated us,

D.G. Addiss, MD, MPH (✉)
Task Force for Global Health, 325 Swanton Way, Decatur, GA 30030, USA

Eck Institute for Global Health, University of Notre Dame, Notre Dame, IN 46556, USA

Center for Compassion and Global Health, 1120 Clifton Rd, NE, Atlanta, GA 30307, USA
e-mail: dgaddiss@gmail.com

© Springer International Publishing AG 2017
L.M. Monteiro et al. (eds.), *Practitioner's Guide to Ethics and Mindfulness-Based Interventions*, Mindfulness in Behavioral Health,
DOI 10.1007/978-3-319-64924-5_12

much less the extent to which aspects of my work depended on those gaps. My awareness of the ethical dimensions of global health emerged gradually.

As a global health practitioner, during the past 5 years I have explored the themes of ethics, compassion, and mindfulness with colleagues from around the world, in the corners of meetings, over meals, and while traveling together. I have been impressed by their willingness to reflect deeply on these themes—and also how infrequently these themes are discussed in the professional literature, conferences, and training programs of global health professionals.

The field of global health ethics is still in its infancy. Rooted in bioethics, global health ethics also concerns itself with the forces of globalization, which fuel both the need and opportunity for global health, as well as with the massive imbalances of power, wealth, and opportunity that separate us as humans. Global health is but one of many fields that have arisen or matured during the past 2 decades, catalyzed by an awareness of our profound interconnectedness and of the impact of globalization on the human condition. What does contemporary mindfulness offer these fields? And how might intentional engagement with these fields inform contemporary mindfulness? Using global health as an example, I explore the essential role of mindfulness in fostering ethical decision-making and in nurturing compassionate, effective action at the global level. I also explore how mindfulness and compassion might contribute to the emerging field of global health ethics.

Mindfulness

The ongoing debate about what constitutes mindfulness reveals a rich tapestry of deeply held perspectives (Monteiro, Musten, & Compson, 2015; Compson & Monteiro, 2016; Mikulas, 2015; Purser, 2015; Baer, 2015). Mindfulness in traditional Buddhism, which evolved over hundreds of years, differs in certain respects from contemporary secular notions of mindfulness and from concepts of mindfulness in other religious and spiritual traditions. Further, the term "everyday mindfulness" is sometimes used to differentiate it from "mindfulness while meditating" (Thompson & Waltz, 2007). Scientific investigation, through the disciplines of psychology and neuroscience, has helped to refine our understanding of mindfulness, while also raising many more questions about its phenomenology, biology, and the robustness of our conceptual frameworks (Baer, 2015; Lutz, Jha, Dunne, & Saron, 2015).

I will refrain from offering yet another definition of mindfulness and will generally use the term in its contemporary sense as offered by Kabat-Zinn (1994, p. 4)—"paying attention in a particular way: on purpose, in the present moment, and non-judgmentally." Both for contemporary ethics and traditional Buddhism, the adverb "non-judgmentally" requires some unpacking, as ethical discernment involves value judgments regarding what is wholesome, ethically responsible, and conducive to right living.

Mindfulness and Ethics

Christian Krägeloh (2016, p. 100) argues that "the purpose of Buddhist mindfulness training is to transform one's deluded ways of thinking into habitual mental states that are associated with wholesome behaviors and that avoid unwholesome ones." Mindfulness practices were traditionally taught in a nuanced monastic context of spiritual and ethical formation (Thupten Jinpa, 2015). Currently offered in secular contexts, there are concerns about extracting the practices from their traditional context and stripping them of explicit ethical and religious content to render them accessible to persons in contemporary western societies with various religious beliefs and backgrounds. However, mindfulness-based interventions such as mindfulness-based stress reduction (MBSR, Kabat-Zinn, 1990) and mindfulness-based cognitive therapy (MBCT, Segal, Williams, & Teasdale, 2002) have provided therapeutic benefit for people with a broad range of clinical and medical conditions (Kabat-Zinn, 2003).

Proponents argue that the impressive benefits of these therapies and training programs, which are now realized by tens of thousands of people, outweigh potential downsides of adapting them for secular societies that value "liberal neutrality" in the public sphere. According to this position, mindfulness-based interventions should avoid being limited by "strong ethical commitments" since they can be beneficial or applicable even "in contexts of controversial moral value" (Schmidt, 2016, p. 1), such as military settings. In other words, contemporary mindfulness-based interventions should not be too strongly linked to a particular view of morality.

Others have questioned the wisdom of extracting meditation and mindfulness practices from their traditional spiritual and ethical foundations. Doing so, they argue, detaches mindfulness practice from a commitment to "right mindfulness" and threatens to reduce it to mere technique, subject to misappropriation (Monteiro et al., 2015; Stanley, 2013).

Several lines of thought and evidence suggest that mindfulness, broadly considered, can enhance ethical motivation, behavior, and decision-making. Shapiro, Jazaieri, and Goldin (2012) recently explored four ways in which contemplative practice, and mindfulness in particular, can improve moral and ethical reasoning. First, mindfulness fosters the ability to shift from a personal, subjective perspective to one that is more objective (Orzech, Shapiro, Warren Brown, & McKay, 2009). Such a shift, known as "reperceiving," is especially important for ethical decision-making when the self feels threatened or when identity is at stake. Second, through the process of reperceiving, mindfulness allows practitioners to more readily consider the perspective of others. This opens them to the possibility of empathy and compassion (Kristeller & Johnson, 2005).

Third, mindfulness can help clarify values. We are often not fully conscious of the values that guide our decisions (Ruedy & Schweitzer, 2010). Mindfulness can reveal subconscious motivations, help us discern whether these motivations reflect our core values, and increase our resolve to embrace values that are wholesome and life-giving (Shapiro et al., 2012). Fourth, nonjudgmental awareness, which is a hallmark of mindfulness meditation, promotes emotion regulation (Chambers, Gullone, & Allen, 2009; Goldin & Gross, 2010). Emotions are a crucial, and often unappreciated, determinant of ethical decision-making (Narvaez, 2014). Substantial research has demonstrated that mindfulness training increases the capacity for healthy, adaptive emotional regulation and lessens the tendency to engage in maladaptive patterns, such as rumination, rigidity, and impulsiveness (Shapiro et al., 2012; Jain et al., 2007; Baer, 2009).

Together, these considerations argue for mindfulness training as a component of educational programs intended to foster ethical decision-making. Yet, with the exception of some clinical settings (Rushton, Kaszniak, & Halifax, 2013; Rushton et al., 2013; Vinson & Wang, 2015; Guillemin & Gillam, 2015), mindfulness and contemplative practice are addressed infrequently in the fields of applied ethics, including bioethics. Little attention is given to how mindfulness should be cultivated, manifested, or brought into ethical deliberation. In part, this may be because the fields of applied ethics assume a certain level of, and capacity for, mindfulness. Such an assumption may not be justified.

Mindfulness and Compassion

Broadly speaking, compassion requires a certain stability of mind. It requires cognitive awareness of suffering, as well as the ability to recognize suffering as suffering. The cognitive basis for compassion involves perspective-taking, insight, and memory (Halifax, 2012). Mindfulness meditation can increase the capacity for taking on perspectives of other people (Shapiro, Schwartz, & Bonner, 1998; Lueke & Gibson, 2015; Baer, 2009).

Compassion also requires emotional attunement or empathy. Empirical studies have shown that mindfulness training increases empathy in medical and health professional students (Shapiro et al., 1998, Shapiro & Izett, 2008; McConville, McAleer, & Hahne, 2016). Upon continued exposure to intense suffering, empathic overload can lead to personal distress, burnout, and so-called "compassion fatigue." Equanimity and emotion regulation are critical to maintaining affective balance and emotional resiliency in such settings (Halifax, 2012; Rushton, Kaszniak, et al., 2013; Ruston et al., 2013; Rushton, 2016; Kearney, Weininger, Vachon, Harrison, & Mount, 2009; Singer & Klimecki, 2014).

Finally, compassion is action-oriented. His Holiness the Dalai Lama notes that compassion "is not just an idle wish to see sentient beings free from suffering, but an immediate need to intervene and actively engage, to try to help" (Dalai Lama, 2002, p. 225). But this is not action borne of a compulsive need to "fix" the situation or alleviate one's own personal distress. Rather, compassionate action requires clarity of intention, awareness of one's own biases, blind spots, and conflicts of interest, and respect for the potential of unintended consequences. It requires wisdom and insight into the causes of suffering. Compassion asks, "What will serve?" It emerges when "the mind is in a state of readiness to meet the world in response to suffering"

(Halifax, 2012, p. 6). Mindfulness practice can help cultivate compassionate responses to suffering (Leiberg, Klimecki, & Singer, 2011; Rosenberg et al., 2015).

To briefly summarize, mindfulness is strongly associated with—and indeed may be essential for—both ethical decision-making and compassion. This does not mean that mindfulness necessarily results in ethical behavior or compassionate action; it is not, in and of itself, sufficient. A host of other co-factors, including our upbringing, culture, physiology, and perhaps even epigenetic factors, play an important role in human moral development (Narvaez, 2014). Nonetheless, the fundamental importance of mindfulness for ethical decision-making and compassion remains unappreciated and overlooked.

Globalization and Ethical Action

We now move to the challenge of ethical action at the global level and the role of mindfulness in guiding such action. The aspiration to achieve a positive or wholesome impact at the global level brings us face to face with the ancient philosophical paradox of "the one and the many." The shift in focus from local to global is accompanied by a transition from the concrete to the abstract, from the individual to the population or system, and from care or compassion to justice. In this transition, the tenor of ethical discourse tends to move from the interpersonal and relational to the legal and transactional.

In our age of globalization, the question of moral status lies at the heart of the ethical endeavor: who or what do we regard as worthy of ethical consideration, and to what extent? Who—or what institution—has the right to confer moral status on individuals or groups of people? In the words of Mother Theresa, how large are we willing to "draw the circle of family" (Reifenberg, 2013, p. 194–195), especially when those within our own group protest that their claims or interests are being ignored or eroded? The process of globalization has so dramatically increased our interdependence—economically, culturally, and politically—that the unintended consequences of apparent ethical action in one setting can inflict injustice or cause suffering for entire populations elsewhere.

Ethical action at the global level requires an uncommon and deep awareness of *both* the "one global" and the "many locals," as well as the interplay between and among them. We turn now to the field of global health to illustrate how these tensions play out and how they might be resolved.

Global Health

Global health is the term given to a rapidly growing, multidisciplinary field that emerged in the 1990s and has its origins in public health, international health, and tropical medicine. It was shaped by a series of global infectious disease pandemics, such as HIV/AIDS; concern for the environment; the forces of globalization; increased funding from private foundations; and the emergence of public–private partnerships to address specific health issues (Brown, Cueto, & Fee, 2006). The purview of global health is broad, including both clinical care and public health, addressing the social as well as biological determinants of health, and involving a wide range of academic disciplines (Koplan et al., 2009).

Given its extraordinary breadth, a precise definition of global health is elusive, even among its practitioners (Beaglehole & Bonita, 2010). A framework definition proposed by Koplan et al. (2009) considers global health to be a notion, an objective, and a discipline.

Global Health as a Notion

Global health is rooted in a deep awareness of the interconnectedness of all things, a recognition that, in the words of Archbishop Desmond Tutu, "My humanity is caught up, is inextricably bound up, in yours" (Tutu, 1999, p. 35). As recent outbreaks such as those caused by Ebola and Zika virus have demonstrated, human disease is no respecter of international borders. Therefore, the notion of global health is not limited or defined by geography. Rather, it is a worldview in which our interconnection and mutual dependency are accepted as given. Global health practitioners work to improve the health of populations, of people they may never meet, separated by vast geographic distances as well as economic, cultural, and political divides. Dr. Bill Foege, former director of the US Centers for Disease Control and Prevention (CDC), referred to this worldview when he said, "Everything is local and everything is global. Global health is not 'over there'—it's right here" (Bill Foege, personal communication, Task Force for Global Health in Decatur, Georgia, April 26, 2012). Global health transcends barriers of time and space, rendering nonessential our usual dichotomies of local and global, here and there, individuals and populations, us and them. As we shall see, effective global health leadership requires mindfulness that can hold the tension and paradox of these dichotomies while guiding ethical action in a global world.

Global Health as an Objective

In practical terms, global health is also a goal. The World Health Organization defines health as "a state of complete physical, mental, and social wellbeing, and not merely the absence of disease or infirmity," and affirms that health is a fundamental human right (World Health Organization, 2006, p. 1). In its pursuit of this goal, criticized for its unattainability (Larson, 1996), global health prioritizes its efforts on behalf of those who are most vulnerable and impoverished, and for whom access to health care is most remote. Thus, the principle of health equity is central to global health (Koplan et al., 2009).

Global Health as an Academic Discipline

Global health is also a rapidly growing field of scholarship and practice, highly popular among students of medicine, nursing, and public health (Landrigan et al., 2011; Macfarlane, Jacobs, & Kaaya, 2008; Battat et al., 2010; Kerry et al., 2013), as well as undergraduates (Hill, Ainsworth, & Partap, 2012). This interest reflects a strong desire among many people to make a difference at a global level, as well as their concern for health disparities (Merson, 2014).

Global Health as a System

The structure of global health is complex, redundant, and somewhat chaotic. It involves a broad range of government agencies and national ministries, both civilian and military; multilateral institutions such as the World Health Organization, UNICEF, and the World Bank; and a host of private sector organizations, including foundations, for-profit corporations, religious institutions, and thousands of non-governmental organizations. These organizations often join together in public–private partnerships or alliances to advance certain health agendas (McCoy, Chand, & Sridhar, 2009; Frenk & Moon, 2013).

Global Health as Compassion

I have made the assertion elsewhere (Addiss, 2015) that global health also is a manifestation and expression of compassion. Global health agencies mobilize vast human and financial resources to relieve human suffering (McCoy et al., 2009). Further, global health seeks to alleviate disease-related suffering of *all* people. In this sense, it embodies the message of universal compassion espoused by spiritual teachers through the ages. Because global health is founded upon an awareness of the deep interconnectedness of all beings, it is radical in its inclusivity. Moral status belongs to all. To realize its vision of health equity, global health emphasizes a "preferential option for the poor." Paul Farmer notes that this is appropriate, since "diseases themselves make a preferential option for the poor" (Farmer, 2013, p. 36).

The universalism of global health places it in tension with the human tendency to reserve compassion for those who are close to us, or who seem worthy of it (Goetz, Keltner, & Simon-Thomas, 2010). In this sense, global health challenges the views of care ethicists, such as Noddings (1984), who argue that the scope of one's responsibility for caring is limited, and that it should be strongest toward close-others, with whom one is in relationship.

Challenges to the Ethic of Compassion in Global Health

The aspirational principles that global health uses to describe itself are not always realized in practice. Global health priorities are often driven by foreign policy, partisan politics, and institutional agendas (Gow, 2002). Practitioners may experience the tension of dual loyalties, divided between the agencies that employ them and the people whose health they seek to improve—and from whom they may be separated geographically and culturally. Those who work in large institutions may find that the work itself is organizational and bureaucratic—even mechanical—in nature. In such settings, global health work becomes abstract and disconnected from the people who are seen as its "recipients." Physician Abhay Bang reminds us that, "global health decisions without compassion become bureaucratic, they become impersonal, they become insensitive. Global health operations without compassion may become autocratic" (Task Force for Global Health, 2011).

Nurturing and maintaining "compassion at a distance" is a challenge for many global health professionals (Addiss, 2015). Awareness of suffering, required both for empathy and compassion, often comes not from a direct human encounter, but from statistics and numbers. Bill Foege highlighted this fundamental challenge in a speech to his CDC colleagues. "If we are to maintain the reputation this institution now enjoys, it will be because in everything we do, behind everything we say, as the basis for every program decision we make—we will be willing to see faces" (Foege, 1984). For many, this was a startling message: what CDC needed was not updated laboratories or improved facilities, but compassion—the willingness of its employees, collectively, to see the faces of suffering.

At times, global health workers are called on to serve in acute situations of overwhelming suffering. The 2014–2015 Ebola outbreak in West Africa was a recent dramatic example. In such settings, empathic arousal can be intense; health and relief workers may be flooded with feelings of inadequacy, fear, helplessness, and anger. Considerable emotional resiliency is required to avoid personal distress and to respond consistently with compassion (Rushton, 2016).

Fear and its political manipulation are among the most serious threats to global health. When the World Trade Center in New York City was attacked on September 11, 2001, the nation was immediately gripped by fear. CDC's top priorities became bioterrorism defense and "homeland security." The ethos within the organization shifted overnight, from public health to civil defense (Altman, 2002). While both public health and civil defense are necessary for national interests, they differ in their fundamental world views.

The power of fear—especially when exploited by politicians and the media—to create chaos, override sensible public health measures, and stifle compassion was demonstrated again during the outbreak of Ebola in West Africa. Anticipating the possibility of patients with Ebola arriving in the United States, Thomas Frieden, Director of the CDC, called on the compassionate impulse of the US public, saying, "I hope that our understandable fear of the unfamiliar does not trump our compassion when ill Americans return to the US for care" (Henry & Stobbe, 2014). His statement highlighted both the power of fear to undermine the compassionate impulse as well as the power of compassion to overcome fear.

Mindfulness and Global Health

The question I now wish to address is not whether mindfulness can enhance ethical discernment, decision-making, and action in global health. It seems difficult, if not impossible, to live out the aspirational values of global health without mindfulness. The landscape and challenges are too complex, the stakes too high. Rather, the relevant question is: What *kind* of mindfulness is needed? Mindfulness of *what*? I suggest that ethical global health practice requires the application of mindfulness in four dimensions or domains. It requires mindfulness of one's own interior landscape and "movements"; global health's core values; the interconnectedness and interdependence of all life; and the external factors (e.g., cultural, economic, historical) that contribute to human health and health inequity. In addition, mindfulness can help overcome dichotomous thinking, which Julio Frenk calls "the greatest threat to global health" (Rosenberg, Utzinger, & Addiss, 2016). We explore these dimensions briefly in this section.

First, global health is extraordinarily complex, requiring collaborations that bridge vast disparities of wealth, privilege, and power, not to mention differences in geography, language, and culture. Without a high degree of self-awareness of one's biases, motivations, limitations, and potential conflicts of interest, it is all too easy for practitioners from "donor" organizations or countries to violate basic principles of solidarity and to impose their own priorities or those of the organizations for which they work. We are often strikingly unaware of the ethical and interpersonal boundaries that we violate. Based on conversations with hundreds of global health leaders, practitioners, and students, I suggest that we also are susceptible to the subtle trap of "compulsion to save the world" (Addiss, 2015). The shadow side of the desire to "make a difference" is over-identification with the righteousness of one's cause and the tendency to cling to specific outcomes, which can lead to defensiveness, over-work, exhaustion, and burnout. Mindfulness is essential to allow space for insight and self-awareness, foster emotional balance, and depersonalize criticism.

Second, as already noted, global health's universal values and its concern with the health of *all* peoples sometimes puts it at odds with the values of nation-states and secular societies. Students entering the field should understand that global health can be perceived as a radical enterprise and they should be well-grounded in its core values. These include solidarity, social justice, equity, respect for all human life, interdependence, humility, introspection, and compassion (Pinto & Upshur,

2009, 2013). Benatar et al. (2003, p. 129; 2014) argue that global health practitioners must cultivate "a global state of mind" and embrace the cosmopolitan virtues of tolerance, curiosity, humility, and generosity. Global health practitioners must be fully mindful of these values, especially during times of crisis and when facing ethical dilemmas.

Third, being rooted in these values is not merely an intellectual exercise. Zen teachers, such as Bernie Glassman, emphasize the importance of a deep *experience* of interconnection (Glassman, 1998). Many successful global health leaders can point to a personal encounter—often an experience with a single patient or individual—that transformed their awareness and set them on a path that eventually became a career (Addiss, 2016a). Such an experience of interconnectedness is accompanied by an invitation to live one's life in accordance with this realization—to participate in it fully. These experiences often provide a renewable source of inspiration for those who dedicate their lives to global health. They also serve as the source of the values that guide the field itself.

Experiences of interconnectedness are inconceivable without mindfulness. Although they may arise unexpectedly, they are conditioned by receptivity and a "particular way" of paying attention to self, others, and one's surroundings, i.e., "in the present moment and non-judgmentally" (Kabat-Zinn, 1994, p. 4). The challenge for those who have been in the field for many years is staying connected to the evocative power of these experiences. Without this, the work of global health, particularly in large government agencies, can become mechanical and dry, and the "faces" fade from view, replaced by "numbers." Mindfulness and contemplative practice can help us remember the experience of interconnection and reignite our imagination. Mindfulness is a pathway to the spiritual "wells" (Gutierrez, 2003) from which we must drink to sustain our spirits and realize the promise of global health.

Fourth, mindfulness of and respect for the complexities, nuances, and particularities of each situation are crucially important. One of the strengths of global health is its focus and insistence on effective action. Good intentions are not enough. Ideally, interventions are based on evidence and guided by people whose lives are affected by them. The fields of international health and development have not always lived up to these principles. "Solutions" from "donor" countries and organizations have often been imposed on "recipients" without regard to historical realities or local priorities, beliefs, or practices (Gow, 2002; Farley, 1991; Caufield, 1997). In a recent example, the understandably high priority given by western medical teams to infection control and cremation during the early stages of the Ebola epidemic did not give adequate consideration to local religious beliefs or traditional burial practices. The epidemic did not begin to subside until the World Health Organization issued guidelines that took these factors into account (Blevins, 2015).

Another example of relative disregard for historical, cultural, and local particularities is the proliferation of short-term missions (Forsythe, 2011) and "voluntourism," which has become big business (Kushner, 2016; Forsythe, 2011). Ostensibly fueled by "compassion," these activities are often characterized by a lack of awareness and mindfulness (Kushner, 2016; Linhart, 2006). They have been criticized as ineffective, misguided, arrogant, and actually harmful. True solidarity and accompaniment must be informed by knowledge of the cultural, political, economic, and historical factors that influence health inequities, and by an awareness of one's own complicity in the systems that underlie the inequities that one is trying to "fix." The Catholic Health Association of the United States (2016) has developed excellent materials that invite those considering short-term global health work into an honest appraisal of motives and a process of mindful reflection regarding what will best serve. Ethical principles and best practices also have been proposed for short-term medical missions (Decamp, 2011; Wall, 2011) and international student training experiences (Crump & Sugarman, 2010).

Of the four domains in which mindfulness is needed for ethical global health practice—one's interior landscape; global health's core values; the profound interconnectedness of life; and the cultural, economic, and historical factors that contribute to health inequity—only the fourth is adequately addressed in schools of public health. However, it is approached as a body of knowledge to be mastered, a set of professional skills to be developed, rather than as a path of mindfulness or of ethical inquiry. As a result, this knowledge is not necessarily or explicitly brought to bear on ethical decision-making.

Leaping Clear of the One and the Many

The primary science that guides and supports interventions in global health is epidemiology, the study of patterns of disease and health across populations. Traditionally, epidemiology tends to view the world in dichotomous categories—healthy or sick, dead or alive, case or control. Epidemiologists seek to understand the causes of—or risk factors for—disease in order to develop effective interventions (Gordis, 2009). Epidemiology has proved to be an extraordinarily powerful tool, and its analytic approach influences the way global health professionals think. In the lived experience of global health, however, the dichotomous distinctions of here vs. there, local vs. global, individuals vs. populations, and us vs. them become blurred. For ethical global health practice, a particularly challenging and pervasive dichotomy is the paradox of "the one and the many," the whole and its parts, or in Bill Foege's words, the "numbers and faces." Effective action at the global level can only be accomplished through attending to the "numbers" through programs and initiatives that operate at scale. But the compassion that motivates and sustains that action is often found in an experience of a particular "face" at the individual level. Both are needed. Foege and Rosenberg (1999, p. 86) wrote, "Successful public health leadership in the next millennium will require…the ability to see the whole and its parts *simultaneously*. Public health leaders…need to scan and to focus and to see relationships. And they need to do these *all at the same time*" (emphasis added).

The paradox of "the one and the many" has been the object of serious reflection at least since the early Greek philosophers (Anderson, 1953; Johnston, 2004). It finds resonance in the Buddhist doctrine of no-self. The whole is qualitatively other than its parts. The self is comprised of non-self elements. And, in the words of Roshi Joan Halifax (2012, p. 229), even "compassion is composed of noncompassion elements." Compassion is enactive, an "emergent process that arises out of the interaction of a number of noncompassion processes" (Halifax, 2012). The paradox of the "one and the many" is also a central concern of public health ethics. A classic challenge in public health is how to weigh the overall good to the whole (i.e., society) provided by interventions against the unintended harm that they cause to a few individuals (Childress et al., 2002; Barrett et al., 2016). The benefit to society is a scant source of solace to the individual who has been harmed. The logic of the whole does not necessarily apply to each of the parts.

Zen masters, too, have contemplated how to hold the tension between the one and the many. Typically, they adopt a non-dual approach. In the thirteenth century, Eihei Dōgen wrote, "the buddha way, is, basically, leaping clear of the many and the one" (Dōgen, 1985, p. 69). Dōgen might suggest to us in our age of globalization that the awakened way, the compassionate way, requires us to leap clear of these dichotomies, to see the faces in the numbers, and to embrace both our deep interconnectedness and our diversity.

More recently, Roshi Bernie Glassman commented on Dōgen's experience and elaborated on his teaching: "The one way to be truly universal is to be very particular, moment by moment, detail by detail. If you are merely 'universal,' you lose the feel of life, you become abstract, facile…But if the emphasis on everyday detail is too rigid, our existence loses the religious power of the universal. To walk with one foot in each world—that was Dōgen's way, and Dōgen's life. In a single sentence, he talked from both points of view, the absolute and the relative, the universal and the particular. He was not only living in both, he was switching so fast between the two that he was in neither! He was entirely free! And this is wonderful, just as it should be!" (Matthiessen, 1985, p. 190).

Glassman's description of Dōgen's ability to live both in the absolute and the relative, the universal and the particular, is reminiscent of the qualities that Foege and Rosenberg (1999, p. 86) maintain are needed for global health leadership, "the ability see the whole and its parts simultaneously…to scan and to focus and to see relationships...to do these all at the same time." How *can* global health practitioners be fully aware of the faces and the numbers, reconcile the local and the global, and stay motivated by a profound sense of humanity's vast interconnectedness while being fully attentive to seemingly endless, minute technical details—all at the same time? Training in mindfulness and contemplative awareness, required to "leap clear of the many and the one," is offered in retreat centers and monasteries of many of the world's religious traditions. It is not often included in the curricula of schools of public health, medicine, or nursing. I believe it should be.

Toward a Global Health Ethics

Having considered the characteristics of global health, explored four domains in which mindfulness can contribute to ethical global health practice, and touched on the challenge of "the one and the many," we turn our attention now to the emerging field of global health ethics. We will begin with a brief description of bioethics and public health ethics, arguing that they provide a necessary but insufficient basis for global health ethics. In particular, we will consider how compassion and the ethics of care might contribute to a mature framework for global health ethics.

Bioethics

As noted earlier, global health ethics is still in its infancy. It is rooted in the field of bioethics, which developed during the 1970s to address ethical issues arising from advances in technology and its medical applications, particularly at the beginning and end of life (Callahan, 2012). The need for bioethics was also highlighted by widely publicized ethical abuses in medical research, particularly the notorious US Public Health Service study on the effects of untreated syphilis among African-American men in Tuskegee, Alabama (Jones, 1981).

Within the field of bioethics, the dominant conceptual framework is known as Principlism, based on the four principles: beneficence, nonmaleficence, justice, and autonomy (Beauchamp & Childress, 2012). The application of these principles to ethical decision-making is often described as a measured, rational process that balances the competing principles, leading to an ethical decision and a clear course of action. In practice, achieving such balance can be difficult. Individuals and societies assign different weights to each of the principles (Page, 2012). The priority assigned to individual autonomy, in particular, has been criticized as inappropriate for some non-western cultures (O'Neill, 2002). Further, preliminary evidence suggests that the degree to which specific principles are valued does not necessarily predict how decisions are made when one is faced with an ethical dilemma (Page, 2012).

Public Health Ethics

In contrast to clinical medicine and nursing, which are focused on individual patients, public health is broader in scope, concerned with the health of populations. Although the four principles are often used to frame and consider ethical challenges in public health, the principle of individual autonomy is tempered by the relational and social dimensions of human interdependence. Similarly, in public health, the principle of justice extends beyond simple distributive justice (e.g., equitable access to health services) to issues such as the social determinants of health (Commission on Social Determinants of Health, 2008) and the responsibilities of the state (O'Neill, 2002).

Once the effectiveness of a particular public health intervention has been demonstrated (the principle of beneficence) and its associated risks are shown to be at least as acceptable as the alternatives (nonmaleficence), attention must be given to the degree to which the intervention would infringe on individual autonomy, whether the benefits and burdens would be distributed equitably (justice), and the degree to which its implementation has been justified to the public with honesty, transparency, and trust (Childress et al., 2002). This leads to several observations.

First, even an intervention with a scientifically acceptable risk–benefit ratio may be considered unethical if it is implemented without respect and concern for the autonomy of those who might benefit from it. Ethics is concerned not only with scientific evidence regarding benefits and risks of a particular intervention (the *what*), but also with *how* it is implemented. For example, surgical sterilization is a safe and effective method of reducing fertility, but is unethical when applied in a coercive manner.

Second, many public health measures, especially when they are compulsory, as with vaccination and seat belts in automobiles, infringe to some degree on individual autonomy; this does not necessarily make them unethical (O'Neill, 2002). Third, ongoing epidemiologic monitoring and evaluation of public health interventions is not only good public health practice; it is an ethical mandate. For example, during the first few years of the onchocerciasis (river blindness) control program in sub-Saharan Africa, its ethical profile was beyond question. Community-directed treatment with the drug ivermectin provided massive relief from suffering, was associated with few adverse reactions, advanced social justice (Bailey, Merritt, & Tediosi, 2015), and established decision-making (autonomy) at the community level (Homeida et al., 2002). The risk–benefit balance shifted radically, though, when monitoring systems established to detect serious adverse events identified cases of neurologic complications, some of which were fatal. These cases occurred in areas that happened to be co-endemic for another parasitic worm, *Loa loa* or African eyeworm. Epidemiologic and laboratory investigation revealed that persons with high-intensity *Loa loa* infection (i.e., more than 8000 organisms per mL of blood) were at risk of serious neurologic complications due to the exquisite sensitivity of that parasite to ivermectin (Twum-Danso, 2003a, 2003b). In areas endemic for *Loa loa*, the river blindness program was halted until safeguards could be put into place to avoid these complications (Addiss, Rheingans, Twum-Danso, & Richards, 2003).

And finally, public health ethics continues to wrestle with the challenge of the "one and the many." Simple utilitarianism ("the greatest benefit for the largest number") does not adequately take into account the one who is harmed or does not benefit. A communitarian approach, in which all voices are invited into the decision-making process, is preferable. However, the communitarian approach assumes a state, government, or community that is both representative of the population and responsive to the needs of its minorities and marginalized persons. This assumption is not always justified.

Global Health Ethics

Global health ethics, in my view, builds on public health ethics, infusing it with a global perspective that transcends borders of nationality, ethnicity, and identity and with certain fundamental values that, while present in public health, are nevertheless more explicitly articulated in global health. These values include human interconnection and interdependence, solidarity, social justice, and the cosmopolitan virtues of tolerance, curiosity, humility, and generosity (Benatar & Upshur, 2014). The principles of solidarity and accompaniment, in particular, have emerged as core values that distinguish global health. They are expressed in a radical inclusiveness that seeks to reduce, if not eliminate, traditional barriers between "donor" and "recipient" and encourages honest appraisal of motives, structures, and practices that are deeply imbedded within the international health and development communities.

These values provide the foundation for a new global health ethics, and as noted above, reveal the tensions inherent in this emerging field. The tensions arise not only from the partisan motivation and self-interest of agencies, organizations, and nations that fund global health work and establish its agenda (Beaumier, Gomez-Rubio, Hotez, & Weina, 2013; Lancet, 2009; Frenk & Moon, 2013), but also because these institutions, particularly the military, tend to appropriate global health as a tactical "tool" (Daniel & Hicks, 2014). Thus, an inherent tension exists between the universal ideals and values of global health and the more limited strategic objectives of some of its funders. In this context, global health workers not infrequently face the challenge of divided loyalties, caught between their commitment to the populations they seek to serve and advancing the goals of the institutions that employ them or fund their work (Briskman & Zion, 2014; London, 2002; London, Rubenstein, Baldwin-Ragaven, & Van Es, 2006; Singh, 2003). When this divergence reaches a critical threshold, the result is moral distress. Within health care, moral distress has been described primarily in the fields of nursing, palliative medicine, and intensive care (Austin, Saylor, & Finley, 2016; Prentice, Janvier, Gillam, & Davis, 2016; Rushton, Kaszniak, et al., 2013; Ruston et al., 2013; Rushton, 2016). Undoubtedly, it is an under-appreciated problem in global health as well (Sunderland, Harris, Johnstone, Del Fabbro, & Kendall, 2015; Ulrich, 2014).

The radical inclusiveness of global health and its commitment to solidarity argue for an ethical framework that addresses the systemic causes of suffering and health inequity while, at the same time, maintains fidelity to the relational, human, and interpersonal foundations of global health practice. On the one hand, the Principlism of bioethics offers a useful tool to identify and balance competing claims, and the human rights approach provides a powerful framework for achieving just social systems. On the other hand, Bill Foege's plea to "see the faces" speaks of the need for global health ethics to embrace the core value of compassion.

Compassion as the Basis for Global Health Ethics

The idea of compassion as a foundation of ethical conduct is not new. According to Chris Frakes, the "pro-compassion camp" includes Aristotle, Adam Smith, Jean-Jacques Rousseau, David Hume, and Arnold Schopenhauer (Frakes, 2010, p. 82). For example, Schopenhauer (1903, p. 213) declared that, "Boundless compassion for all living beings is the surest and most certain guarantee of pure moral conduct" and Albert Schweitzer (1988, p. 11) wrote, "I can do no other than to have compassion for all that is called life. That is the beginning and the foundation of all ethics."

Other thinkers, including Socrates, the Stoics, Immanuel Kant, and Frederick Nietzsche reject compassion as a valid guide for achieving a just society (Frakes, 2010). As an emotion directed at a particular individual or group, they argue, compassion detracts from the reasoned decision-making demanded by equitable and ethical allocation of limited resources. In other words, empathy and compassion interfere with the utilitarian ideal. Supporting this view are findings from a recent study, which suggest that low levels of empathic concern predict utilitarian moral judgment (Gleichgerrcht & Young, 2013). Therefore, compassion and justice are sometimes regarded as being in tension, if not in conflict. If compassion is to be a cornerstone of global health ethics, we will have to resolve this tension.

I believe it is more correct to regard compassion and justice as expressions of the same impulse. In a globalized world, the notion of neighbor—to whom we typically accord moral status, and, if he or she is suffering, offer compassion—must be extended to the entire human family (Addiss, 2016b). In this regard, as a field, global health is in the vanguard, given its concern for "the attainment by all peoples of the highest possible level of health" (World Health Organization, 2006, p. 1).

The notion that compassion and justice are not only interrelated, but that both are required, is not new. The prophet Micah (6:8) wrote, "What does the Lord require of you, but to do justice, to love kindness, and to walk humbly with your God?" Numerous spiritual teachers and philosophers have commented on the interplay and interdependence of justice and compassion. For example, theologians Paul Knitter and Roger Haight (2015, p. 201) argue that "to be compassionate for all requires that we be concerned for justice." Exploring the ethical implications of Ricoeur's dialectic view of love and justice, Van Stichel asserts that, although they operate at different levels (interpersonal and institutional, respectively) and have different logics ("superabundance" and "equivalence," respectively), love and justice need each other. "Love needs justice to be practically embodied, while justice would become more human when inspired by love" (Van Stichel, 2014, p. 505). Referring to Jesus' parable of the Good Samaritan, Maureen O'Connell (2009, p. 205) writes, "When we turn to face suffering persons, we realize that it is no longer enough for individual travelers to step into the ditch and offer emergency aid to the victims of humanly perpetuated violence. Samaritanism calls for a collective response to whole groups of people." Global health is precisely such a collective response.

Ubuntu

A global health ethics could benefit from dialogue with two ethical frameworks that emphasize the personal and relational and that value interconnectedness and compassion. The first of these is the communitarian worldview of Ubuntu, a term found in several Bantu languages of southern Africa (Chuwa, 2014). Archbishop Desmond Tutu describes Ubuntu as "the essence of being human" since it "speaks of the fact that my humanity is caught up and is inextricably bound up in yours. 'I am human because I belong'" (Chuwa, 2014, p. 31). Ubuntu views human life as profoundly interconnected and relational—indeed, the notion of an individual human is inconceivable outside of the relational context of community.

By conceiving of the individual in this way, and through its experience of the deep interconnectedness of human life—which is also a cornerstone of global health (Koplan et al., 2009)—Ubuntu softens the distinction between "the one and the many." The individual is compelled to care for others, since without others one cannot be fully human. Similarly, Ubuntu's profound sense of interconnectedness demands justice, which is both reconciliatory and communitarian. "There is no conflict between the human need for both care and justice. There is not even a separation between the two. Justice and care are concomitant and concurrent. They are perceived as two sides of the same coin" (Chuwa, 2014, p. 135).

Ethics of Care

The second major school of thought that seems philosophically aligned with the core values of global health is the ethics of care. Articulated during the 1980s by Carol Gilligan and Nel Noddings, care ethics takes as its starting point the lived experience of care and caring, upon which human life is absolutely dependent, rather than *a priori* principles based in modern liberalism, which value autonomy, rationality, and self-interest. In contrast to Principlism, care ethics places higher value on connectedness, emotion, relationship, and personal experience. It emphasizes the contextual nature in which moral decisions and actions occur.

Noddings (1984) describes caring relationships as being comprised of the "one-caring" and the one "cared-for." Because the context of relationship is paramount, one's responsibility for caring is essentially limited to persons with whom one is already in relationship. In this view, partiality is virtuous, since caring, as the basis of ethics, is imbedded in relationship. To neglect the care of those with whom one is in relationship for the care of a distant stranger is to neglect one's primary responsibility as the "one-caring." However, the prospect of encountering a needy stranger creates a sense of "wary anticipation" in the one-caring, since, as Noddings writes (1984, p. 9), "aware of my finiteness, I fear a request I cannot meet without hardship. Indeed, the caring person… dreads the proximate stranger, for she cannot easily reject the claim that he has on her."

For global health, this view of care is problematic on two levels. First, the distinction between the "proximate stranger," for whom the one-caring becomes responsible (albeit with "wary anticipation") through a personal encounter, and the "distant stranger," for whom caring is not required or even appropriate, loses its meaning in the context of global health. In practice, global health rejects this dichotomy. The whole point of global health—as well as its prophetic claim—is that we are all, to one degree or another, "proximate strangers," even neighbors. Further, the collaborative interpersonal relationships that sustain the global health enterprise transform "distant strangers" into friends. Thus, global health not only welcomes the "distant stranger," it goes even further to embrace the "global other." As Noddings cautions, however, such an inclusive stance toward care leaves one vulnerable to being psychologically overwhelmed by the magnitude of suffering and by one's inability to address it. We will return to this point shortly.

The second objection to the partiality of care arises from global health's insistence on impartiality, equity, and social justice. Care ethicists since Noddings have wrestled with how to temper the partiality of care, confined within the private, relational sphere, with the ethical demands for impartiality and justice in the public sphere. For example, Halwani (2003) considers care as one (albeit very important) virtue among others. He highlights the importance of moral reasoning for discerning when, in fact, it is virtuous to prioritize care for the suffering stranger (justice) over the claims of care-in-relationship. In this sense, moral reasoning modulates the primacy of care. Others, especially Tronto (1993) and Robinson (1999), hold fast to the primacy of care, not only within close relationships but also as the basis for justice at the societal and political levels. For example, Robinson (2013, p. 137) defines injustice as "those practices, institutions, structures, and discourses which inhibit or subvert adequate care or which lead to exploitation, neglect or a lack of recognition in the giving and receiving of care." Interestingly, this perspective aligns with the Ubuntu worldview, in which "justice is secondary to, and part of, care" (Chuwa, 2014, p. 32).

In accordance with these broader interpretations of care, one could conceive of global health as extending an ethic of care to the global level. In fact, many global health professionals approach their work through a lens of caregiving. They are deeply motivated by an ethic of care and not infrequently inspired by spiritual or religious values, even if these values are not explicit or overtly expressed (Suri et al., 2013). However, scholarship on global health and global health ethics has little to say about the relational one-on-one aspects of caregiving, focusing instead on population-level themes of justice and equity.

At least in part because global health discourse has been largely devoid of content regarding personal values and because its training programs have not addressed self-awareness, emotional resiliency, or mindfulness, global health workers not infrequently find themselves feeling overwhelmed by the enormity of human suffering and by the inadequacy—even futility—of their efforts to address it (Addiss, 2015). By extending their circle of concern (and care) to all humanity, global health workers open themselves not only to Nodding's "wary anticipation of the distant stranger," but also to the lived experience of having failed to care for her. A global health ethic that does not support individuals in their relational caregiving, accompaniment, and solidarity—in addition to addressing the field's central issues of social justice, health equity, and human rights—is, in my view, going to be difficult to sustain. If, as some care ethicists argue, justice is a necessary corrective to the partiality of care, and if an essential value of global health is social justice, what can provide the source of motivation, resiliency, and encouragement for individual practitioners to both enjoin the fight against injustice and to care—for the whole world? Here we return to the theme of compassion and explore its relationship both to care and to justice.

Compassion, Care, and Justice

We are guided in this exploration by Chris Frakes (2010), who worked as a counselor in a domestic violence shelter in the United States. The physical and psychological toll of this work eventually forced her to leave the shelter. Her sustained reflections on this experience led her to conclude that "neither care nor justice adequately motivates attention to the suffering of strangers" (Frakes, 2010, p. 79). Rather, for Frakes, compassion, correctly understood, holds this potential. First, she notes that compassion is more restricted in scope than care, since it is limited to attending to the "negative condition" (Blum, 1980) of suffering. In addition, compassion does not require an intimate or long-term relationship with the person suffering, so it "can be directed not only to those known, but also to those unknown to the agent. Thus although compassion may involve partiality, it can move the agent more generally in the direction of impartiality" (Frakes, 2010, p. 82). So far, this view of compassion aligns more closely with the global health experience than does care as described by care ethicists. Indeed, although global health is also concerned with promoting human flourishing and well-being, it remains largely focused on alleviating the "negative condition" of suffering. Further, relationships in global health, both among individuals and organizations, are often short in duration or low in intensity, circumscribed by particular projects or initiatives. And at times, they would be properly described as transactional.

Along with justice, compassion shares a concern for the unjust suffering of the stranger. However, the aim of compassion "is to alleviate suffering generally, whether or not the one or indeed anyone is responsible for the suffering of its intended target. This is an important distinction from justice, which does not seem to lead automatically to the alleviation of suffering in general" (Frakes, 2010, p. 82). Here again, Frake's discrimination between justice and compassion resonates with global health experience. Global health does concern itself with what john a. powell (2003, p. 103) terms "social" or "surplus" suffering, inflicted by our "social arrangements." In this sense it is grounded in, and intimately allied with, the pursuit of structural justice. But global health also concerns itself with what powell terms ontological or existential suffering, the inevitable suffering inherent in living and dying as a human being.

How then does compassion both modulate the partiality of care and equip us to pursue social justice in the public sphere? Here, Frakes (2010, 85) draws upon the Buddhist virtue of equanimity, which "is specifically directed at overcoming dualism and perceiving fundamental equality." For those who are "compassionate by character," equanimity serves to regulate the emotions and fosters a "disposition that does not mire them in anguish over the enormity and intractability of human suffering, but rather motivates them to perform actions aimed at the alleviation of such suffering" (Frakes, 2010, 87). Frakes' emphasis on emotion regulation and emotional resiliency resonates with recent literature on the psychology and neuroscience of compassion (Halifax, 2011, 2012; Goetz et al., 2010; Klimecki, Leiberg, Lamm, & Singer, 2013). Finally, Frakes (2010, p. 87) defines the virtue of compassion as "the habit of choosing with equanimity the action that is the proper response to the suffering of others." Such a definition seems consonant with global health, which is rooted in the principle of equity and guided by scientific evidence to determine and refine the "proper" response to suffering.

Mindfulness and Global Health Ethics

To briefly recapitulate, we have considered the essential role of mindfulness both for ethical discernment and for compassion at the individual level. Using global health as an example, we also have explored how mindfulness might contribute to global endeavors. We touched on a few of the many ethical challenges in global health, including dual loyalties, "compassion at a distance," inadequate resilience, and fear, and considered four domains, or areas of focus, into which mindfulness might be brought to address some of these challenges. We then addressed the nascent character of global health ethics and explored strands from bioethics, public health ethics, Ubuntu, and care ethics that might contribute toward a more mature conceptual framework for global health ethics. Underlying all of this is the inherent tension between the "one and the many," which permeates global health.

Four Domains of Mindfulness in Global Health

We return now to the four domains of mindfulness that, I suggest, have something significant to contribute to ethical decision-making in global health. One might think of these domains as areas or "objects" of focus or attention, analogous to how one directs one's attention during mindfulness meditation, in turn, to the breath, thoughts, and bodily sensations, for example. Admittedly, to speak of mindfulness as being applied to these four domains extends—and some might argue, distorts— what is commonly meant by mindfulness. Regardless, I suggest that mindfulness, broadly defined, can help address some of the critical ethical challenges in global health.

First, mindfulness brings into awareness one's subconsciously held beliefs, attitudes, assumptions, and emotional triggers, which distort moral judgments. In navigating the complex ethical landscape of global health, the lack of such awareness is a real hazard. Further, mindfulness in this sense must be an ongoing practice, since as Narvaez (2014, p. xxvii) reminds us, "On a moment-to-moment basis, an individual's morality is a shifting landscape. We move in and out of different ethics based on the social context, our mood, filters, stress responses, ideals, goals of the moment, and so on… The trick for most wise behavior is to maintain emotional presence-in-the-moment."

Second, ethical decision-making requires that global health professionals be constantly mindful of, and fully grounded in, the universal values of global health, which sometimes run counter to the values and agendas of funders, employers, and government agencies. Third, being rooted in these values is facilitated by a deep personal *experience* of interconnectedness, whereby the "distant stranger" becomes friend and a commitment is forged to remain, in one way or another, in solidarity. Such a transformative experience can both crystalize a decision to enter the field, and, if mindfully recalled on a frequent basis, sustain a career. The importance of this experiential dimension and the power of mindful fidelity to it are documented in stories from global health practitioners by the Center for Compassion and Global Health (www.ccagh.org). Fourth, to be effective and ethical as a global health practitioner, one must be both knowledgeable about, and mindful of, the cultural, economic, and historical particularities of any situation in which one is working.

Mindfulness and Global Health Practice

How would global health—and global health ethics—benefit if mindfulness were cultivated in these four domains or dimensions? I offer a few speculations. First, mindfulness of one's own internal "landscape," as noted above, would undoubtedly benefit the individual global health practitioner, resulting in improved resilience, self-awareness, and awareness of one's biases and assumptions. This, in turn, could protect against ethical missteps. Second, improved self-awareness and more mindful grounding in the values of global health would provide guidance in navigating divided loyalties. Improved mindfulness in these two domains would also serve to facilitate conversation about shared personal values in global health, in effect ending the current "conspiracy of silence" on this issue. This, in turn, would provide crucial support to global health practitioners and institutions when the flames of nationalism and militarism are stoked by fear, as they were in the United States after the 9/11 attacks on the World Trade Center. In my view, the paucity of such conversations within CDC at that time contributed to its rapid transformation from a premier global health agency to one that, at least for a while, was largely concerned with civil defense.

Mindfulness might also help facilitate a conversation within global health about how individuals and institutions should respond when their well-intentioned interventions result in unexpected harm. The importance of disclosure and apology in cases of unintended injury or wrongdoing is increasingly recognized and practiced in clinical medicine (Wood & Isaac Star, 2007). This is not yet the case in global health. Discerning how these practices might best be brought into global health—where the issues are even more complex—would necessarily begin with mindfulness.

Finally, the underlying challenge of dichotomous thinking, which pervades global health, will never be overcome without mindfulness. As we have seen, a fundamental challenge for the ethics of global health and other global disciplines is the tension between the "one and the many," the faces and numbers. "Think globally, act locally" is an appealing slogan, but in global health, actions and decisions also have global ramifications. An ethic is needed that, in the words of Dōgen, helps global health practitioners leap clear of dichotomy to experience and articulate the "one and the many" in new, integrated ways. In turn, I believe that this would lead to more coherent global health policy and more humane decision-making.

An effort to bring mindfulness training into the global health practice and education would likely be met with challenges similar to those encountered in other public settings, such as schools and hospitals. For global health, mindfulness training would need to be evidence-based, as well as compelling to a largely secular workforce. One of the critiques of bringing mindfulness-based interventions into the secular public sphere is that the practices are stripped from their ethical foundations and taught in a value-neutral context—or some would argue, in an ethical void. This would not be the case for global health. The problem for global health is not that these values do not exist, but that they are inadequately articulated and shared. An intentional welcoming of mindfulness practice could help the field of global health elucidate and express the strong values that it already has. It could also stretch our understanding of mindfulness beyond the individual sense in which it is usually understood to the global level.

This chapter is intended as a prolegomenon, an exploratory foray into new territory. The core values of global health, as described by the leaders of the field, correspond well to those of the spiritual traditions where mindfulness training practices developed. Central to both is compassion. With its explicit core values of compassion, justice, and interconnection, global health could serve as a vehicle for bringing mindfulness into the global arena. In turn, an embrace of mindfulness could significantly influence the emerging field of global health ethics and enable global health to reach its full potential.

References

Addiss, D. G. (2015, December 30). Spiritual themes and challenges in global health. *Journal of Medical Humanities*.

Addiss, D. G. (2016a). Globalization of compassion: The example of global health. In S. Gill & D. Cadman (Eds.), *Why love matters: Values in governance* (pp. 107–119). New York: Peter Lang Publishing.

Addiss, D. G. (2016b, September–October). Compassion in an age of globalization: Who is my neighbor? *Health Progress*, 19–22. Retrieved from https://www.chausa.org/publications/health-progress/article/september-october-2016/who-is-my-neighbor-compassion-in-the-age-of-globalization

Addiss, D. G., Rheingans, R., Twum-Danso, N. A. Y., & Richards, F. O. (2003). A framework for decision-making for mass distribution of Mectizan® in areas endemic for Loa loa. *Filaria Journal, 2*(Suppl. 1), S9.

Altman, L. K. (2002, September 10). At disease centers, a shift in mission and metabolism. *The New York Times*, p. F6.

Anderson, J. F. (1953). *An introduction to the metaphysics of St. Thomas Aquinas*. Washington, DC: Regnery Gateway.

Austin, C. L., Saylor, R., & Finley, P. J. (2016, October 31). Moral distress in physicians and nurses: Impact on professional quality of life and turnover. *Psychological Trauma: Theory, Research, Practice, and Policy*. Advance online publication. Retrieved from doi:https://doi.org/10.1037/tra0000201.

Baer, R. A. (2009). Self-focused attention and mechanisms of change in mindfulness-based treatment. *Cognitive Behaviour Therapy, 38*(Suppl. 1), 15–20.

Baer, R. (2015). Ethics, values, virtues, and character strengths in mindfulness-based interventions: A psychological science perspective. *Mindfulness, 6*, 956–969.

Bailey, T. C., Merritt, M. W., & Tediosi, F. (2015). Investing in justice: Ethics, evidence, and the eradication investment cases for lymphatic filariasis and onchocerciasis. *American Journal of Public Health, 105*, 629–636. https://doi.org/10.2105/AJPH.2014.302454

Barrett, D. H., Ortmann, L. H., Dawson, A., Saenz, C., Reis, A., & Bolan, G. (Eds.). (2016). *Public health ethics: Cases spanning the globe*. New York: Springer Open.

Battat, R., Seidman, G., Chadi, N., Chanda, M.Y., Nehme, J., Hulme, J., Li, A., Faridi, N., & Brewer, T.F. (2010). Global health competencies and approaches in medical education: A literature review. *BMC Medical Education 10*, 94. Retrieved from http://www.biomedcentral.com/1472-6920/10/94

Beaglehole, R., & Bonita, R. (2010). What is global health? *Global Health Action, 3*, 5142. https://doi.org/10.3402/gha.v3i0.5142

Beauchamp, T. L., & Childress, J. F. (2012). *Principles of biomedical ethics* (7th ed.). New York: Oxford University Press.

Beaumier, C. M., Gomez-Rubio, A. M., Hotez, P. J., & Weina, P. J. (2013). United States military tropical medicine: Extraordinary legacy, uncertain future. *PLoS Neglected Tropical Diseases, 7*(12), e2448.

Benatar, S. R., Daar, A., & Singer, P. A. (2003). Global health ethics: The rationale for mutual caring. *International Affairs, 79*(1), 107–138.

Benatar, S. R., & Upshur, R. (2014). Virtues and values in medicine revisited: Individual and global health. *Clinical Medicine, 14*(5), 495–499.

Blevins, J. (2015, November 23). Ebola, Africa, and beyond: An epidemic in religious and public health perspectives. American Academy of Religion, Session A23–315. Retrieved from http://www.podcastchart.com/podcasts/religious-studies-news/episodes/ebola-africa-and-beyond-an-epidemic-in-religious-and-public-health-perspectives

Blum, L. (1980). Compassion. In A. Oksenberg Rorty (Ed.), *Explaining emotions*. Berkeley, CA: University of California Press.

Briskman, L., & Zion, D. (2014). Dual loyalties and impossible dilemmas: Health care in immigration detention. *Public Health Ethics, 7*(3), 277–286.

Brown, T. M., Cueto, M., & Fee, E. (2006). The World Health Organization and the transition from international to global public health. *American Journal of Public Health, 96*, 62–72.

Callahan, D. (2012). *The roots of bioethics: Health, progress, technology, death.* New York: Oxford University Press.

Catholic Health Association of the United States. (2016). A reflection guide for international health activities. St Louis: Catholic Health Association. Retrieved from https://www.chausa.org/docs/default-source/international-outreach/reflection-guide-for-international-health-activities.pdf?sfvrsn=4

Caufield, C. (1997). *Masters of illusion: The World Bank and the poverty of nations.* New York: Henry Holt.

Chambers, R., Gullone, E., & Allen, N. B. (2009). Mindful emotion regulation: An integrative review. *Clinical Psychology Review, 29,* 560–572.

Childress, J. E., Faden, R. R., Gaare, R. D., Gostin, L. O., Kahn, J., Bonnie, R. J., … Nieburg, P. (2002). Public health ethics: Mapping the terrain. *Journal of Law, Medicine & Ethics, 30,* 170–178.

Chuwa, L. T. (2014). *African indigenous ethics in global bioethics: Interpreting Ubuntu.* New York: Springer.

Commission on Social Determinants of Health. (2008). *Closing the gap in a generation: Health equity through action on the social determinants of health. Final Report of the Commission on Social Determinants of Health.* Geneva: World Health Organization.

Compson, J., & Monteiro, L. (2016). Still exploring the middle path: A response to commentaries. *Mindfulness, 7,* 548–564.

Crump, J. A., & Sugarman, J. (2010). Working Group on Ethics Guidelines for Global Health Training (WEIGHT). Global health training and best practice guidelines for training experiences in global health. *The American Journal of Tropical Medicine and Hygiene, 83,* 1178–1182.

Daniel, J. C., & Hicks, K. H. (2014). *Global health engagement: Sharpening a key tool for the Department of Defense.* Washington, DC: Center for Strategic and International Studies.

DeCamp, M. (2011). Ethical review of global short-term medical voluntarism. *HEC Forum, 23,* 91–103. https://doi.org/10.1007/s10730-011-9152-y

Dōgen, E. (1985). Actualizing the fundamental point (Genjō Kōan). In K. Tanahashi (Ed.), *Moon in a dewdrop: Writings of Zen master Dōgen.* New York: North Point Press.

Farley, J. (1991). *Bilharzia: A history of imperial tropical medicine.* New York: Cambridge University Press.

Farmer, P. (2013). Health, healing and social justice: Insights from liberation theology. In M. Griffin & J. Weiss Block (Eds.), *In the company of the poor: Conversations with Dr Paul Farmer and Fr. Gustavo Gutierrez* (pp. 35–70). Maryknoll, NY: Orbis Books.

Foege, W. H. (1984, October 26). *Smallpox, Gandhi and CDC. Fifth annual Joseph Mountin lecture.* Atlanta, GA: Centers for Disease Control.

Foege, W. H., & Rosenberg, M. (1999). Public and community health. In R. W. Gilkey (Ed.), *The 21st century health care leader* (pp. 85–87). San Francisco: Josey-Bass.

Forsythe, R. (2011, September). Helping or hindering? *Volunteer tourism in Ghana and its critical role in development.* Paper presented to Rethinking Development in an Age of Scarcity and Uncertainty: New Values, Voices, and Alliances, for Increased Resilience, University of York, UK. Retrieved from http://eadi.org/gc2011/forsythe-365.pdf

Frakes, C. (2010). When strangers call: A consideration of care, justice, and compassion. *Hypatia, 25*(1, FEAST Special Issue), 79–99.

Frenk, J., & Moon, S. (2013). Governance challenges in global health. *The New England Journal of Medicine, 368,* 936–942.

Glassman, B. (1998). *Bearing witness: A Zen Master's lessons in making peace.* New York: Bell Tower.

Gleichgerrcht, E., & Young, L. (2013). Low levels of empathic concern predict utilitarian moral judgment. *PloS One, 8*(4), e60418.

Goetz, J., Keltner, D., & Simon-Thomas, E. (2010). Compassion: An evolutionary analysis and empirical review. *Psychological Bulletin, 136,* 351–374.

Goldin, P. R., & Gross, J. J. (2010). Effects of mindfulness-based stress reduction (MBSR) on emotion regulation in social anxiety disorder. *Emotion, 10*(1), 83–91.

Gordis, L. (2009). *Epidemiology* (4th ed.). Philadelphia: Saunders Elsevier.

Gow, J. (2002). The HIV/AIDS epidemic in Africa: Implications for U.S. policy. *Health Affairs, 21*, 57–69.

Guillemin, M., & Gillam, L. (2015). Emotions, narratives, and ethical mindfulness. *Academic Medicine, 90*(6), 726–731.

Gutierrez, G. (2003). *We drink from our own wells: The spiritual journey of a people.* New York: Maryknoll.

Halifax, J. (2011). The precious necessity of compassion. *Journal of Pain and Symptom Management, 41*, 146–153.

Halifax, J. (2012). A heuristic model of enactive compassion. *Current Opinion in Supportive and Palliative Care, 6*, 228–235.

Halwani, R. (2003). Care ethics and virtue ethics. *Hypatia, 18*(3), 161–192.

Henry, R., & Stobbe, M. (2014, August 8). American doctor with Ebola arrives in U.S. *The World Post.* Retrieved from http://www.huffingtonpost.com/2014/08/02/american-doctor-ebola_n_5643628.html

Hill, D. R., Ainsworth, R. M., & Partap, U. (2012). Teaching global public health in the undergraduate liberal arts: A survey of 50 colleges. *The American Journal of Tropical Medicine and Hygiene, 87*, 11–15.

Homeida, M., Braide, E., El Hassan, E., Amazigo, U. V., Liese, B., Benton, B., … Sékétéli, A. (2002). APOC's strategy of community-directed treatment with ivermectin (CDTI) and its potential for providing additional health services to the poorest populations. *Annals of Tropical Medicine and Parasitology, 96*(Suppl. 1), S93–S104.

Jain, S., Shapiro, S. L., Swanick, S., Roesch, S. C., Mills, P. J., Bell, I., & Schwartz, E. R. (2007). A randomized controlled trial of mindfulness meditation versus relaxation training: Effects on distress, positive states of mind, rumination, and distraction. *Annals of Behavioral Medicine, 33*(1), 11–21.

Jinpa, T. (2015). *A fearless heart: How the courage to be compassionate can transform our lives.* New York: Avery.

Johnston, W. (2004). *Mystical theology: The science of love.* Maryknoll, NY: Orbis.

Jones, J. H. (1981). *Bad blood: The Tuskegee syphilis experiment.* New York: Free Press.

Kabat-Zinn, J. (1990). *Full catastrophe living: Using the wisdom of your body and mind to face stress, pain, and illness.* New York: Delacorte.

Kabat-Zinn, J. (1994). *Wherever you go, there you are: Mindfulness meditation in everyday life.* New York: Hyperion.

Kabat-Zinn, J. (2003). Mindfulness-based interventions in context: Past, present, and future. *Clinical Psychology: Science and Practice, 10*, 144–156.

Kearney, M. K., Weininger, R. B., Vachon, M. L. S., Harrison, R. L., & Mount, B. M. (2009). Self-care of physicians caring for patients at the end of life: "Being connected. A key to my survival". *JAMA, 301*(11), 1155–1164.

Kerry, V. B., Walensky, R. P., Tsai, A. C., Bergmark, R. W., Rouse, C., & Bangsberg, D. R. (2013). US medical specialty global health training and the global burden of disease. *Journal of Global Health, 3*(2), 20406.

Klimecki, O. M., Leiberg, S., Lamm, C., & Singer, T. (2013). Functional neural plasticity and associated changes in positive affect after compassion training. *Cerebral Cortex, 23*(7), 1552–1561.

Knitter, P., & Haight, R. (2015). *Jesus and Buddha, friends in conversation.* New York: Maryknoll.

Koplan, J. P., Bond, T. C., Merson, M. H., Reddy, K. S., Rodriguez, M. H., Sewankambo, N. K., & Wasserheit, J. N. (2009). Towards a common definition of global health. *Lancet, 373*, 1993–1995.

Krägeloh, C. U. (2016). Importance of morality in mindfulness practice. *Counseling and Values, 61*, 97–110.

Kristeller, J. L., & Johnson, T. (2005). Cultivating loving kindness: A two-stage model of the effect of meditation on empathy, compassion, and altruism. *Zygon, 40*(2), 391–407.

Kushner, J. (2016, March 22). The Voluntourist's dilemma. New York Times Magazine. Retrieved from http://www.nytimes.com/2016/03/22/magazine/the-voluntourists-dilemma.html?_r=0

Lama, D. (2002). Dialogues. In R. J. Davidson & A. Harrington (Eds.), *Visions of compassion: Western scientists and Tibetan Buddhists examine human nature*. New York: Oxford University Press.

Lancet. (2009). What has the Gates foundation done for global health? *Lancet, 373*, 1577.

Landrigan, P. J., Ripp, J., Murphy, R. J. C., Claudio, L., Jao, J., Hexom, B., … Koplan, J. P. (2011). New academic partnerships in global health: Innovations at Mount Sinai School of Medicine. *Mount Sinai Journal of Medicine, 78*(3), 470–482. https://doi.org/10.1002/msj.20257

Larson, J. S. (1996). The World Health Organization's definition of health: Social versus spiritual health. *Social Indicators Research, 38*(2), 181–192.

Leiberg, S., Klimecki, O., & Singer, T. (2011). Short-term compassion training increases prosocial behavior in a newly developed prosocial game. *PloS One, 6*(3), e17798.

Linhart, T. D. (2006). They were so alive!: The spectacle self and youth group short-term mission trips. *Missiology: An International Review, 34*(4), 451–462.

London, L. (2002). Dual loyalties and HIV policy in South Africa – A challenge to the institutions of our professions. *South African Medical Journal, 92*(11), 882–883.

London, L., Rubenstein, L. S., Baldwin-Ragaven, L., & Van Es, A. (2006). Dual loyalty among military health professionals: Human rights and ethics in times of armed conflict. *Cambridge Quarterly of Healthcare Ethics, 15*, 381–391.

Lueke, A., & Gibson, B. (2015). Mindfulness meditation reduces implicit age and race bias: The role of reduced automaticity of responding. *Social Psychological and Personality Science, 6*(3), 284–291.

Lutz, A., Jha, A. P., Dunne, J. D., & Saron, C. D. (2015). Investigating the phenomenological matrix of mindfulness-related practices from a neurocognitive perspective. *American Psychologist, 70*(7), 632–658.

Macfarlane, S. B., Jacobs, M., & Kaaya, E. E. (2008). In the name of global health: Trends in academic institutions. *Journal of Public Health Policy, 29*, 383–401.

Matthiessen, P. (1985). *Nine-Headed Dragon River*. Boston: Shambhala Publications.

McConville, J., McAleer, R., & Hahne, A. (2016). Mindfulness training for health profession students – The effect of mindfulness training on psychological well-being, learning and clinical performance of health professional students: A systematic review of randomized and non-randomized controlled trials. *Explore* (NY). Oct 24. pii: S1550-8307(16)30161-6.

McCoy, D., Chand, S., & Sridhar, D. (2009). Global health funding: How much, where it comes from and where it goes. *Health Policy and Planning, 24*, 407–417.

Merson, M. H. (2014). University engagement in global health. *The New England Journal of Medicine, 370*, 1676–1678.

Mikulas, W. (2015). Ethics in Buddhist training. *Mindfulness, 6*(1), 14–16.

Monteiro, L. M., Musten, R. F., & Compson, J. (2015). Traditional and contemporary mindfulness: Finding the Middle Path in the Tangle of Concerns. *Mindfulness, 6*, 1.

Narvaez, D. (2014). *Neurobiology and the development of human morality: Evolution, culture, and wisdom*. New York: W.W. Norton.

Noddings, N. (1984). *Caring: A feminine approach to ethics and moral education*. Berkeley, CA: University of California Press.

O'Connell, M. H. (2009). *Compassion: Loving our neighbor in an age of globalization*. Maryknoll, NY: Orbis Books.

O'Neill, O. (2002). Public health or clinical ethics: Thinking beyond borders. *Ethics & International Affairs, 16*(2), 35–45.

Orzech, K. M., Shapiro, S. L., Warren Brown, K., & McKay, M. (2009). Intensive mindfulness training-related changes in cognitive and emotional experience. *The Journal of Positive Psychology, 4*(3), 212–222.

Page, K. (2012). The four principles: Can they be measured and do they predict ethical decision making? *BMC Medical Ethics 13*, 10. http://www.biomedcentral.com/1472-6939/13/1/10

Pinto, A. D., & Upshur, R. E. (2009). Global health ethics for students. *Developing World Bioethics*, *9*(1), 1–10.

Pinto, A. D., & Upshur, R. E. G. (Eds.). (2013). *An introduction to global health ethics*. New York: Routledge.

powell, j. a. (2003). Lessons from suffering: How social justice informs spirituality. *University of St. Thomas Law Journal*, *2003–2004*, 102–127.

Prentice, T., Janvier, A., Gillam, L., & Davis, P. G. (2016). Moral distress within neonatal and paediatric intensive care units: A systematic review. *Archives of Disease in Childhood*, *101*(8), 701–708.

Purser, R. (2015). Clearing the muddled path of traditional and contemporary mindfulness: A response to Monteiro, Musten, and Compson. *Mindfulness*, *6*, 23–45.

Reifenberg, S. (2013). Afterword. In M. Griffin & J. Weiss Block (Eds.), *In the company of the poor: Conversations with Dr. Paul Farmer and Fr. Gustavo Gutierrez*. Maryknoll, NY: Orbis Books.

Robinson, F. (1999). *Globalizing care: Ethics, feminist theory, and international relations*. Boulder, CO: West View Press.

Robinson, F. (2013). Global care ethics: Beyond distribution, beyond justice. *Journal of Global Ethics*, *9*(2), 131–143.

Rosenberg, M. L., Utzinger, J., & Addiss, D. G. (2016). Preventive chemotherapy versus innovative and intensified disease-management in neglected tropical diseases: A distinction whose shelf life has expired. *PLoS Neglected Tropical Diseases*, *10*(4), e0004521.

Rosenberg, E. L., Zanesco, A. P., King, B. G., Aichele, S. R., Jacobs, T. L., Bridwell, D. A., … Saron, C. D. (2015). Intensive meditation training influences emotional responses to suffering. *Emotion*, *15*(6), 775–779.

Ruedy, N. E., & Schweitzer, M. E. (2010). In the moment: The effect of mindfulness on ethical decision making. *Journal of Business Ethics*, *95*(Suppl. 1), 73–87. Regulating ethical failures: Insights from psychology. http://www.jstor.org/stable/29789714

Rushton, C. H. (2016). Moral resilience: A capacity for navigating moral distress in critical care. *AACN Advanced Critical Care*, *27*(1), 111–119.

Rushton, C. H., Boss, R., Hallett, K., Hensel, J., Humphrey, G. B., Les, J., … Volpe, R. L. (2013). The many faces of moral distress among clinicians. *Narrat Inq Bioeth*, *3*(2), 89–93.

Rushton, C. H., Kaszniak, A. W., & Halifax, J. S. (2013). Assessing moral distress: Application of a framework to palliative care practice. *Journal of Palliative Medicine*, *16*(9), 1–9.

Schmidt, A. T. (2016). The ethics and politics of mindfulness-based interventions. *Journal of Medical Ethics*, *42*, 450–454. https://doi.org/10.1136/medethics-2015-102942

Schopenhauer, A. (1903). *On the basis of morality*. (trans: Bullock, A. B.). London: Swan Sonnenschein.

Schweitzer, A. (1988). *Place for revelation: Sermons on reverence for life*. New York: MacMillan.

Segal, Z. V., Williams, J. M. G., & Teasdale, J. D. (2002). *Mindfulness-based cognitive therapy for depression: A new approach to preventing relapse*. New York: Guilford Press.

Shapiro, S. L., & Izett, C. D. (2008). Meditation: A universal tool for cultivating empathy. In S. Hick & T. Bien (Eds.), *Mindfulness and the therapeutic relationship*. New York: Guilford Press.

Shapiro, S. L., Jazaieri, H., & Goldin, P. R. (2012). Mindfulness-based stress reduction effects on moral reasoning and decision making. *The Journal of Positive Psychology*, *7*(6), 504–515.

Shapiro, S. L., Schwartz, G. E., & Bonner, G. (1998). Effects of mindfulness-based stress reduction on medical and premedical students. *Journal of Behavioral Medicine*, *21*(6), 581–599.

Singer, T., & Klimecki, O. M. (2014). Empathy and compassion. *Current Biology*, *24*(18), R875–R878.

Singh, J. A. (2003). American physicians and dual loyalty obligations in the "war on terror". *BMC Medical Ethics*, *4*. Retrieved from http://www.biomedcentral.com/1472-6939/4/4

Stanley, S. (2013). 'Things said or done long ago are recalled and remembered': The ethics of mindfulness in early Buddhism, psychotherapy and clinical psychology. *European Journal of Psychotherapy and Counseling*, *15*(2), 151–162.

Sunderland, N., Harris, P., Johnstone, K., Del Fabbro, L., & Kendall, E. (2015). Exploring health promotion practitioners' experiences of moral distress in Canada and Australia. *Global Health Promotion*, *22*(1), 32–45.

Suri, A., Weigel, J., Messac, L., Thorp Basilico, M., Basilico, M., Hanna, B., … Kleinman, A. (2013). Values and global health. In P. Farmer, A. Kleinman, & J. Kim (Eds.), *Reimagining global health*. Berkeley: University of California Press.

Task Force for Global Health. (2011). *Compassion in global health*. Richard Stanley Productions. Accessed March 30, 2017, from https://www.youtube.com/watch?v=ydn0H60K3Nk

Thompson, B. L., & Waltz, J. (2007). Everyday mindfulness and mindfulness meditation: Overlapping constructs or not? *Personality and Individual Differences*, *43*, 1875–1885.

Tronto, J. (1993). *Moral boundaries: A political argument for an ethic of care*. New York: Routledge.

Tutu, D. (1999). *No future without forgiveness*. London: Random House.

Twum-Danso, N. A. Y. (2003a). Serious adverse events following treatment with ivermectin for onchocerciasis control: A review of reported cases. *Filaria Journal*, *2*(Suppl. 1), S3.

Twum-Danso, N. A. Y. (2003b). Loa loa encephalopathy temporally related to ivermectin administration reported from onchocerciasis mass treatment programs from 1989 to 2001: Implications for the future. *Filaria Journal*, *2*(Suppl. 1), S7.

Ulrich, C. M. (2014). Ebola is causing moral distress among African healthcare workers. *British Medical Journal*, *349*, g6672.

Van Stichel, E. (2014). Love and justice's dialectical relationship: Ricoeur's contribution on the relationship between care and justice within care ethics. *Medicine, Health Care, and Philosophy*, *17*, 499–508.

Vinson, A. E., & Wang, J. (2015). Is mindful practice our ethical responsibility as anesthesiologists? *International Anesthesiology Clinics*, *53*(3), 1–11.

Wall, A. (2011). The context of ethical problems in medical volunteer work. *HEC Forum*, *23*, 79–90.

Wood, M. S., & Isaac Star, J. (2007). *Healing words: The power of apology in medicine* (2nd ed.). Oak Park, IL: Doctors in Touch.

World Health Organization. (2006, October). Constitution of the World Health Organization, Basic Documents, 45th ed. Supplement. Accessed March 30, 2017, from http://www.who.int/governance/eb/who_constitution_en.pdf

Part III
Ethics of Mindfulness in Corporate and Military Organizations

Chapter 13
Ethics of Mindfulness in Organizations

Frank Musten

The chapters in this section examine the ethics of bringing mindfulness-based programs (MBPs) into secular settings that do not necessarily embody the ethics typically associated with Buddhism or with Buddhist practice. This has been seen as particularly problematic when the Buddhist practice of mindfulness is introduced into organizational settings (Ronald Purser, 2015; Ronald Purser & Milillo, 2015). The intent of my chapter is to acknowledge their contributions and examine two other ethical issues that require deeper examination.

The first ethical concern I address is the potential for MBPs to result in significantly distressing emotions or experiences. This is usually not what participants expect and thus can be more troubling because it is unexpected. I examine the consequences of negative effects of mindfulness practice through the lens of a duty to care and the process of ensuring safety through appropriate consent to be taught mindfulness practices. The second ethical concern is rooted in the different expectations and impact an MBP has on the employee attending the program and the organization sponsoring the program. This difference in expectations can arise as the participants become more aware of any conflict between sustaining their well-being and meeting the organization's demands; that is, while meeting an individual's needs an MBP may not meet the organizational client's expectations. Issues such as the format of an MBP, clarity of outcomes, and managing the possible divergent expectations of employee and employer are examined.

F. Musten, PhD (✉)
Ottawa Mindfulness Clinic, 595 Montreal Road, Suite 301, Ottawa, ON, Canada, K1K 4L2
e-mail: frank.musten@gmail.com

© Springer International Publishing AG 2017   325
L.M. Monteiro et al. (eds.), *Practitioner's Guide to Ethics and Mindfulness-Based Interventions*, Mindfulness in Behavioral Health,
DOI 10.1007/978-3-319-64924-5_13

Mindfulness Extracted from Its Historical Social Context

In considering why care should be taken in translating a spiritual practice into a secular, organizational context, we can refer to the expectations of practice and the safeguards that were likely inherent in the historical social context where the Buddha shared his teachings. When we contrast those expectations with the expectations modern organizations as well as mindfulness trainers have of their MBPs, two areas emerge where differences between historical and modern social contexts suggest the need for care. The first is the potential risks for modern day participants enrolled in mindfulness programs in organizations that have cultures that are radically different from the historical culture from which the Buddha's practice of mindfulness emerged.

The second is the potential differences between the expectations of mindfulness practices in organizations and the expectations of the followers of the Buddha who were practicing meditation in his sangha.

McMahan (2008) reminds us that the Buddha said he only taught two things, suffering and the end of suffering. The intent of practice was solely to attain the end of suffering by ending the cycle of dependent origination which… "denotes in early Buddhist literature the chain of causes and conditions that give rise to all phenomenal existence in the world of impermanence, birth, death, and rebirth (samsara)" (p. 153). In modern times, the Buddha's idea of dependent origination has come to be a model, for modern Buddhists and others, of an interconnected world. It has become a source of inspiration for the ecology movement as well as a source of inspiration for those of us who see the beauty and wonder in the interconnectedness of all things (McMahan, 2008). Thus, it is important to recognize that Buddhism itself has changed over the centuries so that, at least in the West, it has become oriented more toward reducing the suffering in and of this world than toward following a path of practice that ultimately would allow those who followed his path to escape forever the suffering that was inevitably the consequence of birth.

In the next section, I highlight aspects of the social history of early Buddhism that shaped the intent and expectation of practice at the time. The intent and expectation of practice for those early Buddhists was radically different from the intent and expectation of modern secular mindfulness practice, particularly in organizations. Those differences form the core of our understanding of why there is a need to take care for participants in our MBPs and a need to manage the expectations of organizational clients and program participants.

Much of the next section is based on the work of the historian Richard Gombrich (2006, 2009) who has written extensively on the social history of the Buddha's time. He suggests that the Buddha probably was the son of a leader of a large village that likely did not have a caste system but used other means to rank individuals. According to Gombrich (2006), this is the model the Buddha likely used for his sangha.

While he grew up in a village, he taught in what was likely the beginning of an urban center (Gombrich, 2006). The beginnings of urbanization likely resulted from an agricultural surplus that allowed some people to remove themselves from the land. Some would have been absentee landlords while others would have had a livelihood that was not "derived directly from agriculture" (p. 39).

Gombrich (2006) notes that during the time of the Buddha there was already a counter-culture of individuals who were renouncing the norms of the time. Thus, when he left his own home he stepped into a life that already existed. It is also likely that these renouncers were able to exist also because householders, the heads of families, had the surplus available to support them. Gombrich suggests that the Buddha's message may have resonated with this particular group because, despite their relative material prosperity, they still were subject to the realities that life was often brutal and short. Gombrich (2006) citing McNeill (1998) speculates that the Ganges basin where the Buddha shared his teachings was an ideal environment for producing an agricultural surplus. But because it was warm and damp, it was also a fertile breeding ground for deadly diseases. It was this contrast between the comfort associated with relative wealth and the constant threat of painful illness and death that provided a receptive audience for his teachings.

The Buddha welcomed all into his sangha. As well, his sangha was organized in the manner of his village with no caste system. However, Gombrich's examination of the suttas leads him to conclude that most of the members of the sangha were from the class of householders. There are three aspects of the social history of the Buddha's time that resonated with his teachings and with his decision to create a sangha that was based on his village life. These same three are ones that may not translate well into how mindfulness is presented in secular organizational settings.

The first is the peoples of the time accepted as a reality that life was inherently unsatisfactory. Thus, those who became part of the Buddha's sangha were not expecting to find a way to make life more satisfying but rather to enter a path that would eventually end their cycle of rebirth. This is a very different perspective from that of the modern mindfulness meditator in an organization who expects the meditation to be relaxing and to help manage stress.

Second, the monastic members of the Buddha's sangha viewed meditation as a means to apprehend the wisdom of the Four Noble Truths. That wisdom emerged from a moral life that provided the clarity necessary for the meditator to embody that wisdom. In contrast to secular mindfulness taught in organizations, moral behavior present in a monastic community is not typically taught nor is there the intent that mindfulness practice will lead to wisdom as defined in the Four Noble Truths. However, the participant who begins the practice of meditation may still experience an incongruence between the demands of organizational life and develop an emerging sense of how the demands of their work contrast with their values.

Third, it was likely that only the members of the monastic community who had stepped away from the complexities of living in the world could practice meditation as a means toward the ultimate goal of achieving awakening. There was likely an inherent emotional safety associated with being in the Buddha's sangha removed from many of the stresses that characterized life outside the sangha. It is not clear how a monastic with a pre-existing disorder might have fared in sangha, but it can possibly be presumed that, at least, in some instances the order inherent in sangha life and the Buddha's supportive community would have been therapeutic. The expectations of that historical time included hearing voices, having visions, and so on (Armstrong, 2006). Thus, it is possible to speculate that the sangha would have been accepting of behavior that in modern times would be diagnosed as severe mental illness.

These distinctions between the Buddha's intention for mindfulness practice are a frame against which we can examine the current critiques of mindfulness set in organizational environments.

Critiques and Concerns of Organizational Mindfulness Programs

As MBPs expand in their application into organizations such as corporations and the military, concerns have been voiced that such venues do not necessarily have the commitment to the ethical practices that are at the core of Buddhist practice (Purser & Loy, 2013). The criticisms that have been voiced of secular mindfulness in general and of these specific applications, in particular, are that such secularized, de-ethnicized applications create a risk of causing harm.

The Economist (Schumpeter, 2013) raised a similar concern and added the perspective that perhaps corporate mindfulness programs were really no more useful than, and maybe not even as useful as, a walk in the woods. That suggestion was also addressed in an extensive review by Good and colleagues (Good et al., 2016). While it appears that emerging research suggests there can be benefits from introducing mindfulness into organizations, the research is sparse and the specific nature of those benefits is not yet clear. These observations echo the responses (Choi & Tobias, 2015; Connolly, Stuhlmacher, & Cellar, 2015; Hülsheger, 2015) to a focal article by Hyland, Lee, and Mills (2015).

Monteiro, Musten, and Compson (2015) explored the complexities of bringing mindfulness, a spiritually based practice, into secular settings. A sample of the responses to their article (Baer, 2015; Purser, 2015; Van Gordon, Shonin, Lomas, & Griffiths, 2016) echoed the concern expressed in the Economist (Schumpeter, 2013) and by Choi and Tobias (2015) and Hülsheger (2015). However, these responses from both the secular mindfulness and Buddhist communities also offered an array of possible paths toward addressing those concerns.

Shalini Bahl and Sean Bruyea, authors of chapters in this section, reiterate the concern that MBPs in organizations risk ignoring the ethical intentions that were historically meant to guide mindful practice. Bahl suggests that two ethical paradoxes challenge the trainer who wants to bring mindfulness into organizations. The first is that organizations may be introducing mindfulness practices so that their employees can manage work stress more effectively. However, they may not be altering the working conditions that are the primary source of the stress. The second paradox proposes that corporate cultures, in general, do not embody the same ethic that is integral to the intention of mindfulness practice (Kabat-Zinn, 2011).

Bahl provides a balanced discussion of these paradoxes, focusing on how the mindfulness trainer can navigate them. She refers to "circles of influence" that bring mindful inquiry first into the trainer's personal development, then into the relationship the trainer has with the network of people, potential and actual, who are associated with the trainer's MBP. She suggests that this network be diverse and can include other mindfulness teachers, Buddhist teachers, and the clients themselves. Her final circle includes the processes associated with providing the program.

A detailed description of how to bring mindful inquiry into each of these circles provides a path the mindfulness trainer can follow as they navigate through the ethical challenges associated with bringing mindfulness into organizations. Finally, she introduces the need to bring wisdom and ethical practices into the training processes, engaging the root causes of the problem, and thereby avoiding a myopic approach to mindfulness training.

Bruyea in his chapter describes the complex challenges of bringing mindfulness into a military organization. He chooses to structure his discussion of the ethics of bringing mindfulness into military organizations by first discussing ethics as they are understood by mindfulness trainers. He then gives us a detailed look at the complex nature of the discussion of ethics in the military followed by an insightful look at military culture. Finally, he brings his arguments together into a nuanced discussion of the ethical issues associated with bringing ethics into the military and veteran populations. Bruyea notes that many military tasks require the training in intention and attention that are familiar to mindfulness trainers. Thus, from that perspective mindfulness would not be unfamiliar to military members and thus might facilitate the use of mindfulness as an effective intervention with soldiers and veterans. He discusses the ethical and practical barriers to introducing mindfulness either as resilience training or as a clinical intervention. But he notes that the military culture itself may also pose the most difficult challenge. His discussion of the military culture is insightful. He makes the point clearly that the service-before-self culture of the military and veteran communities may not fit well with the individual approach to practice and awareness that is at the core of many mindfulness programs. He clearly articulates a number of concerns about how mindfulness might be used by the military. However, he also notes that with appropriate cultural awareness, mindfulness trainers can play an important role in helping military members as they are transitioning into civilian life.

Bahl and Bruyea have provided balanced discussions of the ethical challenges associated with extracting a practice like mindfulness from its spiritual context, and specifically from its complex ethical framework. In addition, Bruyea raises the idea that mindfulness trainers may have to recognize there are also cultural challenges they will have to address as they begin to introduce mindfulness as a clinical intervention in military and veteran populations. While his focus is on one population, his insights remind us that all organizations have unique cultures that must be taken into account when mindfulness trainers are considering how they are going to deliver their interventions.

Both authors have clearly laid out a range of ethical challenges we face when we consider bringing mindfulness into organizations. And they have suggested approaches we can take to mitigate against violating the ethical intent of mindfulness as we introduce the practice into organizations. In this chapter, I would like to expand on two areas they touched on. The first, raised by Bahl, is, simply, how can we be assured that our intervention is doing what we say it is doing? The second, raised by Bruyea, is how do we take care of those in the room when we often know very little about who is in the room. That is, we often know very little about the acute and chronic psychological challenges individual participants may be bringing into the MBP sessions. These issues form the first ethical concern that I now address as a duty to care.

The Duty to Care

Bruyea, in his chapter on the ethics of bringing mindfulness into the military, raised the challenges associated with introducing an individually based practice like mindfulness into a culture that puts service before self. His discussion explored the responsibility trainers, who bring mindfulness into organizations, have to know who is in the room. It is possible to generalize from his discussion and acknowledge that all mindfulness trainers have a responsibility not only to know who is in the room. They also have a duty to provide care for those in the room for whom mindfulness is not necessarily a benign intervention. In clinical settings, the question of who is in the room is usually managed through pre-screenings (Dobkin, Irving, & Amar, 2012). The issue of the duty to provide appropriate care for those in the room is addressed in the ethical standards proscribed by the clinician's professional code of ethics.

However, in many organizational settings, codes of conduct, awareness of scope of practice, and ethical guidelines may vary considerably depending on the trainer's own professional training. This level of variation can impact how the iatrogenic effects of mindfulness practice are managed. Evidence is just beginning to emerge that some participants in these programs can experience levels of distress that, at times, can be intense (Creswell, 2017; Lindahl et al., 2017; Lomas, Cartwright, Edginton, & Ridge, 2015; Russ & Elliot, 2017). In part, some distress is a normal consequence of bringing open awareness to the reality of one's life (Coffey et al., 2010); it is a result of the goal of mindfulness training. That distress may not moderate in the early sessions of the program but begins to moderate as mindfulness skills are acquired (Baer, Carmody, & Hunsinger, 2012).

However, some participants may have stronger reactions that may not moderate, or they may experience more serious mental health events during a class. The evidence for these more severe occurrences is often found in anecdotal examples of what has come to be termed "dark night" experiences (Creswell, 2017). There is stronger evidence of significant distress emerging during longer meditation experiences (Lomas et al., 2015; Russ & Elliott, 2017; Yorston, 2001). However, the possibility of a significant distressing experience is acknowledged by the common practice of screening for disorders that are likely to be adversely impacted by mindfulness training (Dobkin et al., 2012). My own experience is that these incidents do occur both in the mindfulness-based programs that are offered generally and in the shorter programs offered in organizations. A model for how these incidents might be managed is offered in a later section.

For the moment, it is important to recognize that most trainers offering these programs in organizations may not be clinicians or may not be experienced in dealing with the distress that could arise in a mindfulness program. Further many trainers may feel that since they are not teaching the program as a clinical intervention, they would not expect anyone to experience significant distress. However, epidemiological studies of the incidence of serious psychiatric disorders within the general population regularly report non-trivial incidence of these disorders (Ahola et al., 2011; Baumeister & Härter, 2007; Norris & Slone, 2014), suggesting there is always a likelihood of someone in the room who is at risk for or experiencing a mental health disorder.

As well, it has been my experience that organizations often have a circumscribed idea of mindfulness as something that will help their employees better manage the stress that seems to be permeating everyone's life and is independent of their overall psychological status (Duxbury, 2008; Duxbury, Stevenson, & Higgins, 2017; Higgins, Duxbury, & Lyons, 2010; Pines, Neal, Hammer, & Icekson, 2011; Toker & Biron, 2012). Thus, both organizations and participants in an organization-sponsored MBP may not have an expectation that distress can emerge as a consequence of participating in a program.

As part of an evaluation of the programs that my colleagues and I at the Ottawa Mindfulness Clinic regularly conduct with organizational clients, we ask participants to complete the Maslach Burnout Inventory, a standard measure of work burnout (Maslach, Jackson, & Leiter, 1997) before they begin the program. It is not uncommon for about half the participants to report levels of emotional exhaustion consistent with burnout. Given the research generally reports high levels of stress in the modern work force, we do not expect other trainers would experience their participants as different from those in our programs. Thus trainers can expect that someone in the room may be experiencing significant psychological distress simply because of the incidence of mental disorders in the general population (Baumeister & Härter, 2007). And, they can also expect that some of their participants will be experiencing significant levels of burnout as a result of their work stress as well as from challenges to work–life balance (Dewa, Lin, Kooehoorn, & Goldner, 2007; Diestel & Schmidt, 2011; Higgins et al., 2010; Watts & Robertson, 2011).

Although there is evidence that mindfulness interventions can mitigate against becoming burned out (Geller, Krasner, & Korones, 2010; Grégoire & Lachance, 2015; Halpern & Maunder, 2011; Hülsheger, Alberts, Feinholdt, & Lang, 2013; Krasner et al., 2009; Wolever et al., 2012), it does not mean everyone in the room will benefit equally or that no one will be distressed by the intervention. Thus, there remains the duty to care for those individuals whose pre-existing distress may be exacerbated by attending a mindfulness program, as well as for those who may experience significant distress as a direct result of attending a mindfulness program.

The potential for unexpected mental health distress related to mindfulness practices means our duty to care begins with informed consent. In clinical settings, it is standard practice to obtain informed consent from participants acknowledging that they are aware of the possibility that the program may include negative experiences or potential exacerbation of present symptoms. Participants also are aware of the support available to them should they feel the need to connect with a trainer who is also usually a clinician. Finally, because participants are regularly screened for pre-existing conditions the trainers typically know who is in the room.

Those same safeguards are not usually available, even for clinicians, offering mindfulness programs in organizational settings. Thus, honoring the duty to care in organizational settings is a common problem for all trainers regardless of their backgrounds. Organizations and participants typically expect mindfulness to help and would not likely understand the need for informed consent. Nor would they likely be particularly comfortable asking their employees to submit to a pre-screening process before signing up for what they believe is a course that will help enhance their sense of well-being. Recognizing those challenges, we have developed a process that we refer to as Affirmed Assent. What I mean by Affirmed Assent is that participants are introduced to both the benefits of mindfulness as well as the challenges that can emerge during practice, typically before enrolling in a program. Thus, when they do enroll they have an idea of what to expect and by signing up they are affirming their assent to take part. In early sessions, the idea that the practice can be difficult and can also be distressing is normalized. And, the program is also offered as one way to increase personal well-being not the only way and for some, not the best way. Thus, the space is left open for a participant to choose another approach at any time during the MBP. This concept may not meet some stringent and rigid perspectives of informed consent, but it does provide a reasonable approach to duty to care that would be acceptable in most organizational settings. (The details of how we introduce Affirmed Consent into our programs, as well as, specific aspects of the inquiry that support Affirmed Consent are discussed in a later section on bringing MBPs into the marketplace.) Having established the need for a duty to care in this section, I address the second ethical concern which is related to issues of evaluating and clarifying outcomes of MBPs.

Outcomes and Expectations

Outcome Evidence

Implicit in the duty to care is the confidence we place in evidence-based outcomes. However, organizational MBPs have yet to produce consistent patterns of effectiveness. Choi and Tobias (2015) noted that there is a lack of longitudinal research confirming that participants who have completed a program actually retain the benefits of mindfulness over the long term. These authors also note there is an absence of controlled studies providing clear support that mindfulness factors rather than, for example, a placebo effect are a likely reason for any observed changes. Hulsheger (2015) suggests there is evidence that mindfulness creates increased awareness. However, he notes that creating increased awareness does not necessarily mean that once an employee is more aware they will therefore be a better employee from the organization's perspective.

Although recent reviews suggest there is significant potential benefit both for individuals and organizations by bringing mindfulness into the workplace (Good et al., 2016; Hülsheger et al., 2013; Hyland et al., 2015; Roche, Haar, & Luthans, 2014), much also remains unknown (Choi & Tobias, 2015; Connolly et al., 2015; Hülsheger, 2015). Thus, it is important for trainers who are developing MBPs in organizational settings to develop clear intentions for their programs that include providing expectations consistent with the current literature. In general, the wise practitioner would be best served by being cautious about the benefits claimed for their MBP.

My colleagues and I have addressed some of these concerns in a program developed to introduce mindfulness as one means of increasing well-being in a public service organization. Recent studies have shown a relationship between mindfulness and well-being mediated by a number of constructs (Bajaj, Gupta, & Pande, 2016; Bajaj & Pande, 2016; Galante, Galante, Bekkers, & Gallacher, 2014; Roche et al., 2014) including Psychological Capital (Roche et al., 2014), a validated measure that has been related to well-being in organizations (Luthans, Avolio, Avey, & Norman, 2007; Luthans, Youssef, & Avolio, 2007; Luthans, Youssef-Morgan, & Avolio, 2015; Roche et al., 2014; Youssef & Luthans, 2012). Based on current research, we felt it was appropriate to assume increased well-being in an organizational setting was a reasonable expected outcome of an MBP. Other researchers (Biron, 2014; Burke, 2009; Singh, Burke, & Boekhorst, 2016) have shown that fostering well being in organizations has a practical, beneficial impact on organizational functioning. Thus, there also seemed to be good reason to expect that connecting mindfulness to organizational effectiveness is likely when the intent of an MBP is to foster employee well-being. As studies are becoming more complex and are including more elegant controls, we are beginning to see that mindfulness remains an effective intervention. However, the degree to which mindfulness is effective depends on many factors (Buchholz, 2015; Good et al., 2016). For example, in clinical settings, where much of the research has been done, it seems that more traditional approaches are as effective (Kuyken et al., 2015; Moon, 2017) and, at times, perhaps more effective (Garland et al., 2014) than a mindfulness intervention.

It becomes more challenging in organizational environments where the challenges of interpreting research findings are compounded by the demands of designing organizational MBPs that suit the organization's infrastructure. Availability of personnel, physical space, participants' schedules—especially in travel-intense companies—often require modifications of standard protocols of MBPs. My own experience is that protocols also are in a constant state of fluidity to meet these organizational realities.

Typical concerns for issues such as time for formal practice can become the least of a trainer's concern. If we take MBSR-informed (Kabat-Zinn, 1990) programs as a model, trainers may be required to decrease the number of sessions from the standard eight-session protocol. Organizational requirements may mean that sessions will have to be shorter than the recommended two and a half hours. That also applies to the length of the meditations themselves which may have to be shortened because of many factors, both organizational and individual. Bahl noted that there is little research that provides direction for knowing if and how protocols can be modified and still be seen as providing the same training. These issues may have a significant impact on the research findings.

As our understanding matures of how mindfulness works, it becomes increasingly important to have a clear expectation of an outcome for a proposed MBP. This problem is not unique to trainers who offer MBPs in organizations, however we will discuss later in this chapter how trainers can provide evidence that their MBP is doing what it is intended to do. Fortunately for our purposes a model, practice-based evidence (Barkham, Stiles, Lambert, & Mello-Clark, 2010; Green, 2012; Jensen et al., 2012), has been developed in response to a similar need among practicing therapists. Much like trainers who structure their MBPs to meet organizational requirements, therapists have the same need to be assured that therapeutic protocols developed in ideal research settings are still valid when translated into the complex interchanges with clients in their real-world offices. I will describe the use of practice-based evidence in an organizational setting below.

Bringing Caring and Efficacy into the Marketplace

The trainer walks a fine line between recognizing that there can be some risk of harm associated with an MBP and not, at the same time, presenting mindfulness as being more harmful than it might be. Coffey, Hartman and Fredrickson (2010) reported a positive though paradoxical relationship between attention and psychological distress. They interpreted this positive relationship as the possible result of paying attention to psychological distress which may make it more salient in the short run but also provide data for better management of those symptoms in the long run. Consistent with these findings and interpretations, some participants in our programs have reported increases in their experience of distress or that, early in the program, the practice does not appear to help them manage their distress. Those expectations are almost always managed through an inquiry process that has the participant beginning to understand mindfulness as a practice of "paying attention to" rather than "getting rid of" one's experience. However, discernment is also required because, in a few instances, we have had participants experience significant emotional distress that increased over the course of sessions. In these cases, it was and is recommended, after an individual session with the participant, that they discontinue in the group in favor of other options.

The trainer can walk a more established line when they make an effort to determine that the MBP they are offering is achieving what it is expected to achieve. In other words, it is an evidence-based practice. Organization representatives, whether they are referring health care providers, disability insurers, or managers want to be assured that the program they are supporting with their referrals or inviting into their organization is a good investment in time and money.

It is often useful to refer back to what the research shows. However, as is the case with psychotherapy (Barkham, Stiles, et al., 2010; Green, 2012; Jensen et al., 2012) most programs evolve to meet the needs of the participants. In many if not most cases, the specific MBP will not completely adhere to the program evaluated in the research study. It thus becomes important to develop an evaluation protocol that can demonstrate that a specific program a trainer has designed achieves the expected results. Clinicians in psychological practice, as well as in health care generally, are beginning to use the evidence they collect from their practice as a means for ensuring that their interventions are achieving what they are meant to achieve. We have adopted this Practice Based Evidence approach to evaluate the efficacy of the programs we offer and have also included Practice Based Evidence in our organizational programs.

In the next two sections, I describe a model for Affirmed Assent as a practical approach for honoring a trainer's duty to care. Following that discussion, an evaluation protocol based on the Practice Based Evidence model is described.

A Two-Stage Approach to Affirmed Assent

The process of Affirmed Assent is a model for honoring the duty to care when the trainer cannot know who is in the room. The two stages include an information session where participants are introduced to the potential challenges they may encounter as they are cultivating a mindfulness practice. The second stage encompasses the first and second sessions of a multiple week program where the inquiry opens the space for those participants who may be having challenges to voice those challenges. There also is an overarching commitment by trainers in the program to ensure that there is an opportunity for those individuals who may feel the need for support or have questions and concerns to have access to the trainers.

Stage One Information sessions are typically offered a week before a program begins. In the information session, in addition to explaining what mindfulness is and how it might be beneficial to participants, we also introduce participants to some of the challenges associated with mindfulness using three experiential exercises. In the first exercise participants are led through a guided meditation where they are asked to intentionally and gently bring their attention first to the objects of their awareness, seeing if it is possible to just know that the objects are present without needing to explore them, then shifting their attention to the breath, and finally bringing awareness to the body.

In the inquiry that follows, some participants will usually share the difficulties they experienced maintaining their attention on the object of their attention; sometimes indicating that they could not turn their mind off. This becomes an opportunity to normalize their experience and to note that the practice, although it sounds simple, is hard, and it is best if they are gentle with themselves. It is also a time to note that the intent is not to change what is happening but to notice what is happening. Often, we then ask participants to offer a single word or a couple of words (popcorn style) that describes why they think it would be important to notice what is going on. In this way, we are beginning to orient participants toward seeing the practice as a way of noticing and then connecting the noticing to taking intentional steps toward the intent of the program which is to foster well-being.

In the second experiential exercise, we introduce participants to the conditions at work that are likely to increase stress at work. Traditionally those have been High Demand, Low Control, and Lack of Support (Karasek & Theorell, 1990; Luchman & González-Morales, 2013; Regehr & Millar, 2007; Shirom, Toker, Alkaly, Jacobson, & Balicer, 2011; Tucker et al., 2008). In the experiential exercise, participants are asked to settle into their breathing, bringing attention just to the breath itself, and then bringing to mind the demands they have in their work and personal life; noticing the physical sensations, emotions, and thoughts that come up. This template is followed for the other two factors related to work stress.

Once the exercise has been completed they are asked to popcorn out a word or two that describes what they noticed when they brought the demands of their work and personal life to mind. This template is repeated for each of the factors associated with work stress.

Participants' responses usually include feeling overwhelmed, exhausted, anxious, and so on. These responses give the trainers an opportunity to note that mindfulness opens up space to see where you are; some time is spent reminding participants that the present moment is not always a pleasant moment. In the last experiential exercise, the three factors that define burnout (Leiter, 2015; Maslach, Schaufeli, & Leiter, 2001), Emotional Exhaustion, Cynicism or Depersonalization, and Loss of a Sense of Personal Efficacy are introduced and explored using the same template. Taken together, these two exercises introduce participants to the reality that what one experiences in a mindfulness course can be distressing. Participants typically only register for a program after the Information Session.

Stage Two In the first and second classes, we open the space for individuals who may be having difficulty sharing their experiences. It can sometimes be challenging as there is a tendency for those who initially share to be ones who have had a pleasant experience with the exercises. Thus, it is sometimes necessary to offer space for other experiences by saying, "That's good. I am sure that not everybody's experience was that pleasant. Could someone share a less pleasant experience they had with the exercise"? That usually opens the space for difficult experiences to emerge and an opportunity to note that too is mindfulness and remind participants that mindfulness is about noticing, not about having a good experience.

Beginning with the first class, we also note in a general way that if anyone is having difficulty understanding the home practice, is struggling with a concept, or is having difficulty with an exercise to contact one of the trainers either by email or by arranging to chat with a trainer either before or after class. Thus, the idea that the experience may not be pleasant is normalized as one of the possible challenges that a participant might encounter.

In summary, starting with the information session participants have an opportunity to explore the ranges of experiences that can arise in meditation. The program is also presented as one, but not necessarily the only, way to foster well-being. Affirmed Assent is a process whereby trainers open the space for potential participants to make an informed decision to enroll in the program and also to continue in the program once they have enrolled.

Are We Doing What We Say We Are Doing?

Most of our programs are offered in public service organizations committed to the well-being of managers and staff. They are also conscious of the public purse and want to ensure that they are getting value for money spent. In one department that was science-based, it was expected that there would be some form of program evaluation that would allow the executive who had championed the program to show the department's senior executives that the program had merit.

There were restrictions that limited the content of the evaluation. First, the program was expected to contribute to employees' well-being with an emphasis on well-being at work. The program was offered in a public service department that required all materials were in English and French. The evaluation had to be brief because there was limited time in the program to administer pre- and post-evaluations.

The evaluation included both standardized assessment instruments that could be scored numerically and thus would provide quantitative measures of pre–post changes. It also included a structured qualitative assessment instrument that examined the processes underlying the changes (Barkham, Hardy, & Mellor-Clark, 2010a). Two primary quantitative measures were chosen, the Maslach Burnout Inventory (MBI) (Maslach et al., 1997) and the Psychological Capital Questionnaire (PsyCap) (Luthans, Avolio, et al., 2007). The MBI scores on Emotional Exhaustion, the factor most often associated with burnout, were used to assess the level of stress experienced by participants pre- and post-program, Scores across the four factors of Hope, Efficacy, Resilience, and Optimism that make up the construct of Psychological Capital (Luthans, Avolio, et al., 2007; Youssef & Luthans, 2012) were used to assess well-being. The qualitative results contributed insight into how individual practitioners were bringing the practices into their work and personal lives. Together these data allowed us to begin to construct a model of how mindfulness was impacting on the participants in this MBP. This model then allowed us to conceptualize how we may want to improve the quality of our interventions.

The evaluation process is important for many reasons. First, it provides evidence that a program is doing what it is intended to do. It provides the data needed to assure the client that the cost of the program was money well spent. The qualitative data provide insight into processes that contributed to the changes in well-being and guide our iterative changes that can improve program effectiveness. Taken together these data allow us to better understand our program and to potentially contribute in a meaningful way to the emerging science around the usefulness of bringing mindfulness into organizations.

Conclusions

My discussion of the trainer's duty to care, as well their need to confirm expectations with outcome evidence, along with the two papers in this section serve as a reminder that much remains to be done before we have a clear picture of how mindfulness impacts organizational life. Shalini Bahl has articulated ethical concerns associated with bringing mindfulness into for-profit organizations. She also notes that trainers are, at times, asked to bring mindfulness into organizations whose practices are not congruent with Buddhist ethics and that mindfulness trainers working in these organization are challenged to maintain their own integrity and the integrity of the teachings.

Sean Bruyea introduces us to the complex field of military ethics. He relates the current discussion of ethics on MBP to the ethical challenges associated with bringing mindfulness into the military particularly when it is intended to improve resilience in hostile environments. Because the organizational culture is not likely to change, the ethics of bringing mindfulness into the military will continue to challenge trainers.

Both authors expand our awareness of the ethical challenges associated with providing MBPs in organizations. However, they do not suggest that trainers not take up those challenges. Instead, they suggest that trainers have an understanding of those ethical challenges. By acknowledging those challenges, they can take the steps that are possible to encourage the practice of wisdom and compassion in program participants.

It is possible for the reader to conclude that, given many, if not most, organizations are not inclined to make structural changes to foster well-being, teaching participants mindfulness to foster individual well-being may be a fruitless or even an inappropriate intervention. However, it is always important to keep in mind that the Buddha accepted the reality of the world he lived in, while he continued to teach the end of suffering (Batchelor, 1998; Gombrich, 2006). In order to facilitate MBPs skillfully, I have outlined how trainers need to be aware of the ethical challenges associated with bringing a practice that was developed in a specific historical sociocultural context into a modern context that is radically different. I suggest that safeguards that were likely present in the historical context are not likely to present in the modern organization where MBPs are now regularly being offered.

Organizations are not the only settings where Buddhist practices are being taught in contexts that are radically different from the historical contexts where the Buddha shared his teachings. As McMahan (McMahan, 2008) has argued, the intent and practice of Buddhism in modern times is radically different from the intent and practice of monastics in the historic Buddhist sangha.

Our model of Affirmed Assent follows from our increasing awareness that mindfulness is not necessarily a benign intervention, and that it is the responsibility of all mindfulness trainers to include protocols in their interventions that honor the common duty to care for participants in our programs.

The need, not only to care for the participants in our MBPs but also to ensure that our programs are doing what we say they are doing, is also not unique to providing intervention in organizations. A protocol referred to as Practice-Based Evidence (Barkham, Hardy, & Mellor-Clark, 2010b; Green, 2012) has been developed to assist practitioners in private practice in insuring that their therapeutic outcomes are consistent with expected outcomes of a specific intervention. The need for this assurance comes from the common experience among therapists and other health care professionals that the clinical research conditions where interventions are developed do not typically reflect the real life clinical conditions under which the treatment is offered. Practice-Based Evidence provides the clinical practitioner with an assurance that the intervention is effective in their own particular real world context.

The divide between expectations and research validation of outcomes is an even bigger concern in organizations where expectations of outcomes may not be supported by available research (Choi & Tobias, 2015; Connolly et al., 2015; Good et al., 2016). Practice-Based Evidence is not intended as a substitute for Evidence-Based Practice with its requirement for randomized assignment to treatment and control groups. However, it does focus the mindfulness trainer in organizations on being able to articulate to a client the potential outcomes expected from an intervention and being able to demonstrate that the intervention had (or potentially did not have) the desired impact on participants completing the MBP.

The chapters in this section remind us how far we have to go to be as confident as we would like that our programs are having the desired impact on individual participants and on organizations. However, the chapters in this section and book also provide the needed direction if we want, finally, to be able to respond to the challenges posed in the Economist article (Schumpeter, 2013): to be more aware of the real impact of what we are doing.

References

Ahola, K., Virtanen, M., Honkonen, T., Isometsä, E., Aromaa, A., & Lönnqvist, J. (2011). Common mental disorders and subsequent work disability: A population-based Health 2000 Study. *Journal of Affective Disorders*, *134*(1–3), 365–372. https://doi.org/10.1016/j.jad.2011.05.028

Armstrong, K. (2006). The great transformation: the beginning of our religious traditions. New York: Alfred A. Knopf, 2006.

Baer, R. (2015). Ethics, values, virtues, and character strengths in mindfulness-based interventions: A psychological science perspective. *Mindfulness, 6*(4), 956–959.

Baer, R. A., Carmody, J., & Hunsinger, M. (2012). Weekly change in mindfulness and perceived stress in a mindfulness-based stress reduction program. *Journal of Clinical Psychology, 68*(7), 755–765. https://doi.org/10.1002/jclp.21865

Bajaj, B., Gupta, R., & Pande, N. (2016). Self-esteem mediates the relationship between mindfulness and well-being. *Personality and Individual Differences, 94*, 96–100. https://doi.org/10.1016/j.paid.2016.01.020

Bajaj, B., & Pande, N. (2016). Mediating role of resilience in the impact of mindfulness on life satisfaction and affect as indices of subjective well-being. *Personality and Individual Differences, 93*, 63–67. https://doi.org/10.1016/j.paid.2015.09.005

Barkham, M., Hardy, G. E., & Mellor-Clark, J. (2010a). *Developing and delivering practice-based evidence: A guide for the psychological therapies.* Chichester, West Sussex; Malden, MA: Wiley.

Barkham, M., Hardy, G. E., & Mellor-Clark, J. (Eds.). (2010b). *Developing and delivering practice-based evidence: A guide for the psychological therapies.* Malden, MA: Wiley.

Barkham, M., Stiles, W., Lambert, M. J., & Mello-Clark, J. (2010). Building a rigorous and relevant knowledge base for the psychological therapies. In M. Barkham, G. Hardy, & J. Mello-Clark (Eds.), *Developing and delivering practice-based evidence.* Malden, MA: Wiley.

Batchelor, S. (1998). *Buddhism without beliefs: A contemporary guide to awakening.* New York: Riverhead Books.

Baumeister, H., & Härter, M. (2007). Prevalence of mental disorders based on general population surveys. *Social Psychiatry and Psychiatric Epidemiology, 42*(7), 537–546. https://doi.org/10.1007/s00127-007-0204-1

Biron, C. a. (2014). *Creating healthy workplaces: Stress reduction, improved well-being, and organizational effectiveness.* Farnham, England: Gower.

Buchholz, L. (2015). Exploring the promise of mindfulness as medicine. *JAMA, 314*(13), 1327–1329. https://doi.org/10.1001/jama.2015.7023

Burke, R. (2009). Working to live or living to work: Should individuals and organizations care? *Journal of Business Ethics, 84*, 167–172. https://doi.org/10.1007/s10551-008-9703-6

Choi, E., & Tobias, J. (2015). Mind the gap: The link between mindfulness and performance at work needs more attention. *Industrial and Organizational Psychology, 8*(4), 629–633. https://doi.org/10.1017/iop.2015.90

Coffey, K. A., Hartman, M., & Fredrickson, B. L. (2010). Deconstructing mindfulness and constructing mental health: Understanding mindfulness and its mechanisms of action. *Mindfulness, 1*(4), 235–253. doi:10.1007/s12671-010-0033-2

Connolly, C., Stuhlmacher, A., & Cellar, D. (2015). Be mindful of motives for mindfulness training. *Industrial and Organizational Psychology, 8*(4), 679–682. https://doi.org/10.1017/iop.2015.99

Creswell, J. D. (2017). Mindfulness interventions. *Annual Review of Psychology, 68*, 491–516. https://doi.org/10.1146/annurev-psych-042716-051139

Dewa, C. S., Lin, E., Kooehoorn, M., & Goldner, E. (2007). Association of chronic work stress, psychiatric disorders, and chronic physical conditions with disability among workers. *Psychiatric Services, 58*(5), 652–658. https://doi.org/10.1176/appi.ps.58.5.652

Diestel, S., & Schmidt, K.-H. (2011). Costs of simultaneous coping with emotional dissonance and self-control demands at work: Results from two German samples. *Journal of Applied Psychology, 96*(3), 643–653. https://doi.org/10.1037/a0022134

Dobkin, P., Irving, J., & Amar, S. (2012). For whom may participation in a mindfulness-based stress reduction program be contraindicated? *Mindfulness, 3*(1), 44–50. https://doi.org/10.1007/s12671-011-0079-9

Duxbury, L. E. (2008). *Work-life conflict in Canada in the new millennium key findings and recommendations from the 2001 National Work-Life Conflict Study: Report six.* Ottawa, ON: Health Canada.

Duxbury, L., Stevenson, M., & Higgins, C. (2017). Too much to do, too little time: Role overload and stress in a multi-role environment. *International Journal of Stress Management.* https://doi.org/10.1037/str0000062

Galante, J., Galante, I., Bekkers, M.-J., & Gallacher, J. (2014). Effect of kindness-based meditation on health and well-being: A systematic review and meta-analysis. *Journal of Consulting and Clinical Psychology*, 82(6), 1101–1114. https://doi.org/10.1037/a0037249

Garland, S. N., Carlson, L. E., Stephens, A. J., Antle, M. C., Samuels, C., & Campbell, T. S. (2014). Mindfulness-based stress reduction compared with cognitive behavioral therapy for the treatment of insomnia comorbid with cancer: A randomized, partially blinded, noninferiority trial. *Journal of Clinical Oncology: Official Journal of the American Society of Clinical Oncology*, 32(5), 449. https://doi.org/10.1200/JCO.2012.47.7265

Geller, R., Krasner, M., & Korones, D. (2010). Clinician self-care: The applications of mindfulness-based approaches in preventing professional burnout and compassion fatigue. *Journal of Pain and Symptom Management*, 39(2), 366–366. https://doi.org/10.1016/j.jpainsymman.2009.11.279

Gombrich, R. F. (2006). *Theravāda Buddhism: A social history from ancient Benares to modern Colombo* (2nd ed.). London: Routledge.

Gombrich, R. F. (2009). *What the Buddha thought*. London: Equinox Pub.

Good, D. J., Lyddy, C. J., Glomb, T. M., Bono, J. E., Brown, K. W., Duffy, M. K., ... Lazar, S. W. (2016). Contemplating mindfulness at work. *Journal of Management*, 42(1), 114–142. https://doi.org/10.1177/0149206315617003

Green, D. (2012). *Maximising the benefits of psychotherapy: A practice-based evidence approach*. Chichester, West Sussex: Wiley.

Grégoire, S., & Lachance, L. (2015). Evaluation of a brief mindfulness-based intervention to reduce psychological distress in the workplace. *Mindfulness*, 6(4), 836–847. https://doi.org/10.1007/s12671-014-0328-9

Halpern, J., & Maunder, R. G. (2011). Acute and chronic workplace stress in emergency medical technicians and paramedics. In J. Langan-Fox & C. L. Cooper (Eds.), *Handbook of stress in the occupations* (pp. 135–156). Northampton, MA: Edward Elgar.

Higgins, C. A., Duxbury, L. E., & Lyons, S. T. (2010). Coping with overload and stress: Men and women in dual-earner families. *Journal of Marriage and Family*, 72(4), 847–859. https://doi.org/10.1111/j.1741-3737.2010.00734.x

Hülsheger, U. R. (2015). Making sure that mindfulness is promoted in organizations in the right way and for the right goals. *Industrial and Organizational Psychology*, 8(4), 674–679. https://doi.org/10.1017/iop.2015.98

Hülsheger, U. R., Alberts, H. J. E. M., Feinholdt, A., & Lang, J. W. B. (2013). Benefits of mindfulness at work: The role of mindfulness in emotion regulation, emotional exhaustion, and job satisfaction. *Journal of Applied Psychology*, 98(2), 310–325. https://doi.org/10.1037/a0031313

Hyland, P., Lee, R. A., & Mills, M. (2015). Mindfulness at work: A new approach to improving individual and organizational performance. *Industrial and Organizational Psychology*, 8(4), 576–602. https://doi.org/10.1017/iop.2015.41

Jensen, D. R., Abbott, M. K., Beecher, M. E., Griner, D., Golightly, T. R., & Cannon, J. A. N. (2012). Taking the pulse of the group: The utilization of practice-based evidence in group psychotherapy. *Professional Psychology: Research and Practice*, 43(4), 388–394. https://doi.org/10.1037/a0029033

Kabat-Zinn, J. (1990). *Full catastrophe living*. New York: Delta.

Kabat-zinn, J. (2011). Some reflections on the origins of MBSR, skillful means, and the trouble with maps. *Contemporary Buddhism*, 12(1), 281–306. https://doi.org/10.1080/14639947.2011.564844

Karasek, R., & Theorell, T. (1990). *Healthy work: Stress, productivity, and the reconstruction of working life*. New York: Basic Books.

Krasner, M. S., Epstein, R. M., Beckman, H., Suchman, A. L., Chapman, B., Mooney, C. J., & Quill, T. E. (2009). Association of an educational program in mindful communication with burnout, empathy, and attitudes among primary care physicians. *JAMA*, 302(12), 1284–1293. https://doi.org/10.1001/jama.2009.1384

Kuyken, W., Hayes, R., Barrett, B., Byng, R., Dalgleish, T., Kessler, D., ... Byford, S. (2015). Effectiveness and cost-effectiveness of mindfulness-based cognitive therapy compared with maintenance antidepressant treatment in the prevention of depressive relapse or recurrence (PREVENT): A randomised controlled trial. *The Lancet.* https://doi.org/10.1016/S0140-6736(14)62222-4

Leiter, M. P. (2015). *Burnout.* New York: Oxford University Press.

Lindahl, J. R., Fisher, N. E., Cooper, D. J., Rosen, R. K., Britton, W. B., & Brown, K. W. (2017). The varieties of contemplative experience: A mixed-methods study of meditation-related challenges in Western Buddhists. *PLoS ONE, 12*(5). doi:10.1371/journal.pone.0176239

Lomas, T., Cartwright, T., Edginton, T., & Ridge, D. (2015). A Qualitative analysis of experiential challenges associated with meditation practice. *Mindfulness, 6*(4), 848–860.

Luchman, J. N., & González-Morales, M. G. (2013). Demands, control, and support: A meta-analytic review of work characteristics interrelationships. *Journal of Occupational Health Psychology, 18*(1), 37–52. https://doi.org/10.1037/a0030541

Luthans, F., Avolio, B. J., Avey, J. B., & Norman, S. M. (2007). Positive psychological capital: Measurement and relationship with performance and satisfaction. *Personnel Psychology, 60*(3), 541–572. https://doi.org/10.1111/j.1744-6570.2007.00083.x

Luthans, F., Youssef, C. M., & Avolio, B. J. (2007). *Psychological capital: Developing the human competitive edge.* New York: Oxford University Press.

Luthans, F., Youssef-Morgan, C. M., & Avolio, B. J. (2015). *Psychological capital and beyond.* New York: Oxford University Press.

Maslach, C., Jackson, S. E., & Leiter, M. P. (1997). Maslach burnout inventory: Third edition. In C. P. Z. R. J. Wood (Ed.), *Evaluating stress: A book of resources* (pp. 191–218). Lanham, MD: Scarecrow Education.

Maslach, C., Schaufeli, W. b., & Leiter, M. P. (2001). Job burnout. *Annual Review of Psychology, 52*, 397–422.

McMahan, D. L. (2008). *The making of Buddhist modernism.* Oxford; New York: Oxford University Press.

McNeill, W. (1998). *Plagues and people.* New York: Anchor.

Monteiro, L. M., Musten, R. F., & Compson, J. (2015). Traditional and contemporary mindfulness: Finding the middle path in the tangle of concerns. *Mindfulness, 6*(1), 1–13. https://doi.org/10.1007/s12671-014-0301-7

Moon, M. A. (2017). Back pain: CBT, mindfulness benefits diminish over time. (NEWS). *Family Practice News, 47*(4), 3.

Norris, F. H., & Slone, L. B. (2014). Epidemiology of trauma and PTSD. In M. J. Friedman, T. M. Keane, & P. A. Resick (Eds.), *Handbook of PTSD: Science and practice* (2nd ed., pp. 100–120). New York: Guilford Press.

Pines, A. M., Neal, M. B., Hammer, L. B., & Icekson, T. (2011). Job burnout and couple burnout in dual-earner couples in the sandwiched generation. *Social Psychology Quarterly, 74*(4), 361–386. https://doi.org/10.1177/0190272511422452

Purser, R. (2015). Clearing the muddled path of traditional and contemporary mindfulness: A response to Monteiro, Musten, and Compson. *Mindfulness, 6*(1), 23–45. https://doi.org/10.1007/s12671-014-0373-4

Purser, R., & Loy, D. (2013). Beyond Mcmindfulness. *The Huffington Post.*

Purser, R., & Milillo, J. (2015). Mindfulness revisited: A Buddhist-based conceptualization. *Journal of Management Inquiry, 24*(1), 3–24.

Regehr, C., & Millar, D. (2007). Situation critical: High demand, low control, and low support in para-medic organizations. *Traumatology, 13*(1), 49–58. https://doi.org/10.1177/1534765607299912

Roche, M., Haar, J. M., & Luthans, F. (2014). The role of mindfulness and psychological capital on the well-being of leaders. *Journal of Occupational Health Psychology, 19*(4), 476–489. https://doi.org/10.1037/a0037183

Russ, S. L., & Elliott, M. S. (2017). Antecedents of mystical experience and dread in intensive meditation. *Psychology of Consciousness: Theory, Research, and Practice, 4*(1), 38–53. https://doi.org/10.1037/cns 0000119

Schumpeter. (2013). The mindfulness business. *The Economist.*

Shirom, A., Toker, S., Alkaly, Y., Jacobson, O., & Balicer, R. (2011). Work-based predictors of mortality: A 20-year follow-up of healthy employees. *Health Psychology*, *30*(3), 268–275. https://doi.org/10.1037/a0023138

Singh, P., Burke, R. J., & Boekhorst, J. (2016). Recovery after work experiences, employee well-being and intent to quit. *Personnel Review*, *45*(2), 232–254. https://doi.org/10.1108/PR-07-2014-0154

Toker, S., & Biron, M. (2012). Job burnout and depression: Unraveling their temporal relationship and considering the role of physical activity. *Journal of Applied Psychology*, *97*(3), 699–710. https://doi.org/10.1037/a0026914

Tucker, J. S., Sinclair, R. R., Mohr, C. D., Adler, A. B., Thomas, J. L., & Salvi, A. D. (2008). A temporal investigation of the direct, interactive, and reverse relations between demand and control and affective strain. *Work & Stress*, *22*(2), 81–95. https://doi.org/10.1080/02678370802190383

Van Gordon, W., Shonin, E., Lomas, T., & Griffiths, M. D. (2016). Corporate use of mindfulness and authentic spiritual transmission: Competing or compatible ideals? *Mindfulness & Compassion*, *1*(2), 75–83. https://doi.org/10.1016/j.mincom.2016.10.005

Watts, J., & Robertson, N. (2011). Burnout in university teaching staff: A systematic literature review. *Educational Research*, *53*(1), 33–50. https://doi.org/10.1080/00131881.2011.552235

Wolever, R. Q., Bobinet, K. J., McCabe, K., Mackenzie, E. R., Fekete, E., Kusnick, C. A., & Baime, M. (2012). Effective and viable mind-body stress reduction in the workplace: A randomized controlled trial. *Journal of Occupational Health Psychology*, *17*(2), 246–258. https://doi.org/10.1037/a0027278

Yorston, G. (2001). Mania precipitated by meditation: A case report and literature review. *Mental Health, Religion & Culture*, *4*(2), 209–213. https://doi.org/10.1080/713685624

Youssef, C., & Luthans, F. (2012). Psychological capital, meaning, findings, and future directions. In K. Cameron & G. Spreitzer (Eds.), *The Oxford handbook of positive organizational scholarship* (pp. 17–27). New York: Oxford University Press.

Chapter 14
Paradoxes of Teaching Mindfulness in Business

Shalini Bahl

Introduction

This chapter is dedicated to exploring the efficacy and ethical considerations of teaching mindfulness in business. The emergence of mindfulness as a popular means of enhancing workplace skills has come under some scrutiny and criticism. Particularly, teaching mindfulness in business without the foundation in ethics and wisdom poses unique challenges and consequences. Drawing from Buddhist teachings, mindfulness research, management theory, and experiences of corporate mindfulness instructors, this chapter looks at two paradoxes of teaching mindfulness in business and its implications for different stakeholders. It offers mindful inquiry of our circles of influence as a comprehensive framework to guide our intentions and work of integrating mindfulness in business to enhance the well-being of all its stakeholders.

Dissatisfaction and Stress in Institutions

Americans' confidence in key institutions continues to dwindle, as indicated by the National Leadership Index (NLI). This nationwide poll measured public attitudes toward leadership across 13 different sectors in the US including business, non-profit, education, religion, and politics. Lead author, Seth Rosenthal, reported, "a vast majority of Americans believe we have a crisis in leadership and that we will

S. Bahl, PhD (✉)
The Reminding Project and Downtown Mindfulness in Amherst, Amherst, MA, USA

Isenberg School of Management, UMass, Amherst, MA 01002, USA
e-mail: Shalini@RemindingProject.com

© Springer International Publishing AG 2017   345
L.M. Monteiro et al. (eds.), *Practitioner's Guide to Ethics and Mindfulness-Based Interventions*, Mindfulness in Behavioral Health,
DOI 10.1007/978-3-319-64924-5_14

decline as a nation unless we do something about it" (quoted in McKiernan, 2012). More recently, the Edelman Trust Barometer, which has been tracking trust in institutions for the past 15 years, reports a similar lack of trust in key institutions—business, government, media, and NGOs (Edelman, 2017). For the first time since the Great Recession, half the countries included in this global survey reported overall trust is below 50% that institutions will do what is right. People believe that leadership has failed to protect them from national and global crises related to issues including health, corruption, refugees, online security, and corporate scandals (Edelman, 2017). The same report reflects an expectation that businesses need to take a broader view of their role in society beyond short-term gains to include doing good work for society.

Looking more specifically at the dissatisfaction within organizations, a majority of employees continue to experience disengagement at work (Mann & Harter, 2016) as job stress continues to impact American adults. For example, since 2007 the Stress in America Survey consistently finds that money and work are the top two sources of stress (APA, 2016). Leaders in organizations are not spared from stress either and CEOs are under pressure to read and adapt to an increasingly complicated business environment. The 19th Annual Global CEO Survey (PwC, 2016) reported highest levels of worry in the past 5 years. Top concerns of CEOs include regulation, geopolitical uncertainty, social instability, readiness to respond to crises, and cyber security. The same survey indicated that most CEOs recognize a fundamental shift from a globalizing world to one with multiple dimensions of power, growth, and threats. CEOs acknowledge that they must address the shifting expectations of their customers and stakeholders who now require CEOs to consider wider stakeholders' needs. My personal experience working with leaders echoes the sentiments of this survey and other consultants like Laloux (2014). Despite their power and their appearance of control, leaders are tired of the pressures to adapt to rapidly changing environment and expectations of multiple stakeholders.

Mindfulness as a Solution to Stress

In a fast-paced culture where stress and dissatisfaction are ubiquitous, mindfulness offers respite in different domains of human life. Mindfulness is rapidly becoming mainstream in medicine, health care, psychology, education, business, and military training (Monteiro, Musten, & Compson, 2015). Although mindfulness traces its roots through many worldviews and religions, it was popularized by Jon Kabat-Zinn in his pioneering Mindfulness-Based Stress Reduction program (MBSR) and based on Buddhist traditions. He defines mindfulness as "the awareness that arises by paying attention, on purpose, in the present moment, and non-judgmentally" (Kabat-Zinn, 2013, p. xxxv).

A common focus in mindfulness trainings is the ability to stabilize attention with the specific attitudes of non-judgment, curiosity, and kindness; these facilitate enhanced awareness. Sustaining this quality of awareness creates conditions for insight into the true nature of life—notably, impermanence, causes of suffering, and transient nature of self—which in turn reduces attachments and aversions and frees people to make more skillful choices (Bahl et al, 2016). In the absence of mindfulness, we react based on past conditioning and habitual patterns that may perpetuate one's own and others' affliction (Goldstein, 2016). Clearly articulates the transformative potential of mindfulness, "At its heart lies a system of training that leads to insight and the overcoming of suffering" (p. 20).

We have growing evidence that mindfulness is associated with greater physical and psychological well-being (for reviews, see e.g., Brown, Ryan, & Creswell, 2007; Holzel et al., 2011; Khoury et al., 2013; Tang, Holzel, & Posner, 2015). Within business contexts, mindfulness offers many benefits including stress-reduction (Narayanan & Moynihan, 2006), better decision-making (Hafenbrack, Kinias, & Barsade, 2014), increased customer satisfaction (Grégoire & Lachance, 2014), self-confidence (Amar, Hlupic, & Tamwatin, 2014), and moral intelligence (Amar et al., 2014; Shapiro, Jazaieri, & Goldin, 2012). Looking at the interpersonal effects of mindfulness, Reb, Narayanan, and Chaturvedi (2012) find a positive relationship between supervisor mindfulness and lower levels of exhaustion and better work-life balance, job performance, and satisfaction. However, the same study also points out that without feelings of autonomy, competence, and connection with other people, employees do not experience the benefits of leader mindfulness. Evidently, mindfulness alone is not enough.

While mindfulness, as a secular body of knowledge and practices, is gaining popularity in business circles, concerns are arising that a superficial form, some call it "McMindfulness" (Purser & Loy, 2013), is taking over. Critics of secular mindfulness argue that decontextualizing mindfulness from its ethical roots harnesses these ancient practices to promote a corporate agenda instead of liberating people from suffering (Purser & Loy, 2013; Schumpeter, 2013). "Mindfulness training has wide appeal because it has become a trendy method for subduing employee unrest, promoting a tacit acceptance of the status quo, and as an instrumental tool for keeping attention focused on institutional goals." (Purser & Loy, 2013). While we stay open to the criticism of secular mindfulness, it is important to note that Purser and Loy do not offer any evidence to support their statements.

Tristan Harris, a former product philosopher at Google and co-founder of the advocacy group, Time Well Spent, also alludes to the hypocrisy of companies in Silicon Valley that provide mindfulness training and meditation spaces to their employees while continuing to develop devices that hijack users' attention by applying psychology of behavior change and persuasion (Bosker, 2016). Clearly, there are increasingly growing concerns from all sectors related to mindfulness training in corporations and its ethical considerations.

As a mindfulness instructor in corporate environments, my colleagues and I encounter some of these ethical concerns and challenges. Taking these ancient practices into secular contexts for the purpose of improving the health and well-being of people, as the MBSR program as well as many other MBIs are designed to do, is consistent with Buddha's use of skillful means to effectively communicate with different audiences (Marx, 2015; Monteiro et al., 2015). According to the Buddhist notion of *upaya* (skillful means), different methods of teaching can be adopted to cater to the different aptitudes and capacities of the audience (Marx, 2015; Monteiro et al., 2015). As such, offering mindfulness in a secular format to ease the suffering of people who may not be open to learning mindfulness if taught as a Buddhist practice is consistent with the Buddhist intention of transforming suffering. However, as we extend these teachings into business contexts, specifically to enhance performance and profitability, we must address the ethical concerns.

Below, I discuss two specific paradoxes of teaching mindfulness in business and explore solutions to maximize the transformative potential of mindfulness for the practitioners while minimizing the possibilities of misuse. These paradoxes are viewed through the lenses of the Buddha's teachings, mindfulness research, business research, and the experience of corporate mindfulness instructors. I propose a framework to explore the efficacy and ethical considerations of teaching mindfulness in business in the hope of providing new perspectives on this very important work.

The Paradoxes

Paradox One: Mindfulness Programs Seek to Reduce Stress at Work Without Changing Work Conditions That Cause Stress

Many businesses are offering mindfulness training at work to reduce stress and build resilience in employees without doing anything about the causes of stress at work. This is a major criticism articulated by Purser and Loy (2013): "Stress is framed as a personal problem, and mindfulness is offered as just the right medicine to help employees work more efficiently and calmly within toxic environments." In other words, without changing the root causes of stress at work, such as long working hours, bad working conditions, and unrealistic goals, businesses are *shifting the responsibility to the workers* to do something about their stress rather than taking responsibility to make deeper changes that promote a healthy work culture. For critics like Purser and Ng (2015), the solution is to change workplaces, and not the employees working there.

Before we explore the role that mindfulness can play in stress reduction at work, let us understand the nature of stress, its prevalence in workplaces, and existing stress-management interventions.

Understanding Stress at Work Few would contest the ubiquitous and debilitating nature of stress (Crum, Salovey, & Achor, 2013). In 2015, Goh, Pfeffer, and Zenios (2015) estimated that 120,000 deaths and 5–8% of annual healthcare costs are associated with management-induced workplace stress. The authors identify ten workplace stressors:

1. Layoffs and unemployment
2. Lack of health insurance

3. Shift work
4. Long working hours
5. Job insecurity
6. Work-family conflict
7. Low job control
8. High job demands
9. Low social support at work
10. Low organizational justice

Critics of secular mindfulness would argue that offering mindfulness as another wellness program without addressing the intrinsic stressors is not going to reduce stress and stress-related problems (Purser & Loy, 2013; Purser & Ng, 2015).

Despite the negative press stress has received, not all stress is bad. From an evolutionary perspective, Crum et al. (2013) explain that adversity can improve physiological and mental functioning to meet the demands and ensure survival. This "good" stress, known as eustress, is beneficial to the person experiencing it and associated with hope, meaning, and vigor (Nelson & Cooper, 2005). Historically, stress researchers focused on the amount—frequency, intensity, and duration—of the external stressor to determine whether stress will be experienced as distress or eustress (Crum et al., 2013). More recently, stress researchers have reported that perception of stress, not the stressor itself, impacts people's health and well-being (Fevre, Kolt, & Matheny, 2006). Variables such as stress mindsets (Crum et al., 2013) and stress hardiness (Kobasa, Maddi, & Kahn, 1982) also influence stress response and outcomes such as health and performance. For example, in a longitudinal study with middle- and upper-managers at a major utility company, Kobasa et al. (1982) found that hardiness, a personality disposition, mitigates the debilitating effects of stressful life events. In a 12-year longitudinal study at Illinois Bell, Maddi (2012) reports that managers who rated higher in hardiness attitude—challenge, commitment, and control—had better performance and health after the disruptive deregulation of their industry. Similarly, Crum et al. (2013) report that people with a "stress-is-enhancing" mindset believe that stress enhances their performance, productivity, health and well-being, and learning and growth, or they can have "stress-as-debilitating" mindset. People's stress mindset influences the extent to which stress is psychologically experienced and behaviorally approached (Crum et al. 2013).

In the context of stress, it is also important to highlight a phenomenon referred to as stress-related growth, in which people fundamentally change for the better as a result of stressful experiences (Crum et al., 2013; Park, Lawrence, & Murch, 1996). Even though people experience distress as a result of stressful events, which has been the focus of much research, contemporary theorists are studying the positive outcomes of surviving difficulty, including the acquisition of wisdom, empathy, meaning, and improved problem-solving abilities (Park et al., 1996).

Stress Management Interventions at Work   The "father of stress," Hans Selye's statement that "stress is an unavoidable consequence of life" (Richardson & Rothstein, 2008) resembles the Buddha's first Noble Truth that life contains unavoidable suffering. Given the inevitability of stress as a part of life, including work, many organizations have adopted stress management trainings to reduce the stress levels experienced by their employees. Broadly, the stress management interventions (SMIs) may be classified as primary when they are focused at the organizational level to alter the source of stress at work and secondary when they are focused at individual employees to train them in managing and coping with stress (Richardson & Rothstein, 2008). Examples of primary preventions include redesigning jobs, processes, workers' decision-making authority, and organizational structures to deal with the sources of stress in the workplace (Fevre et al., 2006). Primary approaches may also attempt to modify organizational culture and tend to be long-term efforts.

Secondary preventions can be divided into three main types: somatic, including relaxation methods such as progressive relaxation and biofeedback (focusing on physiology); cognitive, including mindfulness techniques, techniques to enhance emotional intelligence, and cognitive reappraisal of stress (focusing on individuals' appraisal of and response to stressors); and multimodal, combining somatic and cognitive training benefits to modify both physiological and psychological responses (Fevre et al., 2006).

Primary interventions may be preferable because they proactively alleviate the sources of stress (Fevre et al., 2006). As noted earlier, secondary interventions have been criticized for placing the onus for managing stress on employees and absolving management from their responsibility. There is also a moral appeal that primary interventions should be management's first choice for stress management at work (Fevre et al., 2006). However, there is little empirical evidence to support the efficacy of primary interventions (Fevre et al., 2006; Richardson & Rothstein, 2008). In fact, recent meta-analyses suggest that secondary interventions were more effective than primary interventions and that cognitive techniques were more effective than somatic interventions involving relaxation (Fevre et al., 2006; Richardson & Rothstein, 2008).

A common error made by many people is equating mindfulness, which includes cognitive training, with relaxation, which is a somatic intervention. It is important to note the difference in focus in the two interventions, which may also explain the effectiveness of cognitive techniques over somatic ones. While relaxation aims to refocus attention away from the source of stress and reduce tension in the body by "letting go," cognitive techniques such as mindfulness, invite individuals to confront the dysfunctional thoughts, emotions, and behaviors as they pertain to stress, and to choose more adaptive perceptions and responses (Fevre et al., 2006; Richardson & Rothstein, 2008).

Since stress can be positive (eustress) or negative (distress) and there is insufficient evidence showing primary SMIs to be better than secondary SMIs, we need a more nuanced approach to designing stress management interventions that recognizes the potential of stress to either debilitate or enhance health and performance (Crum et al., 2013; Fevre et al., 2006). A framework to explore this paradox with suggestions is offered later in the chapter.

Paradox Two: Mindfulness Is Grounded in Ethics But Applied in Business Without Ethical Considerations

Traditional Buddhist texts discern between wrong mindfulness and right mindfulness. Right mindfulness combines a "web of factors that give it direction and purpose" (Bodhi p. 31). These go beyond the usual instructions given in secular programs, which focus on awareness of body, feelings, and the mind. The Sattipatthana Sutta (Anālayo, 2004), the Buddha's discourse on the systematic approach to practicing mindfulness (on which most secular programs are based) provides very clear guidance for contemplating the four foundations of mindfulness—body, feelings, mind, and dhammas, which refers to all phenomena of the mind in Pali (the language used for earliest Buddhist teachings).

While most secular programs more directly address mindfulness of body, feelings, and mind, mindfulness of dhammas, which includes contemplation on the ethical and wisdom factors, is barely addressed. The dhammas include contemplation of five hindrances, five aggregates of clinging, six senses, seven factors of awakening, and the four Noble Truths (Goldstein, 2016). The four foundations of mindfulness are depicted in Fig. 14.1. The importance of ethical conduct and wisdom is repeated in the mindfulness of dhammas. More specifically, the fourth Noble Truth lays out the importance of cultivating the mind, wisdom, and ethics as an Eightfold Path to the cessation of suffering. Within the Eightfold Path, mindfulness, along with right concentration and right effort, comprises the domain of mental or meditative development (samadhi). Two other domains are equally important in the Eightfold Path: the wisdom domain (panna) comprising right view and right intention, and the ethical domain (sila) comprising right speech, right action, and right livelihood. A behavior is "right" or "skillful" when it leads to the cessation of suffering by eliminating its roots in three psychological motivations: greed, hatred, and delusion (Monteiro et al., 2015).

Corporate mindfulness, however, is taught in a secular and ethically neutral way and wisdom and ethical conduct, which form such an important foundation of mindfulness in the original teachings, are often missing. As we have already noted, this "McMindfulness" decontextualizes mindfulness from its roots in wisdom and ethical conduct; many commentaries have described the benefits and limitations of secular mindfulness (for example, Marx, 2015; Monteiro et al., 2015; Purser and Mililo, 2015). These commentaries raise important concerns about the purpose, consequences, and efficacy of mindfulness in the absence of ethical considerations. We will focus on three implications of applying mindfulness in business in the absence of ethics and wisdom—the myopic use of mindfulness to benefit business interests, emphasis on acceptance in the absence of wisdom and ethical foundations, and the efficacy of mindfulness in the absence of wisdom and ethical foundations.

Myopic Use of Mindfulness to Benefit the Business A major criticism of teaching mindfulness in the absence of ethical considerations is the application of mindfulness in business to promote the profitability of the business while ignoring the

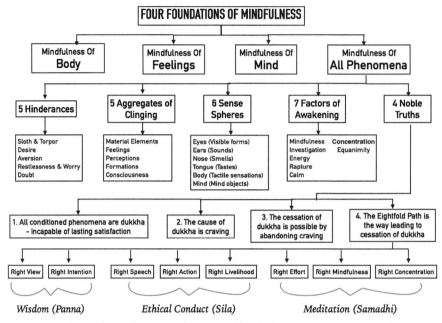

Fig. 14.1 The four foundations of mindfulness

well-being of other stakeholders (Purser and Milillo, 2015). When mindfulness programs narrowly develop skills such as focus and stress-management to improve productivity, employees might experience temporary respite but do not learn to deal with the root causes of suffering—greed, aversion, and delusion. Without cultivating an inquiry into what is wholesome and not wholesome, they may continue to perpetuate suffering for themselves and others.

The inclusion of explicit ethics in Mindfulness-Based Stress Reduction (MBSR), a foundational program on which other secular programs are based, is explained by Kabat-Zinn (2011) as unnecessary because of the presence of an explicit professional code of conduct in the Hippocratic tradition within the context of medicine and healthcare (where MBSR originated). The medical principle of "*primum non nocere*, to first do no harm, and to put the needs of the patient above one's own" is consistent with the ethical foundations of mindfulness and can serve to guide mindfulness teachers within the medical field (Kabat-Zinn, 2011, p. 294).

However, the absence of explicit ethics in mindfulness becomes problematic when it is introduced in professions like business that do not have uniform ethical guidelines and are culturally predisposed to unethical behaviors. Anyone can start a business. Often the founder's values determine the corporate culture and employees' ethical conduct. Even if businesses join professional organizations such as the American Marketing Association that prescribes a code of ethics, the document is "sufficiently vague to allow other interpretations" (Chonko & Hunt, 1985, p. 350).

The existing paradigm on which most business is founded—maximizing shareholder value—also contributes to a corporate culture that can put the interests of the company before those of consumers, environment, and other stakeholders. Ernst and Young's 14th *Global Fraud Survey* (EY, 2016), based on 2800 senior executives in 62 countries, reveals that almost half the executives justify unethical behavior to meet financial targets. Aggressive sales cultures manifest in corporate scandals like Wells Fargo's firing of 5300 employees over phony accounts that employees explained were the result of unrealistic sales quotas. Former Wells Fargo employees discuss "the dichotomy between their ethics training—where they were formally told not to do anything inappropriate—and on-the-job reality of a relentless push to meet sales goals that many considered unrealistic" (Corkery & Cowley, 2016).

Questionable ethics in business professions can also be traced to education. Business students have been known to top cheater's lists. Finance students, in particular, score the highest on traits such as narcissism and materialism, and lowest on empathy, a profile that is related to unethical decision making (Lampe & Lampe, 2012). There is a growing movement that started at Harvard Business School and has spread to other business schools to take an MBA Oath that creates professional accountability within business, just as the Hippocrates oath promotes accountability in the medical profession (Anderson, 2009).

While we are seeing positive trends toward more responsible business, it still remains culturally pre-disposed to ethical transgressions. The absence of an ethical framework leaves corporate mindfulness programs open to myopically serving a narrow group of people with the purpose of maximizing profitability without consideration of other stakeholders. Silicon Valley is often criticized for using mindfulness to narrowly benefit the employees and the businesses (Healey, 2013). A myopic application of mindfulness is creating "'integrity bubbles' that allow employees to reap the benefits of mindfulness while externalizing the problems of fragmentation and distraction" (Healey, 2013). Tristan Harris, a former product philosopher at Google, draws attention to companies like Google, Apple, and Facebook, which are seen as corporate leaders in the mindfulness movement but continue to engineer products that "hijack" users' attention with little consideration of the consequences of their addictive products on their customers (Bosker, 2016).

The lack of an explicit ethical framework in the application of corporate mindfulness can perpetuate institutional blindness and structural inequities that are antithetical to the original purpose of mindfulness to alleviate suffering in oneself and others (Purser & Milillo, 2015). "Such myopia illustrates what can occur when mindfulness training is extracted from a contextual, interdependent, and complex whole" (Purser & Milillo, 2015, p. 15).

While there are good reasons to include ethical foundations in corporate mindfulness programs, there is little research to date on how existing secular programs are impacting ethical behaviors in those businesses. However, early results show that even secular mindfulness programs increase compassionate behavior (Condon, Desbordes, Miller, & DeSteno, 2013), empathy (Shure et al., 2008), and moral reasoning and ethical decision-making (Shapiro et al., 2012).

Researchers (for example, Lampe & Lampe, 2012) are promoting mindfulness as an approach to teaching business ethics because of its potential to develop students' skills such as awareness, self-knowledge, and insight that are needed for ethical decisions. Hoyk and Hersey (2010) describe 45 psychological traps in their book, *The Ethical Executive*, including schemas, biases, and conflicts of interest that lead executives to believe that their unethical decisions are justified. Lampe and Lampe (2012) believe that a Mindfulness-Based Business Ethics Education can teach students the skills to facilitate introspection and a better understanding of their self-deceptive cognitive processes, which are essential for their ethical development. More research is needed to learn how mindfulness can be effectively used to train business professionals in ethical decision-making. Meanwhile, it can be argued that corporate programs, such as Search Inside Yourself, are appropriately applied in organizations because they include compassion practices like loving kindness and cognitive training. These practices can help employees see things from others' perspectives even in the midst of challenging situations, and empower them to take the most skillful actions that benefit all involved. Even in the absence of explicit ethics training, such programs can create safe spaces for people to pause, reflect, and reconnect with their natural empathy.

A skillful combination of scientific evidence, a business case, and experiential learning can be very effective in helping participants learn more skillful ways of dealing with their triggers instead of their default modes of reactivity. The reflections that I have heard people share in corporate mindfulness programs, even after just a short guided-meditation and reflection on making difficult decisions or dealing with triggers, are very promising. As examples, participants shared these observations: "I was embarrassed to see my reaction to the (complaining) client, and if I had paused in that situation, my response would have been very different"; "In pausing I noticed that I am very compassionate towards others but not to myself. I need to pay more attention to me"; "In stopping and seeing things from others' perspectives, I could see the suffering of the other person and what they must be going through. That shifted how I am going to deal with the situation"; "I noticed that my external response was ok but my internal response was unhealthy." Such insights reflecting compassion toward self and others are common in secular mindfulness programs. Even for participants who do not experience compassion, the experience is valuable because it gives them an opportunity to observe their busy minds and reactive hooks, very often for the first time. With careful designing of programs and an understanding of the corporate culture, it is possible to help corporate participants explore compassion toward self and others, even in the absence of direct reference to ethical foundations.

However, there is no existing research that looks at how the shifts experienced by participants in secular programs influence their ongoing ethical dilemmas and actions. Thus, it is hard to say how effective these programs are in shifting people's orientation toward a more ethical orientation that considers the well-being of all stakeholders. The situation for mindfulness teachers is further complicated when they are invited to teach mindfulness in organizations that have been directly criticized for their negative impacts on communities and environments. For example,

Mirabai Bush, one of the pioneering advocates for corporate mindfulness, shares her struggle with the decision to teach mindfulness at Monsanto. Bush's work in the past had involved recovering lands in Guatemala where Monsanto's products had contributed to the land destruction and poverty of the inhabitants (Tworkov, 2001). However, we can all learn from her experience of the judgments that come up in working with different clients and the possibility of letting those be to create spaces for transformation, as was her experience (Tworkov, 2001). Instead of applying a dogmatic approach that blatantly refuses to work with unethical clients, which is counter to mindfulness, each case may need to be considered with fresh eyes. What if mindfulness, even when brought in only for stress reduction, can create a non-judgmental space for people to wake up to their own suffering and how they are creating it for others? What if the employees of the "evil" company are blind to the consequences of their actions, and in their stopping they have a chance to notice that? What if the participants are exposed to other ways of doing business that are compassionate and profitable? What if enough employees in a company wake up to the effects their products are having on their suppliers and customers to make a shift?

No doubt, the main reason mindfulness teachers are invited to organizations is primarily to develop a narrow range of skills, such as stress-management, emotional intelligence, resilience, focus, and creativity to enhance productivity. However, the experience of mindfulness teachers in corporate settings is hopeful because of the complex ways the mindfulness path and practices work. Even though we may not be invited to expand participants' awareness to the consequences of their actions to all stakeholders, a skillful teacher can create space for participants to stop and notice the workings of their minds and their shared humanity, and that can be the start of a transformative experience for someone who has never ventured into a Buddhist retreat. Mirabai Bush eloquently shares her experience of the transformative potential, "Once a person is given a way to explore the inner life, there is no predicting what he or she will find. After a session at Google, one young engineer said: 'Cool. I just defragged my hard-drive!' But another said: 'I saw that all of life was interconnected, not just by the Internet but by something more mysterious'" (Bush, 2015).

To consistently create more of these opportunities for insight and transformation, more work can be done with respect to teachers' own deepening of the practices and the corporate mindfulness curricula, which is discussed in the next section. Meanwhile, these words of the Buddha offer guidance, "The Tathagata has no closed fist of a teacher with respect to the teachings." Bodhi (2011, p. 36) interprets this to mean, "that we can let anyone take from the Dhamma whatever they find useful even if it is for secular purposes."

Emphasis on Acceptance in the Absence of Wisdom and Ethics Secular mindfulness emphasizes the cultivation of attitudes such as acceptance, non-judgment, and self-compassion, which are helpful for working with a self-critical mind (Marx, 2015; Purser & Milillo, 2015). Non-judgment means recognizing the judgments and opinions arising in each moment and having the choice to not act on them or get hooked by them (Kabat-Zinn, 2011). Practicing mindfulness as "non-judgmental awareness" of present-moment experiences develops the capacity in people to quiet the mind and be with their experience without reacting in habitual ways. However, an emphasis on "acceptance of what is" and self-compassion must be balanced with appropriate ethical considerations, discipline, and understanding of the root causes of suffering. Otherwise, practitioners might find themselves ill-equipped to deal with discomfort and unwholesome mental states (Marx, 2015).

The instructions in secular mindfulness programs "to be with whatever is arising" or simply "be with the breath" may be at odds with Buddhist teaching that not all mind states are equal, and to be vigilant to ensure that the mind cultivates wholesome states and is not overtaken by unwholesome states (Marx, 2015). For example, I often hear participants in my mindfulness classes use self-compassion as a reason for not doing the home practices. Self-compassion when not balanced by right intention and understanding (wisdom) and right effort (ethical behavior) can perpetuate the tendency to avoid the discomfort of stabilizing a restless mind. Similarly, sloth and torpor, hindrances to mindfulness can come disguised as self-compassion (Goldstein, 2016). When experiencing a challenging situation or emotion, instead of approaching it with mindfulness, sloth, and torpor may come in with a kind suggestion to take a nap or allow us to fall asleep during meditation as acts of self-care. In the absence of cultivating right understanding of how these unwholesome states perpetuate suffering, secular mindfulness can promote conditions to support unwholesome behaviors. In the absence of wisdom and ethical consideration, self-compassion and acceptance of what is can help perpetuate corporate ideologies that justify unskillful means to achieve the bottom line.

Efficacy of Mindfulness in the Absence of Wisdom and Ethical Foundations In the foundations of mindfulness (see Fig. 14.1), mindfulness is one of the steps on the Eightfold Path and is supported by ethical conduct and wisdom. If mindfulness is not yet strong enough to deal with unwholesome states of mind, wise reflection and a strong ethical foundation can strengthen its hold against those unwholesome states (Goldstein, 2016). Ethical conduct involves investigation of actions, speech, and livelihood that abstain from doing harm to self and others and those that do good. Wisdom involves an understanding of what is wholesome and unwholesome and includes all the intentions and aspirations that lead to wholesome actions. Goldstein (2016), a Buddhist scholar and co-founder of Insight Meditation Center in Barre, explains that a concentrated and collected mind (samadhi) is based on skillful behavior (sila). Without this basis in non-harming, the mind will continue to be agitated by worry, guilt, and regret. We have all engaged in unskillful acts in the past. Instead of forgetting or suppressing unwholesome emotions related to our past actions, we can learn to see with wisdom and draw strength from our commitment to non-harming.

Since the Buddha's teachings are not meant to be dogmas nor accepted blindly, the invitation even with ethical conduct is to reflect on how we feel when we act skillfully and when we do not. The invitation is always to verify the teachings with our immediate experience of reality and whether they contribute to our well-being.

When we can see with clarity that the nature of the mind is to wander and a wavering mind causes dissatisfaction, this kind of wise reflection can provide the right motivation to continue with our practices. In the absence of this training to discern skillful from unskillful, practitioners can be overtaken by their wavering minds and difficult emotions. Similar to the ethical foundation, wisdom, comprising right view and right intentions, is also a vital aspect of mindfulness. Without attending to the direct experience of the unsatisfying, unreliable, and sometimes stressful nature of experience, participants coming to mindfulness programs with the expectations of finding happiness may continue to strive for experiences that feel pleasant. Without a proper understanding of the true nature of experiences, participants may continue to look for peace and a concentrated mind in experiences that are the cause of suffering and distraction.

Shantideva, an ancient Buddhist monk, noted, "We who are like senseless children shrink from suffering but love its causes" (Goldstein, 2016). Secular classes seldom provide an understanding of the first Noble Truth that all conditioned phenomena are dukkha—incapable of giving lasting satisfaction. Secular classes may indirectly allude to this truth by pointing to the impermanence of pleasant and unpleasant events. However, in the absence of directly contemplating on the first Noble Truth, participants are likely to stay stuck in their desire for specific states that feel pleasant. Within organizations too, participants may find temporary release, which comes with the physiological outcomes of bringing attention to the body and breath. But in the absence of cultivating skillful behaviors and right understanding, participants may not be able to reap the transformative benefits of mindfulness and instead never move beyond seeing mindfulness as another form of relaxation. To encourage the path of transformation, the inclusion of ethical and wisdom considerations in designing and teaching mindfulness programs is important and I discuss this below.

Mindful Inquiry of Circles of Influence

A Pragmatic Framework for Corporate Mindfulness

This section utilizes mindful inquiry to address the challenges of teaching corporate mindfulness. Inquiry is a contemplative approach to questioning that is utilized in secular mindfulness programs (Crane, 2009; McCown, Riebel, and Micozzi, 2010). The lens of mindful inquiry is expanded to include not only mindful awareness but also wisdom and ethical considerations. Mindfulness instructors can utilize this expanded framework as a pragmatic approach to navigate corporate mindfulness, without compromising the integrity and efficacy of their programs.

More specifically, mindfulness instructors can systematically direct mindful inquiry to three broad spheres over which they have influence—their personal development, interactions with different groups of people, and processes involved

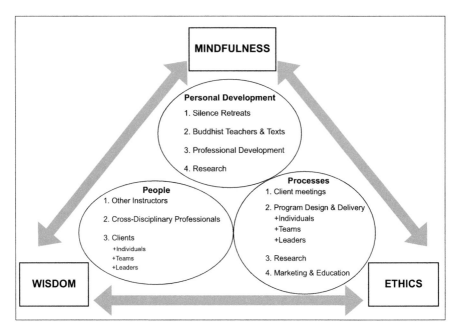

Fig. 14.2 Mindful inquiry of circles of influence for mindfulness instructors

in bringing mindfulness into corporations. The three P's—personal development, people, and processes—can collectively be called circles of influence. As noted earlier, corporate mindfulness has been criticized for its myopic application of mindfulness. Mindful inquiry of "circles of influence" offers a systematic approach for not only instructors, but also organizations and participants, to examine the ripple effects of integrating mindfulness in different domains of activity.

Figure 14.2 depicts the circles of influence for instructors with respect to their personal development, people they interact with, and processes they are involved in to bring mindfulness to organizations. Actions within each of the circles of influence are examined using the process of mindful inquiry. Table 14.1 provides suggestions for applying the lens of mindful inquiry to the circles of influence. Even though the following discussion is primarily exploring solutions from the perspective of mindfulness instructors, organizations can also be invited to examine their circles of influence using mindful inquiry, which is briefly discussed under program design and delivery.

Personal Development The first circle of influence over which mindfulness instructors have control is their own personal development. The responsibility to ensure the "integrity, quality, and standards of practice" of a mindfulness program lies with the mindfulness instructor (Kabat-Zinn, 2011). This responsibility comes not as a burden but is an intention that mindfulness instructors are willing to commit to because of their love for this work and the transformation they have experienced through continued practice. The invitation to mindfulness instructors is to continue

Table 14.1 Circles of influence and mindful inquiry

Circles of Influence: 3 P's	MINDFUL INQUIRY		
	Wisdom Right intentions & understanding	Ethics Right actions, livelihood & speech	Meditation Right effort, mindfulness, concentration
Personal Development	- Deepen understanding of Buddhist teachings - Understand what is wholesome & unwholesome - Contemplate 4 Noble Truth - Examine intentions and align with aspirations for well-being of all - Cultivate wise restrain, loving kindness & compassion	- Examine skillful & unskillful actions - Cultivate strength of mind to abstain from causing harm to self & others - No separation between work and practice - Cultivating attitude of service - Examine complacency in choices: understanding Buddhist psychology & other research - Practice right speech.	- Apply energy to maintain wholesome states & abandon unwholesome states - Maintain regular practice to train mind to be present, open, and quiet - Attend regular retreats - Cultivate steadiness of mind for clarity of 3 characteristics: impermanence, unsatisfactoriness, selflessness
People	- Examine intentions in interactions with other secular and Buddhist instructors, professionals, & clients - Understanding and accepting clients where they are - Exploring what it means to make no distinction between human beings in context of clients - Cultivating loving-kindness & compassion for all clients	- Maintain right speech in all interactions - Noticing emotional tone in mind and heart when speaking - Mindful listening with open mind & heart - Mindful dialog with secular & Buddhist teachers and professionals - Skillful collaborations with other instructors, professionals & researchers - Guided by genuine desire to help clients - Acting with integrity at all times	- Being established in the practices of meditation to show up with wisdom and integrity in all interactions - Apply energy during clients' meetings to arouse wholesome states such as calm, compassion, & equanimity - Apply energy during clients' meetings to abandon unwholesome states such as restlessness, worry, doubt, desires, & aversions.
Processes	- Investigate needs of clients and design program that is conducive to well-being of all involved - Examine if states of greed, aversion, and delusion arise in marketing and working with clients and collaborators - Cultivate wise restraint to grow in concentration and confidence as mindfulness teachers - Cultivate strong wish to alleviate suffering of all beings	- Using skillful methods to design & deliver programs to address challenges of clients - Using skillful means like research and language to help clients see interconnected nature of reality & seek solutions that benefits all stakeholders - Including contemplation of root causes of stress and challenges in order to arrive at skillful means to deal with them - Creating safe spaces for participants to contemplate consequences of their actions on their circles of influence. - Skillful ways to incorporate mindfulness of dhammas in corporate programs - Contemplation on right speech and actions in marketing	- Finding right balance of different practices to cultivate mindfulness and concentration - Helping leadership cultivate calm and collected minds to see interconnectedness of all beings and seek skillful solutions - Developing mindfulness in participants to choose attitudes and actions that are most skillful within each situation - Helping participants learn to integrate mindfulness in daily life - Cultivating right effort in participants to arouse energy for wholesome mindset in all their activities

to integrate mindfulness practices in daily life so that there is no separation between one's practice and one's life (Kabat-Zinn, 2011). However, this integration does not happen automatically and is dependent upon the continued efforts of instructors to deepen their practice and personal development.

All reputable training centers in secular mindfulness such as the Center for Mindfulness in Medicine, Health Care, and Society; and the Search Inside Yourself Leadership Institute have a rigorous application process that requires all participants to have a regular mindfulness practice in conjunction with extended silent retreats to deepen their practice. As any mindfulness instructor would know from personal experience, these requirements do not end with completing the professional development training, but are an ongoing commitment. In the absence of regular silent retreats and daily practice, it is easy for the mind to revert to habitual patterns that seek comfort and avoid discomfort. The silent retreats are intended to help to weaken causes of suffering rooted in desire, aversion, and greed so instructors can embody more fully what they aspire to teach in their programs.

Mindful inquiry as it pertains to right actions involves an examination of skillful and unskillful actions. This inquiry includes investigating ways in which we are complacent about the choices we make (Goldstein, 2016). Mindfulness instructors cannot become complacent about their practice and understanding of Buddhist psychology. As important as internal awareness is for the mindfulness instructor, they need to stay in touch with external awareness such as latest mindfulness research in neuroscience, psychology, and other professional domains. Even as secular instructors it is advisable, if not indispensable, to have a strong grounding in original Buddhist teachings on mindfulness (Kabat-Zinn, 2011). For example, Joseph Goldstein's *Mindfulness: A Practical Guide To Awakening* (2013) clearly explains the Satipatthana Sutta, the Buddha's discourse on the four foundations of mindfulness. This is the foundational sutta not only for MBSR, but also for many other MBI's. It is one of the many sources accessible to secular teachers who do not have extensive training in Buddhist teachings. It is equally important for mindfulness instructors to stay in touch with the latest research related to mindfulness in peer-reviewed journals so they develop a language and understanding to speak with organizational clients in ways that are relevant to them. This work of continued personal development across different domains involving mindfulness can be hard, if not impossible, in the absence of a community of people that can give and get support, which is explored next.

People

Colleagues The next circle of influence within which mindfulness instructors have impact is people including other mindfulness instructors, cross-disciplinary professionals, and organizational clients. In working with corporate clients, mindfulness instructors can face challenges involving ethics and/or efficacy. Since it is unrealistic for instructors to have a depth of understanding and experience in the broad range of knowledge that includes Buddhist psychology, secular mindfulness, and the diverse professional domains within which they are teaching, it is advisable for instructors to interact with other professionals with diverse experiences and backgrounds in formal and informal ways.

In light of some of the nuances and ethical issues involved in teaching mindfulness in corporate environments, it would be beneficial for secular mindfulness instructors to have dialogue with Buddhist teachers as well as researchers studying mindfulness in contexts relevant to corporations. There is no one program or approach that is best for all clients. We need more opportunities for open dialogue between Buddhist scholars and corporate mindfulness instructors in order to challenge and clarify the mindfulness concepts and applications in secular contexts (Monteiro et al., 2015). With mindful inquiry, Buddhist scholars can gain a better understanding of organizational contexts and challenges and corporate instructors can deepen their understanding of the dharma. These interactions can take many forms. Some of the interactions can be informal like those between cohort members of professional mindfulness training or mindfulness instructors coming together in a geographic region to discuss the ethical considerations coming up for them. Other interactions can be given a more formal structure. For example, conferences can be organized around issues related to ethics in corporate mindfulness such as the Academy for Contemplative and Ethical Leadership organized by the Mind and Life Institute in 2015.

Another way to formalize these interactions is by collaborating with domain experts on specific projects or with the experts within the clients' organization. For example, I have a marketing background and do not need as much external help in creating mindfulness programs for sales and marketing professionals. However, when the corporate program involves team assessments and organizational change, I collaborate with mindfulness practitioners who have expertise in these areas. A notable example of such a collaboration is between The Dalai Lama, a Buddhist teacher and spiritual leader, and Laurens van den Muyzenberg, a management consultant. Their book, *The Leader's Way, The Art of Making the Right Decisions in Our Careers, Our Companies, and the World at Large* (Lama & Muyzenberg, 2009), integrates Buddhist teachings on mindfulness, wisdom, and ethics in dealing with leadership dilemmas. The authors skillfully apply Buddhist principles of right view and right action in combination with three aspects of reality—impermanence, interdependence, and dependent origination—to decision-making. The Buddha's teachings provide a framework to find happiness by eliminating the root causes of suffering. And because businesses cannot survive without happy employees, customers, and shareholders, the insight and practices provided by Buddha can be applied in corporate contexts to ease suffering, albeit using language and examples relevant to businesses. This book exemplifies how Buddhist ethics and practices can provide a pragmatic framework for decision makers to help them see the consequences of their decisions on all stakeholders so they can take skillful actions to ensure the well-being of all who are impacted by the decisions. It also builds credibility for incorporating an ethical and holistic approach promoted in Buddhist teachings of mindfulness by pointing out that the Buddhist concepts of impermanence and interdependence are also the basis for systems thinking in the West. Here we see a helpful coming together of Buddhist teachings with management theory made possible by collaboration between people with diverse backgrounds.

I also want to highlight the need for corporate mindfulness instructors to collaborate with researchers to explore the benefits of the different aspects of mindfulness for different corporate audiences and contexts. Much of the existing research is based on the MBSR program that involves meditations of 40 min. Corporate audiences are typically taught much shorter meditations, often because of the limited time available to them. It would be helpful to see the efficacy of the shorter meditations, with and without apps, using rigorous research methods. Being a highly experiential program with many benefits accruing in the long run, we may need to design longitudinal studies involving mixed methods—qualitative and quantitative.

Clients Another essential group of people within mindfulness instructors' circles of influence is clients. Mindfulness instructors have a direct impact on clients not only through the delivery of programs but also through other interactions with them. It is expected that mindfulness instructors embody the work they are teaching their clients. However, it is very easy in the absence of continual reminding, to be swayed by judgments of the client, aspirations of impressing the client, and other distractions. Bringing wise attention to unwholesome thoughts and habitual tendencies can support instructors in being fully present with an open mind and heart. It can be very useful before every client interaction to take a few minutes to notice what is arising. This creates the space to realign one's intention to alleviate suffering in the people one interacts with.

Being established in the practices of wisdom, ethical conduct, and concentration trains corporate instructors to show up with confidence and humility, with compassion and a non-wavering mind, with knowledge and the ability to let go of what is known in favor of what is most alive and necessary to address in the present moment. This is not meant to create an ideal that creates striving. There will be times when things do not go as expected when we are most likely to resort to our habitual ways of dealing with discomfort. However, the more we ground ourselves in the practices of wisdom, ethical conduct, and mindfulness in our daily lives, the easier it will be for us to recognize and accept our default behaviors so we may choose the more skillful options. Challenging situations are perfect opportunities for instructors to demonstrate what it means to act with integrity, authenticity, and transparency in difficulty. It is here that corporate participants can be exposed to alternative models of working that are based on a calm and collected mind that provides clarity, courage, and compassion to take right action that supports the well-being of all involved.

The other aspect of interactions with clients that is relevant to our discussion is meeting clients where they are. As pointed out earlier, the question of working with clients with an unethical reputation deserves a non-judgmental assessment that will differ from case to case. However, it is essential for instructors to remain open, curious, and equanimous in their discussions with clients so we avoid falling on either extremes of the spectrum, from refusing to work without any consideration to agreeing to work for the wrong reasons and wrong here would include situations where the mindfulness program is knowingly being used in deceitful ways to pacify employees as described by Purser and Milillo (2015). The other consideration in working with clients with different backgrounds and responsibilities is to be sensitive to their needs and use language and practices that honor their unique challenges and concerns. It is said that the Buddha used 84,000 methods that were tailored for people with different capacities and aptitudes (Marx, 2015).

Processes This category includes mindful inquiry of the wide spectrum of activities that instructors engage in. Processes include work-related activities such as client-specific work, which includes meetings, designing and delivery of programs, and post-program actions to support the ongoing work of cultivating mindfulness in organizations as well as the ongoing work of research, marketing, and education. Suggestions are offered within each category to address some of the concerns raised within the paradoxes discussed above with respect to addressing root causes of stress and the ethical aspects of mindfulness.

Client Meetings This is the most critical step upon which rests the program design and delivery. Most clients have some preliminary ideas of what they want based on what they have experienced personally or read about. Listening to clients and asking questions to learn about the participants is important so that programming solutions are offered that address the systemic issues perpetuating the challenges. For example, a private preschool whose CEO had attended a popular mindfulness program that I am trained in wanted me to offer that program to its teachers at their annual retreat attended by 500 teachers. Upon exploring the demographics and challenges of the teachers with the management, it was clear that the program they wanted would not be most appropriate because of its emphasis on neuroscience and business applications. That focus would not be relevant to a group of teachers with varied educational backgrounds and facing challenges that were very specific to being teachers. Rooted in the foundations of mindfulness, corporate mindfulness instructors can listen with a calm and collected mind to offer mindfulness-based solutions that are best for the participants rather than a program that maximizes returns for the management or is being preferred by the client for the wrong reasons.

Given an opportunity, mindfulness instructors can share research to educate clients about the benefits of skillful and compassionate actions that consider all stakeholders. For example, the longitudinal study by Sisodia, Sheth, and Wolfe (2014) reveals that conscious businesses (who have a purpose beyond maximizing profitability and look to maximize well-being of all stakeholders and not just shareholders) featured in their research outperformed the S&P 500 by 14 times and Good to Great Companies by 6 times over a period of 15 years. Other market trends such as the shift in more than 50% of U.S. population from mindless to mindful consumption (Rider, 2016) are also opportunities for companies to incorporate a more responsible mindset that can be promoted in mindfulness programs. Tying latest research outcomes and market trends to Buddhist teachings of interdependence, cause and effect, and impermanence can help business leaders see how their actions impact their stakeholders with whom they coexist in their communities.

Design and Delivery of Programs Based on information received from the clients, the mindfulness instructor can make proposals for the right program to meet the particular audience characteristics and needs. As discussed earlier, primary interventions focusing on organizational change should be considered only if the organization has already tried secondary or employee-level interventions that have failed. In the case of organizational change, mindfulness instructors would be expected to have cross-disciplinary expertise to help design the change process and its implementation in collaboration with management. Examples of frameworks involving mindfulness in organizational change are Reinventing Organizations by management consultant, Laloux (2014) and Theory U by Otto Scharmer (2009) who is a Senior Lecturer at MIT and co-founder of the Presencing Institute. Adaptive leadership (Heifetz, Linsky, & Grashow, 2009) is another management theory that has a natural fit with mindfulness. Mindfulness can help leaders meet adaptive challenges by letting go of habitual patterns and engaging with uncertainty in new and sophisticated ways (Hunter and Chaskalson, 2013).

Similarly, mindfulness can provide a foundation to explore other disciplines in business like marketing (Bahl et al. 2016), finance, and operations. Bahl et al. (2016) explored the transformative potential of mindfulness on consumers, environment, and society within the marketing discipline. At the practical level, mindfulness instructors can collaborate to work with different functional teams in organizations. Team-level programs can be designed not only to improve the team performance but their collective wisdom and awareness of consequences on their circles of influence.

In designing employee-level interventions, due consideration should be given to unique causes of stress across different professions and organizations. For example, the main stressors for preschool teachers, financial advisers, and leaders are different. In the full-day retreat for preschool teachers, mindfulness-based practices and strategies for self-care and self-management were included to deal with teachers' physical and emotional burnout. The main cause of stress for financial advisers was the high rates of failure, common in that industry, which required emotional and cognitive resilience training. For the group of leaders that I worked with, managing uncertainty and constant change was the main source of stress for which the adaptive leadership framework (Heifetz et al., 2009) was useful.

As previously noted in the discussion on SMIs, cognitive trainings were found to be more impactful than relaxation trainings (Richardson and Rothstein, 2008). While we teach participants mindfulness-based practices for cultivating inner calm, for most participants it will also be helpful to provide cognitive training to shift their perception of stressors and work with stress in skillful ways. For example, Kobasa et al. (1982) highlight three dispositions essential to stress hardiness—commitment, control, and challenge. Each of these dispositions can be carefully nurtured with mindfulness. Employees can learn to shift their perspective to transform feelings of alienation into commitment, helplessness into hope that comes with control over what we can change, and threat into a challenge that pushes us to utilize our ingenuity and resources to figure out a solution. Similarly, many corporate programs utilize resilience frameworks offered by Seligman (2006) that can help people train in cognitive resilience.

The issue of myopic application of mindfulness can be addressed in program design and delivery by including exercises inviting participants to create their circles of influence and explore how the mindfulness skills learned can be applied in interactions with each group within their circles of influence. This exercise can be done individually and in groups. I have found that giving people time to work in groups to explore ways they are going to integrate mindfulness into their work and beyond to be a very useful and fun activity for them. Depending upon whether the instructor is working at the level of individuals, teams, or leadership, their circles of influence will look different and the impact they have on each is also different. For example, the focus for individual employees may be integrating mindfulness in their own lives and how they might be able to incorporate this work in their interactions with other people they work with as well as people outside the organization that they have contact with like suppliers and customers. In working with teams, there are more opportunities to formalize how mindfulness can be incorporated in teamwork and collectively how they can make their interactions with suppliers and clients more mindful. They can spend time creating a common vocabulary, processes, and spaces to support the deepening and integration of mindfulness skills they found useful to deal with their frequent and critical challenges of working as a team. It is important to highlight that individual emotional intelligence does not automatically translate into team emotional intelligence (Druskat & Wolff, 2001). Leaders' circles of influence extend to include other stakeholders like their community and environment. Leaders can benefit most from learning Buddhist concepts in the mindfulness of dhammas that speak to interdependence, impermanence, and causality to help broaden their lens used in strategic thinking and decision-making to consider all stakeholders and not just shareholders. Using existing research, market trends, and management frameworks there are ways to integrate mindfulness of dhammas into strategic planning and implementation in a pragmatic way. This of course depends on the teachers' personal development and grounding in the foundations of mindfulness as well as familiarity with management theory and frameworks. Such a meeting of Dharma and management creates many opportunities for collaborations like the one we saw manifest in the book, *The Leader's Way* (Lama & Muyzenberg, 2009).

The ethical and wisdom dimensions of mindfulness are essential not only for pragmatic reasons highlighted above but also to maximize the efficacy of mindfulness programs. For example, consider a mindfulness instructor who is hired by a manufacturing company to develop focus in its employees to minimize accidents caused by lack of concentration. The employees can be taught basic mindfulness practices such as "Awareness of Breath" and the "Body Scan." However, if the root causes of distraction are not addressed, simply teaching the meditations can be a hit or miss approach. In addition to the practices, if employees are invited to explore their challenges to stabilizing their minds, then solutions can be offered to deal with the root causes of distractions. A useful framework here could be contemplation of the five hindrances to mindfulness—desire, aversion, sloth and torpor, restlessness or worry, and doubt. By helping the employees learn to pay wise attention to the underlying energy and factors keeping them distracted, they can learn to skillfully address those challenges. If sloth and torpor is the main challenge to staying focused, then paying attention to their diet, sleep, physical activity, and working environments can offer solutions. If people are being laid off, which is causing worry and restlessness in employees, then the employees and management may have to work individually and collectively to address employees' anxiety that is leaving them distracted. Similar explorations of other hindrances can provide appropriate solutions that meditation alone cannot provide.

To address the pitfalls of focusing on attitudes that promote non-judgment, acceptance, and self-compassion, instructors can present other mindfulness attitudes to balance self-serving outcomes and complacency. For example, self-compassion can be balanced with curiosity for what are wholesome and unwholesome mind states. Further, inviting participants to contemplate on their circles of influence can encourage them to make skillful choices that ease suffering for themselves and others affected by their decisions. If there is insufficient time given to mindfulness instructors to provide a deeper contemplation of the wisdom and ethical factors, at least they can give resources to the participants so they know there is more they can do to deepen their mindfulness practice and what are some ways they can continue to learn and grow.

Post-Program Actions It is essential for mindfulness teachers to make a note of the observations made during the mindfulness workshops. It is usual in such trainings for organizational processes that are working and those that are dysfunctional to come up in participants' discussions. To the extent participants' confidentiality is maintained, a summary of the observations and insights can be shared with management so they can adjust practices and processes to meet the changing needs of their employees and other stakeholders.

To reap the benefits of the mindfulness training, it is essential that management support the participants in continuing with the mindfulness practices on an ongoing basis. They can do this in several ways. It is helpful to provide a physical space and facilitators who can lead the practices on a regular basis. Online communities, such as gPause at Google, are effective ways for employees to share mindfulness resources such as apps, articles, and discussion forums. It is also helpful to integrate the practices and strategies that participants found useful in the mindfulness training into their daily functioning. A common way participants integrate mindfulness is starting their meetings with a couple of minutes of mindfulness meditation. Richard Fernandez, co-founder of Wisdom Labs and former Google executive at the leading edge of bringing mindfulness in organizations, shared his experience working with Fortune 500 manufacturing, retail, and pharmaceutical companies (Fernandez, 2017, personal communication). In working with the leadership in one such company to cultivate compassion by seeing similarities, mindful listening became the operating style, which focuses on understanding rather than problem solving. He also confirmed the importance of finding "ambassadors" within the company to take the lead for organizing regular on-site meditations.

Mindfulness Marketing, Education, and Research Another way that mindfulness instructors impact the world is through marketing of their mindfulness programs. Mindful inquiry, using the lenses of wisdom, ethics, and mindfulness, provides a good framework to assess the intentions, actions, and consequences of our marketing efforts. Looking at the marketing plans through the lens of wisdom can remind instructors to contemplate on their intentions and consequences on different populations who may be exposed to their marketing messages.

Much of corporate mindfulness, including programs, books, and apps, is focusing on improving productivity, happiness, and other positive states of mind. While this can be considered a skillful means to engage corporate audiences and may have opened many doors for mindfulness in corporations, are we considering the unintended consequences of marketing mindfulness as a productivity and happiness-enhancing tool? Thich Nhat Hanh notes that "the art of happiness is also the art of suffering well" (Hanh, 2014). If we are only speaking about mindfulness in association with positive outcomes without speaking about the inherent unsatisfactoriness in all conditioned phenomena, we may be perpetuating the causes of suffering—desire, aversions, and delusions. People attending these programs may be provided with opportunities to contemplate on what is wholesome and unwholesome. However, for people who are not attending programs, the blogs and media coverage of mindfulness as a way to increase happiness and productivity may strengthen the root causes of suffering that right mindfulness is seeking to weaken.

Contemplating on right action and speech can further help to examine the integrity of the words, language, and research used in marketing. In our enthusiasm for mindfulness, it is easy to want to overpromise or offer mindfulness as a panacea for all problems that a client has. Mindfulness of our body, mind, and feelings can provide an inner compass to assess if our marketing actions feel appropriate and wholesome. The body never lies. If we are planning to do or say anything that is not skillful, checking in with the body can bring awareness to that, even if the mind thinks it is a good idea.

Marketing channels like blogs and videos can be utilized as a way to educate people about the deeper meaning of mindfulness when practiced with wisdom and ethical considerations. It would be interesting to do a content analysis of all the online blog posts and media content for mindfulness. My guess is that much of the focus is on benefits of mindfulness to be better at something and achieve success and positive states of mind with little reference to the transformative potential of mindfulness to liberate all beings from suffering. Especially, in the context of business, there is a big opportunity for mindfulness instructors to blog about the ways in which mindfulness can support leaders and other professionals see the interconnected nature of reality and provide frameworks using mindfulness, wisdom, and ethics to support organizational strategy and functions.

Conclusion

This chapter was designed to draw attention to some of the common criticisms and challenges pertaining to teaching mindfulness in corporations. Exploration of these issues using the lenses of Buddhist teachings, psychology, and management research and practices uncovers many opportunities to expand the scope of impact that mindfulness can have on business and make this world a better place for all beings. We've come a long way from the time I tried to introduce some of these ideas as a marketing professor and was called a "new-age hippie." Emerging research in neuroscience, psychology, and other disciplines has established that mindfulness practices offer tangible benefits in different domains of human well-being. The focus of many corporate programs has been on improving skills including focus, stress-management, and emotional intelligence, and corporate mindfulness programs have skillfully combined research findings with mindfulness teachings to create a set of practices, strategies, and skills that can develop different workplace competencies.

The courage, ingenuity, and resilience of the instructors introducing mindfulness in secular domains such as business are noteworthy. Mindfulness instructors may have stepped into this new domain with necessary caution and are now at a place to take a new direction with more resolve. They can work in cross-disciplinary teams to expand the scope of mindfulness benefits into corporate strategy and processes. The impact of their commitment can be deeper if we include the wisdom and ethical dimensions of mindfulness. With the experience and knowledge that we now have, is it possible for mindfulness instructors and practitioners to imagine bigger and bolder applications of mindfulness that fulfill its transformative potential to alleviate suffering in all beings. Can mindfulness provide a foundation for new management thought and leadership? How can it contribute to creating a corporate paradigm that maximizes not only shareholder but also all stakeholders' value?

Martin Luther King Jr. said, "We are caught in an inescapable network of mutuality, tied in a single garment of destiny. Whatever affects one directly, affects all indirectly" (King, 2000, p. 65). This interconnectedness and interdependence in human beings is also alluded to in mindfulness teachings. It is not a moral or religious fact, but people's experience, which is reflected in emerging trends. Some of these trends noted earlier include people having broader expectations from business, consumers' movements toward mindful consumption, environmental awareness, and new technologies making this world more connected. The shifting trends are making it impossible to ignore the consequences that businesses have locally and globally. As we navigate our circles of influence, let us continue to ask ourselves how we can effectively guide and push the boundaries of what is possible: What role can mindfulness play to support businesses in seeing the interconnected reality of all beings and finding creative solutions to enhance the quality of life of all beings?

References

Amar, A. D., Hlupic, V., & Tamwatin, T. (2014). Effect of meditation on self-perception of leadership skills: A control group study of CEOs. *Academy of Management Proceedings*, *2014*(1), 14282. https://doi.org/10.5465/ambpp.2014.300
American Psychological Association (APA). (2016). *Stress in America: Impact of discrimination*. Retrieved from http://www.apa.org/news/press/releases/stress/2015/impact-of-discrimination.pdf

Anālayo, B. (2004). *Satipatthāna: The direct path to realization*. Birmingham: Windhorse.

Anderson, M. (2009). *Why we created the MBA Oath*. Retrieved March 31, 2017, from https://hbr.org/2009/06/why-we-created-the-mba-oath

Bahl, S., Milne, G. R., Ross, S. M., Mick, D. G., Grier, S. A., Chugani, S. K., ... Boesen-Mariani, S. (2016). Mindfulness: Its transformative potential for consumer, societal, and environmental well-being. *Journal of Public Policy & Marketing, 35*(2), 198–210. https://doi.org/10.1509/jppm.15.139

Bodhi, B. (2011). What does mindfulness really mean? A canonical perspective. *Contemporary Buddhism, 12*(1), 19–39. https://doi.org/10.1080/14639947.2011.564813

Bosker, B. (2016). *The binge breaker*. Retrieved March 31, 2017, from https://www.theatlantic.com/magazine/archive/2016/11/the-binge-breaker/501122/

Brown, K. W., Ryan, R. M., & Creswell, J. D. (2007). Mindfulness: Theoretical foundations and evidence for its salutary effects. *Psychological Inquiry, 18*(4), 211–237.

Bush, M. (2015). Awakening at work: Introducing mindfulness into organizations. In J. Reb & P. W. Atkins (Eds.), *Mindfulness in organizations: Foundations, research, and applications* (pp. 333–354). Cambridge: Cambridge University Press.

Chonko, L. B., & Hunt, S. D. (1985). Ethics and marketing management: An empirical examination. *Journal of Business Research, 13*(4), 339–359. https://doi.org/10.1016/0148-2963(85)90006-2

Condon, P., Desbordes, G., Miller, W., & DeSteno, D. (2013). Meditation increases compassionate responses to suffering. *Psychological Science, 24*, 2125–2127. https://doi.org/10.1037/e578192014-060

Corkery, M., & Cowley, S. (2016, September 16). *Wells Fargo warned workers against sham accounts, but 'they needed a paycheck'*. Retrieved March 31, 2017, from https://www.nytimes.com/2016/09/17/business/dealbook/wells-fargo-warned-workers-against-fake-accounts-but-they-needed-a-paycheck.html

Crane, R. (2009). *Mindfulness-based cognitive therapy: Distinctive features*. London: Routledge.

Crum, A. J., Salovey, P., & Achor, S. (2013). Rethinking stress: The role of mindsets in determining the stress response. *Journal of Personality and Social Psychology, 104*(4), 716–733. https://doi.org/10.1037/a0031201

Druskat, V. U., & Wolff, S. B. (2001). *Building the emotional intelligence of groups*. Retrieved March 31, 2017, from https://hbr.org/2001/03/building-the-emotional-intelligence-of-groups

Edelman, R. (2017). *Edelman TRUST BAROMETER reveals global implosion of trust*. Retrieved March 31, 2017, from http://www.edelman.com/news/2017-edelman-trust-barometer-reveals-global-implosion/

Ernst, & Young. (2016). *EY publishes 14th global fraud survey—Corporate misconduct: Individual consequences*. Retrieved March 31, 2017, from http://www.ey.com/ie/en/newsroom/news-releases/press-release-2016-ey-publishes-14th-global-fraud-survey---corporate-misconduct--individual-consequences

Fevre, M. L., Kolt, G. S., & Matheny, J. (2006). Eustress, distress and their interpretation in primary and secondary occupational stress management interventions: Which way first? *Journal of Managerial Psychology, 21*(6), 547–565. https://doi.org/10.1108/02683940610684391

Fernandez, R.M. (2017, March 8). Phone interview.

Goh, J., Pfeffer, J., & Zenios, S. A. (2015). The relationship between workplace stressors and mortality and health costs in the United States. *Management Science, 62*(2), 608–628. https://doi.org/10.1287/mnsc.2014.2115

Goldstein, J. (2016). *Mindfulness: A practical guide to awakening*. Boulder, CO: Sounds True.

Grégoire, S., & Lachance, L. (2014). Evaluation of a brief mindfulness-based intervention to reduce psychological distress in the workplace. *Mindfulness, 6*(4), 836–847. https://doi.org/10.1007/s12671-014-0328-9

Hanh, T. N. (2014). No mud, no lotus: The art of transforming suffering. Parallax Press.

Hafenbrack, A. C., Kinias, Z., & Barsade, S. G. (2014). Debiasing the mind through meditation. *Psychological Science, 25*(2), 369–376. https://doi.org/10.1177/0956797613503853

Healey, K. (2013). *Searching for integrity: The politics of mindfulness in the digital economy*. Retrieved March 31, 2017, from http://nomosjournal.org/2013/08/searching-for-integrity/

Heifetz, R. A., Grashow, A., & Linsky, M. (2009). *The practice of adaptive leadership: Tools and tactics for changing your organization and the world*. Boston: Harvard Business.

Hölzel, B. K., Lazar, S. W., Gard, T., Schuman-Olivier, Z., Vago, D. R., & Ott, U. (2011). How does mindfulness meditation work? Proposing mechanisms of action from a conceptual and neural perspective. *Perspectives on Psychological Science, 6*(6), 537–559. https://doi. org/10.1177/1745691611419671

Hoyk, R. & Hersey, P. (2010). *Ethical executive: Becoming aware of the root causes of unethical behavior*. Stanford: Stanford University Press.

Hunter, J., & Chaskalson, M. (2013). Making the mindful leader: Cultivating skills for facing adaptive challenges. In H. S. Leonard (Ed.), *The Wiley-Blackwell handbook of the psychology of leadership, change, and organizational development* (pp. 195–219). Malden, MA: Wiley-Blackwell.

Kabat-Zinn, J. (2011). Some reflections on the origins of MBSR, skillful means, and the trouble with maps. *Contemporary Buddhism, 12*(1), 281–306. https://doi.org/10.1080/14639947.201 1.564844

Kabat-Zinn, J. (2013). *Full catastrophe living: How to cope with stress, pain and illness using mindfulness meditation*. London: Piatkus.

Khoury, B., Lecomte, T., Fortin, G., Masse, M., Therien, P., Bouchard, V., … Hofmann, S. G. (2013). Mindfulness-based therapy: A comprehensive meta-analysis. *Clinical Psychology Review, 33*(6), 763–771. https://doi.org/10.1016/j.cpr.2013.05.005

King, M. L. (2000). *Why we can't wait*. New York: New American Library.

Kobasa, S. C., Maddi, S. R., & Kahn, S. (1982). Hardiness and health: A prospective study. *Journal of Personality and Social Psychology, 42*(1), 168–177. https://doi. org/10.1037//0022-3514.42.1.168

Laloux, F. (2014). *Reinventing organizations: A guide to creating organizations inspired by the next stage of human consciousness*. Brussels: Nelson Parker.

Lama, D., & Van Den Muyzenberg, L. (2009). *The leader's way: The art of making the right decisions in our careers, our companies, and the world at large*. New York: Crown Business.

Lampe, M., & Engleman-Lampe, C. (2012). Mindfulness-based business ethics education. *Academy of Educational Leadership Journal, 16*(3), 99.

Maddi, S. R. (2012). *Hardiness: Turning stressful circumstances into resilient growth*. New York: Springer.

Mann, A., & Harter, J. (2016). *The worldwide employee engagement crisis*. Retrieved March 31, 2017, from http://www.gallup.com/businessjournal/188033/worldwide-employee-engagement-crisis.aspx

Marx, R. (2015). Accessibility versus integrity in secular mindfulness: A Buddhist commentary. *Mindfulness, 6*(5), 1153–1160. https://doi.org/10.1007/s12671-014-0366-3

McCown, D., Reibel, D., & Micozzi, M. S. (2010). *Teaching mindfulness: A practical guide for clinicians and educators*. New York: Springer.

McKiernan, P. (2012). *Americans' confidence in leaders rises, remains low*. Retrieved March 31, 2017, from https://www.hks.harvard.edu/news-events/news/press-releases/nli-2012

Monteiro, L. M., Musten, R., & Compson, J. (2015). Traditional and contemporary mindfulness: Finding the middle path in the tangle of concerns. *Mindfulness, 6*(1), 1–13. https://doi. org/10.1007/s12671-014-0301-7

Narayanan, J., & Moynihan, L. (2006). Mindfulness at work: The beneficial effects on job burnout in call centers. *Academy of Management Proceedings, 2006*(1). https://doi.org/10.5465/ ambpp.2006.22898626

Nelson, D., & Cooper, C. (2005). Stress and health: A positive direction. *Stress and Health, 21*(2), 73–75.

Park, C. L., Cohen, L. H., & Murch, R. L. (1996). Assessment and prediction of stress-related growth. *Journal of Personality, 64*(1), 71–105. https://doi.org/10.1111/j.1467-6494.1996. tb00815.x

Purser, R., & Loy, D. (2013, July 01). *Beyond McMindfulness*. Retrieved March 31, 2017, from http://www.huffingtonpost.com/ron-purser/beyond-mcmindfulness_b_3519289.html

Purser, R. E., & Milillo, J. (2015). Mindfulness revisited. *Journal of Management Inquiry*, *24*(1), 3–24. https://doi.org/10.1177/1056492614532315

Purser, R., & Ng, E. (2015). *Corporate mindfulness is bullsh*t: Zen or no Zen, you're working harder and being paid less*. Retrieved March 31, 2017, from http://www.salon.com/2015/09/27/corporate_mindfulness_is_bullsht_zen_or_no_zen_youre_working_harder_and_being_paid:less/

PwC. (2016). *19th Annual global CEO survey: Redefining business success in a changing world*. Retrieved March 31, 2017, from https://www.pwc.com/gx/en/ceo-survey/2016/landing-page/pwc-19th-annual-global-ceo-survey.pdf

Reb, J., Narayanan, J., & Chaturvedi, S. (2012). Leading mindfully: Two studies on the influence of supervisor trait mindfulness on employee well-being and performance. *Mindfulness*, *5*(1), 36–45. https://doi.org/10.1007/s12671-012-0144-z

Richardson, K. M., & Rothstein, H. R. (2008). Effects of occupational stress management intervention programs: A meta-analysis. *Journal of Occupational Health Psychology*, *13*(1), 69–93. https://doi.org/10.1037/1076-8998.13.1.69

Rider, K. M. (2016). Consumer consumption & brand strategy: From mindless to mindful marketing. In *CMO technology news*. Retrieved March 31, 2017, from http://www.cmotechnews.com/index.php/CMO-Challenges/consumer-consumption-brand-strategy-from-mindless-to-mindful-marketing

Scharmer, C. O. (2009). *Theory U: Leading from the future as it emerges*. San Francisco, CA: Berrett-Koehler.

Schumpeter. (2013). *The mindfulness business*. Retrieved April 01, 2017, from http://www.economist.com/news/business/21589841-western-capitalism-looking-inspiration-eastern-mysticism-mindfulness-business

Seligman, M. (2006). *Learned optimism: How to change your mind and your life*. New York: Alfred Knopf.

Shapiro, S. L., Jazaieri, H., & Goldin, P. R. (2012). Mindfulness-based stress reduction effects on moral reasoning and decision making. *The Journal of Positive Psychology*, *7*(6), 504–515. https://doi.org/10.1080/17439760.2012.723732

Shure, M. B., Christopher, J., & Christopher, S. (2008). Mind-body medicine and the art of self-care: Teaching mindfulness to counseling students through yoga, meditation and qigong. *Journal of Counseling and Development*, *86*, 47–56.

Sisodia, R., Sheth, J. N., & Wolfe, D. B. (2014). *Firms of endearment: How world-class companies profit from passion and purpose*. Upper Saddle River, NJ: Pearson Education.

Tang, Y., Hölzel, B. K., & Posner, M. I. (2015). The neuroscience of mindfulness meditation. *Nature Reviews Neuroscience*, *16*(4), 213–225. https://doi.org/10.1038/nrn3916

Tworkov, H. (2001). *Contemplating corporate culture*. Retrieved April 01, 2017, from https://tricycle.org/magazine/contemplating-corporate-culture/

Chapter 15
Mindfulness and Minefields: Walking the Challenging Path of Awareness for Soldiers and Veterans

Sean Bruyea

Introduction

Following a relatively recent and rapid expansion, mindfulness practices have been embraced not only by medicine but also by business, management studies, schools, and the legal profession (Poirier, 2016; Purser & Loy, 2013). Mindfulness has also been employed in the military and veteran context to treat posttraumatic stress disorder (PTSD) (Reber et al., 2013; Rees, 2011) as well as to build soldiers' resilience (Jha et al., 2015; Jha, Morrison, Parker, & Stanley, 2017; Stanley, Schaldach, Kiyonaga, & Jha, 2011). (Unless otherwise indicated, the use of "soldier" in this text refers to all members who wear a military uniform, regardless of service, environment or element-army, navy, and air force personnel as well as marines. Soldier for the purposes of this paper is a term of convenience and respect with no offense intended.). Such resilience-building measures are not only intended to "immunize against stress" but mindfulness has been "operationalized" to "optimize" soldier performance (Stanley & Jha, 2009).

The application of mindfulness in the military context has raised ethical questions and concerns (Monteiro, Musten, & Compson, 2015; Purser, 2015; Purser & Loy, 2013; Senauke, 2016). This debate reflects some fundamental differences between military and mindfulness worlds that have applicability to not only employing mindfulness in the military context but also within the veteran population and stimulates a subsequent "curiosity" inherent to mindfulness (Bishop et al., 2004, p. 232). What are the differences between mindfulness and military practices and ethics? Are these differences relevant to teaching and/or practicing mindfulness? Is there some common ground between these two worlds? Are there dark conse-

S. Bruyea, MA (✉)
Independent freelancer, Nepean, Canada
e-mail: seankis@rogers.com

© Springer International Publishing AG 2017   373
L.M. Monteiro et al. (eds.), *Practitioner's Guide to Ethics and Mindfulness-Based Interventions*, Mindfulness in Behavioral Health,
DOI 10.1007/978-3-319-64924-5_15

quences or illuminating hope in introducing mindfulness to military personnel and veterans?

In making a modest attempt to answer some of these questions, we require some basis upon which to compare and contrast military and mindfulness approaches. Since the ethical debate sparked concerns about employing mindfulness in the military, looking at the two ethical worlds will be the first step. Since ethics do not always reflect practices, the second step considers a practical or "operational" (Kabat-Zinn, 2011) understanding of the way things are done in the two environments. Finally, salient aspects of military and mindfulness ethics and practices will be studied for commonalities and differences, with a hope that there is a place for the two worlds to meet on common, enlightened grounds. The intention of separating the two worlds until the final section is that readers can appreciate the unique and rich nature of both cultures separately, with the hope that much of the comparison and contrasts will become self-evident. Teachers of mindfulness provide the greatest value to practitioners when they understand both themselves and the practitioner. This is central to a teacher's "authenticity, or ultimate relevance" (Kabat-Zinn, 2003, p. 150) and provides the foundations of a "well-trained and highly experienced and empathic teacher" (Kabat-Zinn, 2011, p. 292). Otherwise, teachers and practitioners will be unaware of (and unprepared for) the minefields both may encounter when walking the path from military experience to mindfulness.

This discussion is both a theoretical and a practical study of the manner in which mindfulness and military worlds may collide or cooperate. This analytic process also includes some helpful insight into military practices and cultures, and as such, this discussion has relevance for teachers, practitioners, and researchers both within the mindfulness world but also for military leaders as well as for practitioners employing other therapies treating or hoping to treat military and veteran populations.

Teaching Mindfulness to the Military: Awakening Teachers and Practitioners

This chapter traces a winding path through the two worlds: mindfulness first, followed by the military. Both worlds are complex, multivalent, grounded in rich traditions, and embroiled in somewhat fierce ethical debates. Any written study of these worlds must fall short. One cannot practice mindfulness nor can one truly comprehend the awesome demands of military duty or the monstrosity of war merely through reading. However, reading is a good first step to becoming aware of what these two cultures share and how they are often diametrically opposed.

Culture can act as a barrier to "cross-cultural counseling" (Sue, 1981). Since counseling and psychotherapy "can be viewed as a process of interpersonal interaction and communication," effective counseling requires that the counselor and the client "must be able to *appropriately* and *accurately send* and *receive* both *verbal* and *nonverbal* messages" (Sue, 1981, p. 27, original italics). Breakdowns in communication are frequent between members of the same culture and the greater the differences between the two cultures, the greater the opportunity for breakdowns in communication. As such, "different cultural and subcultural groups require different approaches" (Sue, 1981, p. 99).

The discussion herein demonstrates the potentially harmful mistake practitioners would make if they were to assume that the military culture is *not* at least as comprehensive and influential upon soldiers as the impact ethnic cultures have upon members of their respective groups. Furthermore, we must consider the enduring effect military culture has upon soldiers even when they leave the military and become veterans. This impact expanded upon in this chapter reveals that military service itself, and not only trauma resulting from that service, can create immense obstacles to rejoining not just civilian life but reconnecting with themselves. "Mindfulness is about *relationality*" Jon Kabat-Zinn (2013) writes, emphasizing that "[m]eaning and relationship are strands of connectedness and interconnectedness" and this connectedness "may be what is most fundamental about the relationship of what we call *mind* to physical and emotional health" (p. 271, original italics). Military culture profoundly disconnects individuals from themselves and civilian society. Bringing *connectedness and interconnectedness* to soldiers and veterans can therefore pose multiple challenges. As such, teaching mindfulness to this culturally unique population requires much consideration, to which this chapter contributes.

When conducting mindfulness, "if it is to be effective in treating clinical problems, [it] is best conducted by [teachers] who have adequately formulated views of the disorders that they seek to treat and of the ways that mindfulness training can be helpful to clients with those disorders" (Teasdale, Segal, & Williams, 2003, p. 157). Military service, as well as its potent and enduring cultural influences, limits a veteran's ability to reintegrate into and connect (or reconnect) with civilian life in ways characteristic of clinical disorders (Bruyea, 2016; Segsworth, 1920; Smith & True, 2014; Waller, 1944). As such, from a clinical as well as a cultural perspective, mindfulness teachers would be most *helpful* to military and veteran clients if they were to have *adequately formulated views* as to the profound impact military service and culture have upon individuals who serve in uniform. Kabat-Zinn (2011) tells us teachers should have a "direct authentic full-spectrum first-person experience" (p. 292) of mindfulness. However, understanding oneself is not enough. Kabat-Zinn (2003) asks how can teachers

> …ask someone else to look deeply into his or her own mind and body and the nature of who he or she is in a systematic and disciplined way if one is unwilling (or too busy or not interested enough) to engage in this great and challenging adventure oneself, at least to the degree that one is asking it of one's patients or clients? (p. 150)

Asking soldiers and veterans *to look deeply into his or her own mind and body and the nature of who he or she is* requires not only an awareness of oneself on the path of mindfulness, but also an awareness of the military experience and how it impacts these individuals wishing to walk a similar path. This is my rationale for presenting the two worlds separately and then meeting at the end to discuss the nature of compatibility and/or conflict between the two worlds.

Mindfulness: Definition, Practice, and Ethics

Mindfulness is not practiced with universal consistency, has not been defined consistently, nor does it have a universally applicable and articulated ethical code. Bishop et al. (2004) observe "[t]here have been no systematic efforts to establish the defining criteria of [mindfulness'] various components" (p. 231), while "mindfulness…enjoys a multiplicity of definitions" (Monteiro et al., 2015, p. 4). These inconsistencies should not limit our attempts to capture as much commonality between definitions, ethics, and practices of mindfulness where possible.

Defining Mindfulness John Kabat-Zinn (2005), the founder of the modern Western mindfulness movement, defines mindfulness as "the awareness that arises from paying attention, on purpose, in the present moment, and non-judgementally" (p. 180). This definition includes three essential and widely (but not universally) accepted, elements or "axioms" of contemporary mindfulness practice: "'On purpose' or intention, 'Paying attention' or attention, [and] 'in a particular way' or attitude", i.e., "non-judgmentally". These three axioms are "interwoven aspects of a single cyclic process and occur simultaneously" in a "moment-to-moment process" (Shapiro, Carlson, Astin, & Freedman, 2006, p. 375).

The above definition as well as other commonly cited ones (Bishop et al., 2004; Grossman, 2015) allow wide interpretations by practitioner, teacher, and researcher. The result: contemporary mindfulness practices can be as elaborate and rich with moral implication or they can be "denatured" (Grossman, 2015, p. 17) to the bare essence of a robotic meditation or become synonymous with merely paying attention (Grossman, 2015; Monteiro et al., 2015; Purser & Loy, 2013; Van Gordon, Shonin, Griffiths, & Singh, 2015). Nevertheless, Kabat-Zinn's (2005) definition remains one of the more prevalent and widely accepted definitions of mindfulness (Shapiro et al., 2006). Hence, it will serve as the definition to be used throughout this chapter when looking at the compatibility of mindfulness and military worlds.

Practice of Mindfulness Since contemporary mindfulness concepts were first introduced by Jon Kabat-Zinn 30 years ago, a dizzying diversity of practices has emerged (Purser & Loy, 2013; Tisdale, 2016). In a conventional healthcare context, which has produced most of the research on the efficacy of mindfulness, there is likewise a plethora of mindfulness approaches. They include two of the "most commonly known and established modalities" (Monteiro et al., 2015, p. 4): mindfulness-based stress reduction (MBSR), "the root program from which most mindfulness-based interventions (MBIs) are derived" (Monteiro et al., 2015, p. 2) and mindfulness-based cognitive therapy (MBCT) (Baer, 2003; Coronado-Montoya et al., 2016).

Typically, the clinical MBIs consist of a group setting with eight or more individuals who meet on a weekly basis for 8–12 weeks (Baer, 2015; Monteiro et al., 2015). Mindful or purposeful meditation, as opposed to "relaxation or mood management" techniques, is central to the practice as a form of "mental training" (Bishop et al., 2004, p. 229). Consistent with the definitions above, MBIs typically include an "attentional component" that helps develop the "ability to intentionally regulate attention" through practices to cultivate "deliberate and sustained observation of thoughts, feelings, physical sensations, and other stimuli as they occur in the present moment" (Coffey, Hartman, & Fredrickson, 2010, p. 236). These practices include "body scans," "awareness of breath," and "mindful movements" complemented with regular "dialogues" between teacher and participant "that explore the experiential aspects of these practices" (Monteiro et al., 2015, p. 5). For MBIs, the intention is to reduce the "mental dispersal" while "cultivating the wisdom" to take responsibility for our "unfolding experience" (Monteiro et al., 2015, p. 4).

One component of this wisdom is to develop acceptance of the inner and outer world of each participant. As feelings arise and senses take note of the participant's *unfolding experience*, participants are encouraged to maintain "an attitude of openness and receptivity to these experiences, rather than judging, ignoring, or minimizing them, particularly when they are unpleasant" (Coffey et al., 2010, p. 236). Some of those goals could include: minimizing "rumination and brooding" wherein minds enter circular processes focusing upon feelings, senses, or thoughts that take the participant away from the present moment into a path that provokes feelings of anxiety or depression, and reducing "*emotional avoidance*," wherein thoughts or feelings that are incongruous with our self-image, or are painful, are suppressed, effectively shutting off the awareness of the here and now (Gilbert & Choden, 2014, p. 135, original italics). Bishop et al. (2004) underscore that "mindfulness is not a practice in thought suppression; all thoughts or events are considered an object of observation, not a distraction" (p. 232).

Bhante Gunaratana (2015) describes 11 attitudes to guide successful mindfulness including don't expect anything, don't strain, don't rush, don't cling to anything, and don't reject anything, let go, accept everything that arises, be gentle with yourself, and investigate yourself (p. 34) while Thich Nhat Hanh (1976) offers insight:

> ...is relaxation then the only goal of [mindful] mediation? In fact the goal of meditation goes much deeper than that. While relaxation is the necessary point of departure, once one has realized relaxation, it is possible to realize a tranquil heart and clear mind....to take hold of our minds and calm our thoughts, we must also practice mindfulness of our feelings and perceptions. To take hold of your mind, you must practice mindfulness of the mind. You must know how to observe and recognize the presence of every feeling and thought which arises in you. (p. 37)

Monteiro et al. (2015) stress that for traditional mindfulness practices, "the cultivation of attention and concentration through meditative practices is viewed as necessary but not sufficient for right mindfulness to develop." What is necessary for right mindfulness is the cultivation of "discernment, wise action, or wisdom" (p. 3).

Ethics in Mindfulness and Defining Terms Just as there are diverse and varied definitions and practices of MBIs, there are concomitantly just as many ethical approaches to conducting MBIs. This diversity continues to fuel a persistent ethical debate in the field of mindfulness (Baer, 2015; Grossman, 2015; Kabat-Zinn, 2011; Monteiro et al., 2015; Purser & Loy, 2013; Van Gordon et al., 2015).

However, such diversity in the world of MBIs is dwarfed by the immense world of philosophical ethics, which lies beyond the scope of this discussion. It is helpful, nonetheless, to provide a clear definition of ethics and morals upfront. Some ethical models are prescriptive as to one's character, such as the field of positive psychology (Baer, 2015). Paul Grossman (2015) in his commentary on ethics in mindfulness draws upon definitions originating in moral or philosophical theory to include the concepts of "rightness and wrongness of certain actions", "goodness and badness of the motives and ends", as well as "an internal and literally embodied set of attitudes and values" (pp. 17–18). Such definitions can be more problematic than helpful. How does one agree upon rightness, wrongness, good, or bad? Who defines what attitudes and values are the ones to have?

A simpler definition will be more helpful here. The word "moral" originates from the "Latin *mores*, which means custom or habit, and it is a translation of the Greek *ethos*, which means roughly the same thing," which in turn is the origin of the term "ethics" (Hare, 2014, para. 2). Central to any code of ethics or morality is essentially a "set" of "do's or don'ts" (Donagan, 1977, p. 54) for the "conduct of human life" (Rendtorff, 1986, p. 33). Since both morals and ethics dictate how we do things or should do things, ethics and morals are interchangeable. Both are more easily understood if defined as how we conduct ourselves or *should* conduct ourselves. Hence, ethical codes provide the rules for accepted and desired conduct.

Mindfulness Ethics: A Practical Approach Considering this simpler definition, we can see that even the brief discussion of the practices outlined above include an inherent ethic as to how to conduct mindfulness. Most, if not all, participants and arguments in the debate on mindful ethics agree there must be an ethical code as to how to conduct mindfulness (Amaro, 2015; Baer, 2015; Greenberg & Mitra, 2015; Grossman, 2015; Kabat-Zinn, 2011; Lindahl, 2015; Magrid & Poirier, 2016; Monteiro et al., 2015; Poirier, 2016; Purser, 2015; Purser & Loy, 2013; Van Gordon et al., 2015). Considering that we are talking about practical ethics, i.e., how to conduct mindfulness, and considering that Kabat-Zinn's definition (2005) is the most widely accepted, an understanding as to the commonalities in how to conduct mindfulness can be advantageously developed through a deeper understanding of Kabat-Zinn's (2005) "operational" definition of mindfulness: "the awareness that arises from paying attention, on purpose, in the present moment, and non-judgementally" (p. 180). This definition offers an ethics-in-practice guideline for how to conduct mindfulness, which we can use to compare general approaches to mindfulness with military ethics and practices. Let us look in greater detail at the five elements of his definition: paying attention, on purpose, in the present moment, non-judgmentally, and awareness.

Paying Attention *Attention* is the starting point for most, if not all, forms of mindfulness practice. However, paying attention to music, television, traffic, work meetings, or other daily activities "do not necessarily characterize acts of mindfulness" (Grossman, 2015, p. 18). In mindfulness practice, paying attention is something much more and focusing attention is central to most, if not all, practices of "meditative concentration" (Van Gordon et al., 2015). As Monteiro et al. (2015) as well as others emphasize, meditation is not mindfulness, although it is a foundational component of mindfulness. The reduction of mindfulness into meditation has raised concerns that even some "popularized notions of mindfulness [have] become denatured to an extent that the practice loses its innovative, radical meaning, and becomes just another word for attention" (Grossman, 2015, p. 17). Nevertheless, it is important to note that even the most *denatured* program calling itself mindfulness requires paying attention.

However, to *pay attention* in most conceptions of mindfulness has two commonly accepted foci. First, mindfulness does not require that one merely pay attention to anything. One should pay attention to something stable, something non-stimulating, non-distracting, something that grounds and centers us in the present moment. Gunaratana (2015) tells us, "Therefore we must give our mind an object that is readily available every present moment. One such object is our breath" (pp. 45–46). The second focus of the mind is to pay attention to what one's senses perceive *in the present moment.*

In the Present Moment Once the mind is centered or anchored upon the breath, the second focus of attention comes into play. The centering on the breath puts "out the welcome mat for whatever arises" (Kabat-Zinn, 2011, p. 297) as it arises in that moment, resulting in an awareness of "the constantly changing nature of sensations, even highly unpleasant ones" (Kabat-Zinn, 2011, p. 298) or the "unfolding of experience moment by moment" (Kabat-Zinn, 2003, p. 145). By being aware of the spontaneously emerging moment by moment sensations, thoughts, and feelings, one should take "notice" (Bishop et al., 2004, p. 232), "see," "observe," "watch" (Gunaratana, 2015), or *pay attention* to them but not necessarily *attend to* them by ruminating or dwelling upon the emerging sensations, thoughts, and feelings. Instead, one returns one's attention back to the breath. Paying attention to, or noticing, the emergent moment by moment experience can be understood as the more practical aspect of awareness. Being in the present moment is a goal in itself wherein the "intention" is "to understand rather than to judge, in full acceptance of whatever may emerge." The resulting "intelligence is the door to freedom and alert attention is the mother of intelligence" (Nisargadatta Maharaj as cited in Kabat-Zinn, 2011, p. 300).

Non-Judgmentally Shapiro et al. (2006) contend that "[h]*ow* we attend is also essential" and, central to how we attend is the attitude one brings to mindfulness practice (p. 376, original italics). Some contemporary approaches to mindfulness have reduced non-judgment in the mindfulness context to a mechanical mental process "so easily achieved" (Grossman, 2015, p. 18) as if the human mind can robotically shut off all judgment and feelings. Kabat-Zinn (2003) concurs that mindfulness practice is never "mechanical" (148). He further explains that "[n]on-judgmental does not mean to imply…there is some ideal state in which judgments no longer arise" (Kabat-Zinn, 2011, p. 291). Opinions and judgments will naturally arise but "we do not have to judge or evaluate or react to any of what arises, other than perhaps recognizing it in the moment of arising as pleasant, unpleasant, or neutral" (p. 292). Consequently, this non-judgmental approach then allows the practitioner "in any moment either to cling and self-identify or not" (p. 292).

Often used synonymously or in conjunction with *non-judgmentally* or *without judgment* is the concept of acceptance. The "acceptance-based" component of mindfulness, along with the attentional-based component are "common to most definitions of mindfulness" (Coffey et al., 2010, p. 236). Acceptance for some approaches to mindfulness has been or could be interpreted as "passivity" (Monteiro et al., 2015, p. 6) or more benignly, as a detached and unconcerned observer of one's own unfolding internal and external experience, albeit to be performed with gentleness with oneself (Gunaratana, 2015). However, even the more sanitized descriptors for how to interpret *acceptance* often include concepts of "curiosity, experiential openness," and "receptivity" (Bishop et al., 2004) as qualifiers or conjoined concepts with that of acceptance. For others, acceptance is performed with generosity, kindness, and respect for our mortality (Monteiro & Musten, 2013) as well as "empathy, gratitude, gentleness, and loving kindness" (Shapiro & Schwartz, 2000, p. 253) while mindfulness awareness is "generally agreed to be open, accepting, curious, compassionate, and kind" (Baer, 2015, p. 957). As Grossman (2015) argues, "attention to experience is never emotionally neutral or devoid of attitudes toward what we are observing in any situation" (p. 19). Grossman notes that it is common in mindfulness practices to take on the following "attitudinal stance":

> …supplant the judging mind with an attitude of kindness, curiosity, generosity and patience toward these sensations, which already exist and which we may not be able immediately to change. We might even be able to generate a subtle feeling of compassion toward this unstoppable unpleasant process that is unfolding within our own bodies, as well as the courage to stay tuned in to this unpleasant experience for the moment. (p. 20)

For Grossman (2015), this "benevolent orientation" or "stance toward our experience reflects… an internally consistent ethical value system aimed not only to one's own perceptions and thoughts but also to all objects of perception and thought" (p. 20) to be perceived with "an affectionate, compassionate quality… a sense of openhearted, friendly presence and interest" (Kabat-Zinn, 2003, p. 145). Thus, non-judgment in a mindfulness context requires a highly benevolent attitude that is, in spite of the seemingly neutral valence of nonjudgment, more benevolent, compassionate and kind than devoid of any attitude.

On Purpose and Awareness One of the more overlooked components of mindfulness is the component of "on purpose" that becomes, at the most aspiring levels of mindfulness, synonymous with awareness. Fundamentally, "[t]he practice of mindfulness begins with the creation of an intention to pay attention" (Monteiro &

Musten, 2013, p. 27). In mindfulness practice, there is "an intentional effort to observe and gain a greater understanding of the nature of thoughts and feelings" (Bishop et al., 2004, p. 234). This is intention at its most basic interpretation of *on purpose*, an almost mechanical process. However, like each of the components of Kabat-Zinn's definition, there are multiple interpretations of *on purpose*. After decades of personal practice, Kabat-Zinn (1990) would later identify the need for "some kind of personal vision" (p. 46). This vision can evolve and change as well as include multiple intentions ranging from short-term tangible changes in behavior such as self-regulation all the way to a revolutionary change in *weltanschauung* or worldview. Shapiro et al. (2006) provide an example at the behavioral end: "a highly stressed businessman may begin a mindfulness practice to reduce hypertension. As his mindfulness practice continues, he may develop an additional intention of relating more kindly to his wife" (p. 375). However, mindfulness for Kabat-Zinn and its 2500-year-old experience with the human condition was ultimately about developing greater personal insight as to how each of us fits in with the universe but also an intention of alleviating suffering, not merely for those who practice mindfulness, but alleviating suffering for all humanity, a view shared by other teachers (Monteiro et al., 2015; Purser, 2015; Van Gordon et al., 2015). These are indeed lofty goals that are not always achievable for teachers or practitioners. However, in setting more modest personal goals, those practitioners who identified an *intention* for their mindfulness practice at a personal level tended to achieve those intended goals (Shapiro et al., 2006).

Mindfulness is not the "end in itself," but instead mindfulness is "grounded in a clear formulation of the origins and cessation of suffering" and "has always been used as only one of a number of components of a much wider intervention" to address suffering with the sum of the impact of these components being greater than "the sum of their parts" (Teasdale et al., 2003, p. 159). Mindfulness may not be an end itself but in the context of *on purpose*, developing a larger *awareness* of our interconnectedness with ourselves and others becomes a worthy end. In this context, *on purpose* and *awareness* become nearly synonymous, while *awareness* takes on its second component, more spiritual than the first component of merely *paying attention* to what arises:

> …it is inevitably the personal responsibility of each person engaging in this work to attend with care and intentionality to how we are actually living our lives, both personally and professionally, in terms of ethical behaviour. An awareness of one's conduct and the quality of one's relationships, inwardly and outwardly, in terms of their potential to cause harm, are intrinsic elements of the cultivation of mindfulness… (Kabat-Zinn, 2011, p. 294)

Kabat-Zinn's (2011) intentions regarding the practice of mindfulness are indeed far richer than a face-value interpretation of his definition of mindfulness. Nevertheless, the range of interpretations currently in mindfulness practice is indeed multivalent. The question for this discussion is how compatible are some of the above mindfulness ethics-in-practice with the ethics and practices of the military and veteran world?

Military Ethics and Culture

Ethics: Fragmented and Vague or Internationally Monolithic and Clearly Articulated?

There is something universal about military service in that "[t]he figure of the warrior is truly cross-cultural" (Fields, 1991, p. 3). Both Fields (1991) and French (2003) have tracked and expanded upon a code, both explicit and implicit, that has characterized soldiers and militaries throughout documented history. These codes are often an overlap and melange of professional ethics and character virtues expected and desirable for soldiers. They include, but are not limited to, the chivalric concepts of sacrifice, courage, loyalty, respect, integrity, and honor (Fields, 1991; French, 2003; Moelker & Kümmel, 2007). Over time, these codes, at least in Western civilization, have influenced and indeed "simultaneously transformed in systems of law, on the one hand, and in codes of interpersonal behavior on the other" (Moelker & Kümmel, 2007, p. 293). Such codes came to influence not just how war was conducted in the Middle Ages but, along with the works of those who studied the conduct of war, can be "counted among the intellectual roots of present day humanitarian law" (Mader, 2002 cited in Moelker & Kümmel, 2007, p. 293).

Missing in the above rather praiseworthy account of the influences of warrior codes is the question of why were the codes necessary if a virtuous character was demanded for military service. Virtuous character traits are inherently ethical. The reality is that soldiers operate in a realm of humanity's darkest experience: the willful taking and giving of lives. In measuring and applying the use of force to this end, "[m]ost warriors will err on the side of excess" (Challans, 2007, p. 40). As such, these codes were created to save society and civilians from warriors, but also to save warriors from themselves and the horrors of war (Challans, 2007; French, 2003). French (2003) elaborates upon the codes of honor in militaries throughout history:

> In many cases this code of honor seems to hold the warrior to a higher ethical standard than that required for an ordinary citizen within the general population of the society the warrior serves. The code is not imposed from the outside. The warriors themselves police strict adherence to these standards; with violators being shamed, ostracized, or even killed by their peers….The code of the warrior not only defines how he should interact with his own warrior comrades, but also how he should treat other members of his society, his enemies, and the people he conquers. The code restrains the warrior. It sets boundaries on his behavior. It distinguishes honorable acts from shameful acts….Accepting certain constraints as a moral duty, even when it is inconvenient or inefficient to do so, allows warriors to hold onto their humanity while experiencing the horror of war…(pp. 3, 10)

Nevertheless, such influential and apparently unobstructed ancient origins as well as the widespread presence of warrior codes throughout societies may lead one to believe that such ethical codes are firmly codified and universal among modern militaries. This is not the case. Most militaries in OECD (Organization for Economic Co-operation and Development) nations developed explicit ethical codes of conduct only in the latter part of the twentieth century, often created on an ad hoc basis, one exception being Japan (Ota, 2008). Only recently did these nations establish such codes as part of "any pragmatic, workable education program" (Robinson, 2008, p. 1).

Robinson, De Lee, and Carrick (2008) brought together studies of the ethics programs of the militaries from ten OECD nations in an attempt to find both commonalities and differences. Their work reveals much inconsistency between not only various nations' approaches to military ethics but also ethical codes between various services (army, air force, navy, marines) within the same nation. In this aspect, the world of military ethics and that of mindfulness ethics, although both having ancient origins, are currently practiced in both an inconsistent and multivalent manner.

Most of these nations have only recently begun drawing upon ethical theories to develop their professional codes. Given the wide-ranging, longstanding, and conflicting approaches to ethical theory, as well as the similarly characterized philosophical debates in how to conduct war, it is not surprising that using ethical theory models to develop codes would result in different approaches by different nations in codifying military ethics. Nevertheless, of the ten nations studied in the edited volume by Robinson et al. (2008), all identify values, virtues, and/or principles as the basis for their respective military ethical codes. For instance, and not surprisingly, courage and/or selfless service have been adopted by seven of the countries studied. While integrity and the related overlap of the values, virtues, and/or principles of honor, respect, responsibility, and credibility are included in the formal codes of eight of the nations studied (Robinson, 2008, p. 7).

Such values, virtues, and principles leave much open to interpretation: "loyalty, for instance, will be interpreted as loyalty to the group and not to others, or at least to the group first and others second" (Robinson, 2007b, p. 267). What is a more militarily effective value or virtue: brotherhood, comradeship, friendship, or teamwork? (Verweij, 2007; see also Robinson, 2008). Is courage to be moral, to be physical, or both? Is fighting to the death or surrendering courageous? Can an enemy be courageous? Does intention, as Aristotle wrote, have any bearing on evaluating courage? Can one remain loyal to the group while demonstrating courage and integrity sufficient to speak against group actions when those actions violate laws or codes? The reality is, like most virtues and values, courage can be "elusive and mysterious" (Olsthoorn, 2007, p. 276). The interplay of all of these values can make even a professional philosopher dizzy.

Perhaps the most important question remains: are these ethical lessons and/or codes internalized by military members sufficiently to change their minds, let alone their characters? It is unclear whether military recipients internalize any of these codes or approaches to ethics, especially if they conflict with more prevalent cultural influences within the military. How can soldiers weigh such profound and sometimes contradictory demands upon their character, judgment, and behavior in the midst of life-threatening combat? Aristotle would tell us that the developing that ability, known as *phronesis* (practical wisdom or discernment) is crucial to being a good citizen (Robinson, 2007a, 2008). However, "military educators tend to be poor at instilling...*phronesis*" (Robinson, 2008, p. 8). For most militaries, ethical codes that seek to change character and instill virtues and values are aspirational. Unlike a military mission with practical and achievable goals, ethical codes seeking internal changes are a wish list that remains unachievable. They require "critical ethical reflection against a backdrop of so much rote learning and uncritical sloganeering" (Cook, 2008, p. 65).

To find out how soldiers behave outside of the philosophical classroom, or as veterans once the uniform comes off, we must look not only at explicit ethical guidelines, but the deeper, and often unarticulated, military culture and its potent psychological dimension.

Military Culture: The Basics

If all nations' militaries and the individual services within each nation have adopted differing ethical codes, does that not imply that the culture of each service and their respective nations' militaries will likewise differ? Irrespective of differences, what influence does military culture have upon individuals in uniform?

Defining culture is difficult. There exist at least 250 definitions (English, 2004). Being an organization, military culture can be understood in terms of Edgar H. Schein's (1992) widely accepted and helpful definition of organizational culture:

> A pattern of shared basic assumptions that the group learned as it solved its problems of external adaptation and external integration that has worked well enough to be considered valid and, therefore, to be taught to new members as the correct way to perceive, think, or feel in relation to the problems. (p. 12)

First and foremost, we cannot forget that military service is not merely a job or profession; it is a way of life. Central to understanding military culture is to recognize a military's most significant *problem* not faced by any other occupation or profession: how to fight and win wars. Central to fighting and winning wars is the willingness to sacrifice one's life, and the taking of other lives. Certainly, militaries are engaged in other operations such as peacekeeping, domestic and international disaster relief as well as humanitarian operations. However, the principal mandate of the military remains to prepare for and to fight wars (Burk, 2008; Loomis & Lightburn, 1980).

However, in the medical field there is a dearth of research on the nature, forms of inculcation, and effects of military culture, except for limited studies on how military culture contributes to mental health stigma in the military, the transition experience, or mental health problems (Bryan & Morrow, 2011; Haynie & Shepherd, 2011; Smith & True, 2014). Much of our current understanding of the nature and effects of military culture come from sociological studies. Although not focused upon military culture specifically, Schein's (1992) work on organizational culture provides a template that helps us to understand why military ethics may have a limited impact upon the soldier's way of doing things.

Organizational "culture can be analyzed at several different levels, where the term *level* refers to the degree to which the cultural phenomenon is visible to the observer." There are three levels according to Schein. The first, "artifacts… include all the phenomena that one sees, hears, and feels" (Schein, 1992, pp. 16–17). The military is unlike any other culture in this respect as it is replete with artifacts such as uniforms, ranks, badges, medals, parades, salutes, and ceremonies, as well as the multitudinous weapons and equipment of their trades. The second level is that of "espoused values, which predict what people will *say* in a variety of situations but which may be out of line with what they will actually *do* in situations where those values should, in fact, be operating." (Schein, 1992, pp. 20–21, original italics). For example, most if not all Western militaries that allow females in uniform have established codes prohibiting sexual harassment. Yet, in both the United States and Canada, widespread sexual harassment continues, seemingly unabated (Deschamps, 2015; Turchik & Wilson, 2010).

The final level operates deep within the culture are the "values in use" also known as "basic assumptions." These are implicit assumptions that actually guide behavior, that tell group members how to perceive, think about, and feel about things." Basic assumptions "tend to be those we neither confront nor debate and hence are extremely difficult to change" (Schein, 1992, p. 22). As such, they are difficult not only to see, but also participants acting upon them on a daily basis, as well as onlookers, typically cannot articulate basic assumptions. This deeper level is where espoused ethical codes are superseded by the potent beliefs, values, and reflex actions of basic assumptions. In the military, one obvious example is the prevalent ethical code to report wrongdoing and offenses. However, reporting an offense by a unit member, such as sexual harassment or an infraction of an ethical code cannot violate a basic assumption, i.e., that a soldier does not jeopardize group cohesion by *ratting* on another. As a result, infractions and harassment can remain unreported and continue with some degree of impunity. Vehement mistrust of outsiders, another basic assumption, prevents outsiders from investigating infractions, let alone making changes.

Another prevalent, but little researched or debated, conflict exists between the universally espoused military ethic of upholding the values of the society they serve while respecting civilian control and direction of the military. In many militaries, this ethic confronts the basic assumption that military service and its members are morally superior to civilian organizations and civilians in general (Robinson, 2007a). A 2003 survey of American military personnel revealed that two-thirds of those polled "said they think military members have higher moral standards than the nation they serve" (Bacevich, 2005, p. 24). In Canada's military, the worst insult is to be accused of marching like a "civvy" (derogatory term for civilian) being undisciplined like a *civvy*, or being lazy like a *civvy* (Rose, 2015). The Damoclean sword that terrorizes those who wish to remain in the military is the threat to unilaterally expel them as detestable civilians once again.

Certainly, militaries have operated in secretive cultures and environments for national security reasons, and their training and equipment require isolation from civilian societies (Fotion & Elfstrom, 1986). Soldiers are deployed overseas, away from their families, friends, and communities and train to fight an enemy *out there*. This can only serve to further isolate military members from their respective civilian societies and much of the accompanying social innovation and changes that occur therein. We know little as to how this isolation impacts military members' abilities to embrace civilian values. We do know such isolation is key to replacing individual identity with a collective military identity.

The potent sense of belonging to the military family often takes on a far greater priority than the conjugal family. Kraft (2007) is a clinical psychologist who served with the American forces during the Iraq war. She concluded that she "would be unable to function in Iraq if my children stayed at the forefront of my consciousness…I decided I could not be a combat psychologist and mother at the same time. I had to be one or the other" (p. 35). She decided to end communication with her family during her deployment. Further understanding the cultural gap between civilians and military will assist our understanding of this decision, which is unthinkable for most people.

The Civilian-Military Cultural Gap In spite of recent trends to roll back progress in social programs and attitudes, all Western nations have experienced social advancements post-World War II. Militaries likewise have progressed. However, civilian culture has been changing much faster than military culture in "postmodern" nations (Nuciari 2007, p. 226). This gap has widened considerably faster in some nations than others in the past 20 years (Pew Research Center, 2011). All militaries of the post-World War II period have become smaller (Moskos, Williams, & Segal, 2000). In America's case, Andrew Bacevich (2013) refers to an economic elite that profited disproportionally during the latest wars in Iraq and Afghanistan. Concurrently, a relatively small volunteer professional military was used to fight wars of luxury versus wars of necessity. He labels these two groups "the two one-percents" (Bacevich, 2013, p. 40–44). Whereas the economic elite have been "enriching" themselves at the expense of the remaining 99%, the 99% who do not wear a military uniform have likewise benefitted from the sacrifices of the 1% who serve in a small and increasingly isolated military population. Meanwhile, this isolation encourages an apathy in the general public that often fails to understand what soldiers endure on their nation's behalf. As Thompson (2011) writes, "the military community has been drifting away from mainstream American society" (p. 38). One Navy Captain interviewed by Thompson (2011) said, "U.S. political elites didn't view the military so much as part of the greater American society but as their own private army" (p. 39). The result has been a removal of the military from wider civilian democratic decision-making leaving U.S. soldiers to become "the forgotten 1 percent" (Bardenwerper, 2011).

What cultural elements characterize this gap? Military sociologists in Canada noted a growing international awareness, that between nations, militaries shared fundamental commonalities known as the "military way" (Cotton, 1982/3, p. 10). Later, sociological studies indicated "[t]his supranational military culture is more collectivistic, more hierarchy-oriented, and less salary-driven than the average civilian working culture" (Soeters, Poponete, & Page, 2006, p. 16). Notably, this *supranational military culture* allows military members to function in certain situations with international counterparts more easily than military operating with civilians, even from the same country (Soeters et al., 2006, p. 17).

One of the more prominent aspects of military culture is a collectivism that replaces one's individual identity with that of the military institution. Morris Janowitz (1959) noted that in placing immense demands upon soldiers to identify completely with the institution, "[m]ilitary life is, in short, institutional life" (p. 25). Goffman (1961) identified the military as a "total institution" wherein through "a series of abasements, degradations, humiliations, and profanations" the self is "systematically…mortified" resulting in "radical shifts in his *moral career*" (Goffman, 1961, p. 317, original italics). The stripping down and figurative death of the individual's identity makes way for the individual soldier to not only identify with the military institution at large, but also through institutional socialization to identify with "shared norms, values, and beliefs" with "the goal being to create an individual whose conception of self is largely defined by the organization" (Haynie & Shepherd, 2011, p. 503). Ultimately, the individual comes to accept that the highest calling for the military members is the accomplishment of the military's mission. Complete and total identification with the military is reinforced with strict military codes of conduct and immense socialization pressures to conform and perform along with "an obedience to authority that is woven into the service member's identity." The result is that "very little free will remains" (Smith & True, 2014, p. 152). The consequence of this new identification with the *military way* is an impaired ability to identify with the civilian world.

Not only is the *military way* a daily performance of professional duties, the military way is formed at a far deeper level of the soldiers' psychological makeup. Once we understand the powerful tools and how they are used to inculcate the *military way*, we begin to understand the degree and intensity of the civil-military gap, as well as the difficulty soldiers may have in accessing an identity separate from the collective institutional identity, a phenomenon that can endure long after serving soldiers become veterans.

Psychological Demands of Modern Militaries

As early as 1920, a Canadian researcher into rehabilitation of military members noted "[m]ilitarization almost ranked as a disability itself." (Segsworth, 1920, p. 67). Later, American sociologist Willard Waller (1944) wrote, "Every Veteran Is at least Mildly Shell-Shocked" as a chapter title to his ground-breaking book, *The Veteran Comes Back* (p. 115). Modern psychiatry and psychology have led many of us to believe that only a minority of military members ever suffer such psychological conditions. However, neither Segsworth nor Waller were talking necessarily about diagnoses that met a clinical threshold, but a marked tendency of many military members to suffer subthreshold conditions that may not qualify for a clinical diagnosis, but that nevertheless prevented optimal reintegration into civilian society.

However tempting, we cannot dismiss such views merely because they were written almost a century ago. The psychological demands of military service in an advanced technological age require not only more education but also greater psychological pressures and stresses. Whereas pre-1950s era militaries used external "arbitrary, informal methods of punishment" to instill discipline (Capstick, 2003, p. 51), post-modern militaries have moved toward encouraging self-discipline through "greater reliance on manipulation, persuasion, and group consensus" (Janowitz, 1960, p. 8). Soldiers in modern warfare must often operate independently; fulfilling the military mission, without the supportive group cohesion or the physical presence of authoritarian leadership relied upon in previous times. As such, modern militaries are placing greater psychological demands upon individuals to more deeply internalize the military culture, while simultaneously suppressing individual will and needs.

The ethical bible of the Canadian Forces, *Duty with Honour*, emphasizes;

> Discipline among professionals is fundamentally self-discipline that facilitates immediate and willing obedience to lawful orders and directives while strengthening individuals to cope with the demands and stresses of operations. It instils self-assurance and resiliency in the face of adversity and builds self-control. (*Duty*, 2003, p. 27)

Such internal discipline is only possible when one has a powerful sense of group belonging that transcends the psychologically immense time and distance of modern battlefields. The emphasis upon internal discipline is not unique to Canada and has been increasingly emphasized among all Western militaries over the past six decades (Janowitz, 1960).

To instill self-discipline, the military employs powerful indoctrination and socialization techniques to ensure the institutional goals become intertwined with and inseparable from one's individual identity. Indoctrination is synonymous with brainwashing (Farber, Harlow, & West, 1957). There is little difference between the techniques used in ideological cult-like indoctrination, and military indoctrination except the military instills "more traditionally accepted standards of conduct and socially accepted values" (McGurk, Cotting, Britt, & Adler, 2006, p. 15).

Military indoctrination is, in short, an "*intensely extreme form of persuasion*" (Bruyea, 2011, original italics) that convinces civilians volunteering for military service to "engage in behaviors that represent a radical departure from their prior experiences and worldview" (McGurk et al., 2006, p. 15). The two most important *behaviors* demanded of military service are: "(1) killing someone else in the service of a mission to protect one's country, and (2) the willingness to subordinate self-interests, including survival, in the service of group goals" (McGurk et al., 2006, p. 15).

Perhaps the most popularly known vehicle for indoctrination tools utilized by the military is that of basic training or *boot camp*. Sleep deprivation, disorientation, constant bombardment of the military's demands and expectations, demanding physical regimens, repetitive activities, compressed time schedules, as well as strict and comprehensive codes of dress and deportment are part of the "information over-load" and immense stressors placed upon every military member during this initial boot camp stage (Baron, 2000, pp. 241–7). The goal is an "assault on an individual's attitudes, beliefs, and values" (Baron, 2000, p. 241) while separating him or her from "previous achievement, family, and individuality" (McGurk et al., 2006, p. 19). The goal is to replace these parts of the individual with the military family, its expectations, values, status, and standards.

Immense peer pressure and other socialization techniques are used to reinforce the military's expectations. Modern militaries do not necessarily need to use the proverbial abusive Drill Sergeant as even polite and "more subtle procedures…pre-pare individuals for effective indoctrination" (Baron, 2000, p. 241). Not surprisingly, "stereotypical depiction of nonmembers as evil or misguided" as well as inculcation of a "messianic group purpose" (Baron, 2000, p. 241) such as defending a nation's honor, values, constitution, etc., solidify the self-identification of the reformed civilian as a full-fledged military member.

It would be a mistake to think such pressures are exerted only during basic train-ing. Less overt or extreme measures can follow basic training, further reinforcing initial indoctrination. The often-isolated work environments away from civilians and being dressed markedly different from civilians solidify the soldier's attach-ment to the military. Unique and often oppressive military disciplinary codes that punish infractions of dress, deportment, and socialization would be unthinkable in a civilian world. Symbols of achievement such as medals, badges, and unit honors for participating in battles and wars underscore a sense of belonging while internal-izing a military identity replete with military expectations. One Canadian woman observed profound changes in her air force spouse during peacetime pilot training:

> And when I first met Pete, I said to him one day, "Could you fly over a village and bomb?" 'Cause I'm kind of a peacenik. … And he said to me, "No, I couldn't do that." And about midway through fighter weapons school, I noticed this wall—not towards me or towards anybody—but I noticed something changing. And he was becoming this fighting machine. And I don't know how they did it, but they did it. And I said to him, "Could you fly over a village and bomb?" He said, "If I was ordered to, yes." That cold and simple. And I went, "My God, what have I married?" (Harrison & Laliberté, 1994, p. 20)

Even in peacetime, military members are subjected to constant messaging and rhet-oric from peers as well as in the forms of orders, ethical codes, codes of honor, mission goals, regulations, voluminous operational procedures, exercises, multiple career-long training courses with role-playing, etc. This is all enforced by the threat of exclusion and exile from the highly interdependent military community, where even questioning of how things are done can invite social condemnation of being disloyal or even traitorous. The result is "profound changes to internal psychology and cognitive processing" consequentially resulting in changes to "perceptions, atti-tudes, and beliefs" of the soldier (Bruyea, 2016, p. 72). Smith and True (2014) observed that in the United States military "high levels of social integration, regi-mentation and social control" strip each military member of "his or her individuality and agency" (p. 152). In this environment "attitudes and beliefs …become solidi-fied, more extreme over time, integrated into other aspects of self and, as a result, relatively impervious to change" (Baron, 2000, p. 245); this transformation can last long after the soldier leaves the military to return to civilian life as a veteran.

It would, however, be glib to assume that today's military members and veterans are not highly resourceful and intelligent. Popular culture, including mental health professionals, "think that the military turns previously free-thinking people into aggressive, unthinking automatons with crew cuts: [s]uch misunderstandings have potentially negative effects on the process of psychotherapy and can leave a service member feeling isolated and misunderstood." (Christian, Stivers, & Sammons, 2009, p. 31). Military members may not be automatons, but there is much automatic, and polarized thinking that may not mesh with the civilian world, let alone mindfulness practices. Thus, any mindfulness program that is to be complementary or assistive to military members has these above-mentioned obstacles to overcome. How will these profound internal changes in soldiers and veterans complement or collide with mindfulness practices? Can mindfulness provide opportunity for soldiers and veterans to see the world once again as a civilian?

Mindfulness and the Military: Complement or Collision

Military Mindfulness: An Oxymoron?

Mindfulness in the military context has been frequently categorized as one of a number of meditative practices "which induce a state of consciousness enabling increased focus, increased awareness, and deep relaxation" (Elwy, Johnston, Bormann, Hull, & Taylor, 2014, p. S76). Much of the research into and application of mindfulness in the military context has been in response to the "high incidence of post-traumatic stress disorder (PTSD), suicides, and other adverse events" from soldiers returning from operations in Iraq and Afghanistan (Rees, 2011, p. 1232) as well as attempts to enhance resilience by building mental fitness for possible future exposure to traumatic situations (Rothschild, Kaplan, Golan, & Barak, 2017). Nevertheless, the use of meditation in the military has been referred to as an "oxymoron" (Rock, 2009). Are mindfulness techniques antithetical to military culture and practices? Or does there exist some common ground between the two?

Much attention has been directed at the U.S. military adoption of mindfulness, termed "Warrior Mind Training" or "Samurai Mind Training" (Rochman, 2009). At first glance, the Samurai image may seem appropriate. Popular perception would have us believe that Samurai warriors were devout practitioners a mindful-like meditative practice. Unfortunately, this popular perception is based largely on a myth (Benesch, 2016) that accompanied a nationalistic reaction to the disempowerment of the Samurai warrior class in the late nineteenth century. Ironically, the template for a reawakened Japan-centric Samurai warrior image was to model Western feudal virtues of the knighthood and nobility such as the "English conceptions of the gentleman" (Benesch, 2016, p. 9). There is little indication that Samurai warriors were any more mindful than modern professional militaries because Samurai, like their modern professional counterparts, sought to suppress the self by "controlling unconscious emotional functions" (Ohnishi & Ohnishi, 2009, p. 177), not to be mindful of them. The creators of the "Warrior Mind Training" chose the "mythic Japanese fighter…after careful deliberation" as "it was certifiably anti-sissy" (Rochman, 2009).

The provenance of popular perceptions must be considered when attempting to import practices into the military setting without evaluating their efficacy or suitability to the unique nature of military cultures. Given the immense stress of military service and combat as well as the psychologically and morally charged demands of sacrificing and taking lives, *careful deliberation* should employ more than superficial marketing techniques and hasty experimentation which seek to minimize offending military members. Based upon the work of former American Psychological Association (APA) president, Martin Seligman and others (Eidelson, 2011), the United States military has implemented a model of resilience-building, which also includes funding to study and potentially incorporate mindfulness training, for more than 1.1 million soldiers largely as an experiment carried out during regular military training without having conducted any randomized controlled trials (Eidelson, 2011; Lester, McBride, Bliese, & Adler, 2011; Purser, 2014; Senauke, 2016). If mindfulness is to be implemented in the military or veteran setting, it would be beneficial for practitioners and military to anticipate possible interactions of mindfulness practices and culture with military culture and practices.

Military Practices Complementary to Mindfulness?

On a more grounded basis (versus myth-perpetuating and rashly considered), mindfulness and the military do have certain similar approaches. Let us return to John Kabat-Zinn's (2005) definition of mindfulness practice: "the awareness that arises from paying attention, on purpose, in the present moment, and non-judgmentally" (p. 180). As discussed, this definition contains both explicit and implicit guidelines for the practice of mindfulness. How do the explicit guidelines interact with military culture and practices?

Mindfulness in requiring the focusing of attention upon something stable, in the present moment, is not unlike the demands placed upon the individual soldier. Recruits are constantly drilled to focus upon marching, deportment, standing at attention, all while not letting the mind wander. It is not a coincidence that the first guideline for mindfulness practice, *paying attention*, is also one of the first practices of military training, *standing at attention*. Most practices, including those in the military setting, requiring concentration or the focusing of the mind also require the mind *pay attention*.

The purpose of focusing the military mind and body through practices such as standing at attention is to train the military mind to *pay attention* to the task at hand and not let the mind become distracted. An unfocused mind in the military can translate into careless practices that can lead to serious injury, loss of life, and/or mission failure. Aircrews working with jet engines must be highly vigilant, a form of mindfulness, to not leave tools scattered about or be careless with any objects lest these be ingested into the engine. Squadron personnel are regularly called upon to walk hangar aprons, taxi-ways, and runways to search for debris to prevent FOD (foreign object damage) to jet engines. Sailors are constantly and regularly drilled to be ever mindful of anything or any situation that may initiate a fire onboard. Such fires can be devastating in their rapid spread and degree of destruction. Army soldiers must be highly focused on patrol or when operating complex modern equipment or even simple, yet lethal, firearms. A commonly cited example of mechanically interpreted mindful practice is the controlled yet relaxed breathing techniques utilized by all riflemen, but especially for snipers (Amaro, 2015; Monteiro et al., 2015; Purser, 2014) attempting to *neutralize a target*.

Given the mission-oriented culture of the military, *paying attention* is a decidedly conscious function, a parallel to "an intention to pay attention" in mindfulness practice (Monteiro & Musten, 2013, p. 27). As such, paying attention in the military is clearly *on purpose*. As discussed, *on purpose* for Kabat-Zinn (1990) would come to include "some kind of personal vision" (p. 46). The military institution replaces one's personal identity, beliefs, and goals with the institutional identity, beliefs, and goals. For military members, on a deeply personal level, mission accomplishment, while protecting their peers with their lives, is the most important personal goal. This institutional goal becomes the *personal vision* for most, if not all, soldiers in whatever role they are assigned. Powerful socialization enforced by the vigilance of authorities and peers are ever-present and develop a "unanimous group consensus" (Baron, 2000, p. 245). This environment reinforces the internalization of the institutional goals as *personal vision*.

Due to complex weapon technology, constantly changing nature of the battlefield, unpredictability of the enemy, and/or the life and death implications of each and every soldier's action, military operations require an ongoing, constant, and highly disciplined *awareness* of one's environment unlike any other employment or profession. The military places great emphasis on "situational awareness" in the military role (Jha et al., 2015, 2017; Stanley & Jha, 2009). The rote learning and constant reinforcement of skills, tasks, goals, and unit cohesion through training and exercise develops quick reflexive reactions and rapid processing of information through cognitive shortcuts known as heuristic processing (Gigerenzer & Gaissmaier, 2011; Giner-Sorolla & Chaiken, 1997). This heuristic processing bypasses the more complex mental pathways (Giner-Sorolla & Chaiken, 1997) developing mechanical reactions that can be free of judgment.

The *fog of war,* its accompanying unknowns, the uncertainty as to how one's capability and intent will interact with the enemy's capability and intent as well as other confounding environmental factors have long characterized military operations. Militaries have compensated for these unknown's by ensuring the *knowns* are controlled. Training, attention to detail and precision, rote learning, role-playing, exercises, and more training are what the military can control. When many actions and reactions can become instinctual or reflexive, then the military can devote attentional resources to being aware of the battlefield, the enemy, and the environment. This all contributes to mission success while hopefully minimizing friendly losses. Thus, the military *appears* to fit criteria for a mechanically mindful organization. Military operations demand that all soldiers develop an acute and astute *awareness* by *paying attention* in a *most purposeful manner*, by focusing, without life-threatening or other distractions, *in the present moment* in an automatic, potentially *non-judgmental*, manner.

Mindfulness and Military Minefields: Clash of Cultures

The above comparison of military culture and practices to Kabat-Zinn's (2005) definition is clearly a minimalist and rather mechanical template for mindfulness. This minimalist approach to mindfulness appears to establish the basis for mindfulness programs created for the military (Jha et al., 2015; Stanley & Jha, 2009). The main goal in Jha et al.'s (2015) study is to promote a "*mind 'at attention'*" (Introduction, para. 1, original italics) in order to reduce "mind wandering" and "attentional lapses" so as to ultimately "protect against associated performance costs" (last para.). The second study (Stanley & Jha, 2009) introduces mindfulness to "promote resilience against stress and trauma so that warriors can execute their missions more effectively" (para. 4), a form of "mental armour" to "enhance warrior performance" so that "warriors will be ready, willing, and able to deploy again when needed" (last para.).

Kabat-Zinn (2011), intended mindfulness to be accessible "as commonsensical, evidence-based, and ordinary, and ultimately a legitimate element of mainstream medical care" (p. 282). He avoided concise, definitive, or comprehensive definitions. Rather he provided "*operational* definitions" (original italics) that did not seek "absolute accord" with "classical teaching" (p. 291). However, his intention was not to limit mindfulness to these sanitized *operational* definitions. Mindfulness was always intended to be a rich, multi-contextual, and evolving experience, as testified by Kabat-Zinn's (2011) assertion that his "entire" 600 plus page book, *Full Catastrophe Living* is, "in some sense…a definition of mindfulness" (p. 291).

Those implementing mindfulness with a more mechanical approach that principally serves institutional goals may respond with a collective, *so what?* If mindfulness, even in its most minimalist form, benefits someone or something (and there is no policing such limited interpretations), then why not provide mindfulness to the military, thereby, indirectly or directly benefitting soldiers and veterans? Baer (2015) claims that "mindfulness is inherently ethical" and that mindfulness teachers "are bound by professional codes" (p. 958). However, resilience-building programs that already, or will come to, include mindfulness are not necessarily being introduced by medical professionals, but instead by "non-commissioned officers who are required to serve as 'Master Resilience Trainers'" (Eidelson, 2011, para. 7). Non-commissioned officers are rarely, if ever certified, medical professionals.

The American Psychological Association (APA) (2011) stipulates a "competency benchmark" that could guide the introduction of mindfulness into the military setting in a less minimalist manner. The second component of "Professionalism," titled "Individual and Cultural Sensitivity" requires "awareness, sensitivity and skills in working professionally with diverse individuals, groups and communities who represent various cultural and personal background and characteristics defined broadly." Psychologists are required to recognize "Others as Shaped by Individual and Cultural Diversity and Context" (APA, 2011, p. 2). However, mindfulness practitioners may see culture as having a purely ethnic origin and may see military culture as merely unique working conditions. A United States Veterans Administration (VA) resource seeks to address the need for mindfulness practitioners to understand military culture. Although this resource guide was limited to treatment of retired military, the book interprets culture principally through the perspective of the complex medical conditions suffered by veterans, especially those suffering PTSD. The resource guide noted that veterans did "express the desire for mindfulness teachers who have a better understanding of Veteran culture" (Kearney et al., 2015, p. 88). What veteran practitioners meant by culture is not made entirely clear, nevertheless this oversight can constitute an obstacle to teaching mindfulness in the military and veteran context. Other obstacles are discussed next.

Military Barriers to Mindfulness

Service Before Self That the VA resource overlooked salient features of veteran culture is not surprising due to the above noted dearth of scientific research in this area. One particularly challenging aspect of military culture poses difficult to surmount obstacles to the teaching and practice of mindfulness: subjugation of the self. In Robinson, De Lee, and Carrick's (2008) study of international military ethics, the subjugation of the individual to the military's goals, beliefs, and expectations is universally required in the various militaries studied. Subjugation of the self is the one ethic that is solidly established in both *espoused values* as well as the deeper subconscious construct of *basic assumptions*. A deeper analysis of espoused military virtues reveals the following all require subjugation of the self: "loyalty," "duty," "responsibility," "discipline," "solidarity," "professionalism," "fraternity," "teamwork," " can do' attitude," "humility," "unity," "unselfishness," "cheerfulness," "selfless commitment," and "service before self" (Robinson, 2008, p. 7).

Suppression of the self through obedience, loyalty, etc., is universally inculcated and socialized at a deep cultural and individual psychological level. Both the British and the Canadian military enshrine sacrifice of the self to all things military in the concept of "unlimited liability" (Mileham, 2010), a term coined by General Sir John Hackett in 1983. Canada has taken this retrospective and prospective ethical commandment to heart, perhaps more than any other nation (Mileham, 2010). "Unlimited liability and service before self" (*Duty*, 2003, p. 20) requires that all military members place the mission first, their fellow soldiers second, and their personal needs last. Like Britain, Canada views unlimited liability as a one-way contract completely subjugating the life of the soldier to the service of the state without any reciprocal contract stipulating legal duties of the state toward the individual soldier. All other nations studied in Robinson et al.'s book (2008), although perhaps not professing so explicitly blatant an ownership of the soldier's life, operate very similarly at the basic assumption level: selfless service is deeply indoctrinated at all stages of military service (Bruyea, 2016).

Haynie and Shepherd's (2011) study of wounded American Marines leaving the military noted that "while such extreme socialization serves the needs of a combat force, it is mutually exclusive with the development of a strong sense of 'individual self'" (p. 504). This phenomenon was common to all soldiers studied, irrespective of individual differences. These "dimensions of military identity…conflict with many dimensions of an integrated civilian identity" (Smith & True, 2014, p. 153) and, as noted above, are extremely resistant to change.

Subjugation of the self is perhaps mindfulness' greatest obstacle and challenge when dealing with military personnel and veterans. How does an individual soldier pay attention to the feelings, sensations, and thoughts that arise within, when the most powerful socially acceptable indoctrination and socialization tools have been imposed from without, often 24 h a day and throughout one's military career to thoroughly suppress and diminish the importance of all that is the *self* that does not serve or contribute to the military's goal?

In general, warrior cultures with their focus upon strength, discipline, self-sacrifice, courage, can-do, or *cheerfulness* attitudes, already "clash" with mental health cultures, which "tend to talk almost exclusively in clinical language of 'disordered' behavior associated with illness" (Bryan & Morrow, 2011, p. 17). Surely then, warrior cultures similarly would clash with mindfulness practices with their language of compassion, non-judgment, feelings, sensations, acceptance, "tranquil heart" (Hanh, 1976), "loving kindness" (Monteiro & Musten, 2013), or "loving friendliness" (Gunaratana, 2015) meditations, and "spontaneous compassion toward others and toward oneself" (Kabat-Zinn, 2011, p. 293).

Placing oneself first is repugnant for most soldiers with "obedience to authority…woven into the service member's identity" (Smith & True, 2014, p. 152). There also exists a "pervasive mental health stigma among military personnel" (Bryan & Morrow, 2011, p. 16), while military culture discourages self-advocacy (Smith & True, 2014). Meanwhile, soldiers are required to self-report their need for mental health services (Smith & True, 2014). How can soldiers or veterans seek out mindfulness or other mental health services when soldiers deeply identify with values of strength, stoicism, and self-denial, as well as with a culture that comprehensively discourages identification and expression of self-needs? If they do enter a mindfulness course, how difficult will *paying attention* to themselves be, let alone developing the *awareness* of the multifaceted nature of their humanness? One journalist in Iraq observed the common process soldiers employed to prepare for combat in an account of behavior immediately before a battle: "It's best to shut down, to block everything out. But to reach that state, you must almost give up being yourself" (Smith & True, 2014, p. 154). To do otherwise could jeopardize themselves, but more importantly, failure to suppress one's own feelings, needs, and awareness could result in the deaths of their comrades, or equally abhorrent for the soldier and the military, mission failure.

Mindfulness and "Tyranny of the Mission" Anticipating enemy intentions and actions, protecting fellow soldiers, and awaiting orders are constant companions to the ultimate goal: mission success. Some have referred to this as "tyranny of the mission" (Axinn, 2009, p. 63). Soldiers may develop keen survival instincts through situational awareness, but such awareness is single-mindedly focused upon the mission, often to the exclusion of all else. Training and battlefields may unfold moment-to-moment, but soldiers' awareness is thoroughly goal-oriented. Practitioners of mindfulness, from the "very beginning," are encouraged to "let go of their expectations, goals, and aspirations for coming" to mindfulness practice and "to simply 'drop in' on the actuality of their lived experience and then to sustain it as best they can moment by moment" (Kabat-Zinn, 2003, p. 148). Of course, it is common for individuals to come to mindfulness with agendas and goals. Kabat-Zinn (2003) asks "how will a teacher skillfully reconcile their motivation to achieve these perfectly sensible goals with the orientation of nonstriving, nondoing, and letting go that must inform the meditation practice and the entire program if it is to be mindfulness?" (p. 150).

For soldiers and veterans, how can teachers help them break thorough the deeply socialized and indoctrinated need to see the world in terms of threats, situational awareness, mission accomplishment, and a tireless vigilance that sees life and death implications in the most benign situations? One Canadian Forces veteran summarized a common difficulty with letting go in the civilian world: "There was just an overwhelming sense that nothing mattered. Either nothing mattered or everything mattered way too much" (Rose, 2015, p. 71). Such typically polarized thinking thoroughly developed through the military experience presents a tragic interpersonal obstacle, but also an opportunity for teachers to guide the soldier or veteran in developing *awareness, moment by moment.*

Nonjudgment and Distortions of Connectedness Smelling the roses or appreciating the moment appears an impossible goal for soldiers and veterans. Thich Nhat Hanh (1976) describes one of his walking meditations: "I like to walk alone on country paths, rice plants, and wild grasses on both sides, putting each foot down on the earth in mindfulness, knowing that I walk on the wondrous earth" (p. 12). Living in the moment non-judgmentally and feeling connected with one's environment can be anathema to soldiers who view the environment in life-threatening or mission-enhancing terms. Judgment of the outside world has long been taught as a survival mechanism to not only distinguish friend from foe, but also how to use the surrounding environment to diminish or deny the effectiveness of the enemy while enhancing one's ability to defend oneself or multiply the effectiveness of one's resources against the enemy.

Forever spoiled is the unjudging appreciation of one's environment. Valleys no longer become beautiful green sanctuaries with heart stopping vistas, but killing zones to concentrate fire upon the enemy. Pastoral or tropical island paradises become obstacle courses in which to play cat and mouse with ships and submarines, while attacking from the sun and clouds can optimize fighter jet effectiveness. Quaint and meandering urban alleyways can conceal an ambush; any road can harbor an improvised explosive device. Training and combat that necessitates automatic reflexes optimize survival in war but also such reflexes are persistent and, therefore difficult to shake. Soldiers become deeply connected to their environment, but not in a manner that allows them to appreciate the environment on its own terms.

Kabat-Zinn (2013) tells us that "at its core, mindfulness is about relationality" and that "when you feel connected to something, that connection immediately gives you a purpose for living" (p. 271). The military also fosters a form of connection through deep bonding among soldiers and within military units. Cohesion (group bonding) is fundamental to military culture (Burk, 2008). Indoctrination reinforces this cohesion by fostering close in-group identification among military members, while fomenting deep mistrust of out-group members (McGurk et al., 2006).

Since civilians are widely mistrusted, and soldiers can find it difficult to open up to uniformed practitioners, building therapeutic alliances is problematic: veterans view civilians with "suspicion and distrust" (Bryan & Morrow, 2011, p. 17) and perceive them "as being naïve, misinformed, or even worse, judgmental" (Smith & True, 2014, p. 155). Yet mindfulness is practiced in a group setting involving open dialogue (Kabat-Zinn, 2011). If group members are military or veterans, then military culture can loom large, potentially inhibiting open sharing and dialogue. Similar inhibition can be expected when soldier and veteran practitioners guide military groups. Considering the deeply inculcated subjugation to authority, especially if it wears a uniform, a mistrust of all that is non-military, and a powerful repression of the self, reaching the "connectedness and interconnectedness of mindfulness" (Kabat-Zinn, 2013, p. 271) appears impossible:

> When people are willing to communicate with honesty and candor, and at the same time with mutual respect, an exchange of perspectives can take place that may lead to new ways of seeing and being together for the people involved. We are capable of communicating far more than fear and insecurity to each other when our emotions become part of the legitimate scope of our awareness. (Kabat-Zinn, 2013, p. 480)

Deep distrust of civilians by military, and misunderstandings of the military by civilian practitioners, can complicate or hinder therapeutic progress. Practitioners, however, can develop "credibility" (and therefore connectedness) with culturally different clientele by understanding their worldviews (Sue, 1981). Importantly, therapists would benefit by understanding how military culture fosters perturbations in concepts otherwise understood differently outside of the military experience.

Soldiers have long confused friendship with comradeship: "Veterans try to regain such feelings [stemming from comradeship], but they fall short" (Hedges, 2003, p. 116). Friendship takes work, unlike comradeship where "[t]here are fewer demands if we join the crowd and give our emotions over to the communal crusade" (Hedges, 2003, p. 116). Friendship is integral to moral life and encourages moral growth (Wadell, 1989), whereas the "ecstatic" nature of comradeship does not seek moral growth but leaves comrades to "rest on their emotional bliss" (Gray, 1998, pp. 90–91). This persistent misconception by military culture of comradeship as friendship coupled with military distrust of civilians can lead veterans to frequently report struggling with developing friendships outside the military (Black, 2007). Intense, ecstatic relationships formed in a military world, cannot be replicated in any other environment. The veteran can be left with a sense of a gaping loss after leaving a distorted notion of interconnectedness inherent in the *military family*. The consequence of which leaves veterans feeling civilian life has let them down, leaving them disconnected from the very society for which they were willing to sacrifice their lives.

The disconnectedness inculcated by military authority and reinforced by the horrors of combat, can be replaced by the intimate process of developing mutually respectful interconnected friendships that allow individuals to be themselves. This is a difficult task for many veterans, but developing true friendships is critical to successful civilian integration (Haynie & Shepherd, 2011; Rose, 2015; Smith & True, 2014). Nonetheless, mindfulness, incompatible with many areas of military practices and culture, offers hope. Interconnected and interdependent notions of friendship are not unlike the precepts of mindfulness, which accepts others as they are without forcing them into a mission-goal, friendly enemy, insider–outsider highly polarized template for life.

Non-Judgment and Killing A military exists, predominantly, to fight wars. To fight wars, soldiers must be taught to overcome "an inherent reluctance to kill" through indoctrination and socialization techniques that "shape attitudes toward killing" (McGurk et al., 2006, p. 21). The goal is to develop a reflexive response to kill, "without hesitation," on command (Moore, Hopewell, & Grossman, 2009, p. 310). This training is so deeply ingrained through processes that, like learning "how to ride a bike," are "virtually resistant to decay" (Moore et al., 2009, p. 320). Obedience, immense socialization pressures, suppression of self, and comprehensive *artifacts*, *espoused values*, and *basic assumptions* constantly reinforce one's subjugation to the military collective that "ritualize the violence of war" (Snider, 1999, p. 15). Ultimately, these complex and comprehensive normative guidelines in turn reinforce "discipline [which] reassures soldiers in combat and defines when and how they are 'authorized' to violate the normal societal prohibitions against killing and violence" (Snider, 1999, p. 15). In doing so, they overcome the "universal human phobia [to] *interpersonal human aggression*" (Moore et al., 2009, p. 309, original italics).

In this context, there appears little room for mindfulness to coexist with the operational military world other than in a perverted, *denatured* form that may increase survivability, but also allows further psychological and moral burdens placed upon soldiers to more efficiently and repeatedly carry out the military mission, and potentially *neutralize* more targets.

Can we claim a practice that further detaches soldiers from their moral selves or places additionally unthinkable moral burdens as some form of mindfulness? In the context of mindfulness practice, non-judgment is neither robotic nor is it ever "mechanical" (Kabat-Zinn, 2003, p. 148). As noted above, non-judgment has been variously interpreted as including concepts of acceptance, curiosity, generosity, gentleness with oneself, openness, kindness, respect for our mortality, empathy, gratitude, loving-kindness, patience, and compassion. Most, if not all, of these concepts cannot be found in either espoused military ethics or the more subconscious world of military culture's basic assumptions. Having said that, Israel is the only nation of nine studied (Kasher, 2008; Robinson, 2008) that includes a mindful-admirable virtue required of its military: "respect for human life." Nonetheless, military service deeply inculcates a "black-and-white, dichotomized framework of enemy/ally, superior/subordinate" that is fundamentally at odds "with a more autonomous, even anomic, civilian identity" (Smith & True, 2014, p. 158). This polarized *Weltanschauung* is not only anathema to the "intrinsic relationality" of relationships encouraged by mindfulness practice (Kabat-Zinn, 2013, p. 480), it is also anathema to mindfulness *non-judgment* in all but its most mechanical, minimalist connotations.

Unintended Consequences of (Mis)using Mindfulness Increasing the capacity of soldiers to deploy on more missions than they would have been otherwise capable and thereby engage in more combat (and ostensibly more killing) raises fundamental moral questions. In this light, the U.S. military, featuring the Samurai myth as the macho mascot for its mindfulness program to build resilience and effectiveness in soldiers, has some ironic implications. The Samurai myth led to Japan's coopting of Japanese Buddhist Zen teachers and schools to participate in the "appropriation" and distortion of Zen for "narrow societal (and especially military) ends" that contributed prominently in "concocting a witch's brew of violent nationalism" (Senauke, 2016, p. 77). The result was a half-century of aggressive military expansionism and war atrocities rivaling the horrors of World War II Europe. As ethicist Daniel Dwyer (2003) points out, "spiritual development does not necessarily go hand in hand with moral development" (p. 64). The current-day employment of mindfulness in the military context to optimize the efficacy and availability of the soldier resource is in direct opposition to developing not just a moral, but a mindful and aware military. Mindfulness teachers of military personnel, should be, if they are not already, facing the ethical dilemma of *dual-use* similar to the moral issues arising in neuroscience where drugs are being weaponized; that is, used to push the physical limits of soldiers in "maintaining alertness", "combating fatigue", and "improving cognitive functions" (Tracey & Flower, 2014).

There is a growing awareness that the psychological cost of combat, and potentially military service in general, can extend beyond the commonly accepted clinical diagnoses of PTSD and depression. Moral injury has received growing attention thanks to the pioneering work of individuals like psychiatrist Jonathon Shay (2002). Moral injury has been defined as "Perpetrating, failing to prevent, bearing witness to, or learning about acts that transgress deeply held moral beliefs and expectations" (Litz et al., 2009, p. 700). More recently, Andrew Bacevich (2013) has captured moral injury in the umbrella concept of "*Breach of Trust*" as the title of his book. Even those who do not meet a clinical threshold of PTSD can suffer the debilitating effects of moral injury. Those who do not kill, because of the military collective identity, can suffer the same burdens of those who do kill (Grossman, 2009). Moral injury has been under-studied but as one soldier notes "It's the moral injury over time that really kills people. Soldiers lose their identity. They don't understand who they are anymore" (Sherman, 2015, p. 7). Edward Tick (2014), psychiatrist and founder of the non-profit organization, *Soldiers Heart*, argues that the "wounding" from moral injury "can be so painful and disillusioning that it leads to the veteran's loss of the will to live and can even haunt a veteran on his deathbed" (p. 121).

When we use mindfulness to pursue goals that, even if intended to increase survivability in the modern battlefield, but that nevertheless result in a further distancing of soldiers from themselves, are we complicit in worsening the longer term moral and psychological burden of soldiers that already endure far too much? Since we are all interconnected and soldiers serve and die at our whim, are we all not complicit in pushing their limits beyond the soldier's humanity?

Military ethics has experienced a fierce debate as to whether there are *just wars*. "Wars are rarely just" and that "'the myth of the just war' is that if we believe that war is easily justified, we will tend to fight more wars" (Fiala, 2010). The employment of pharmacology and eventually mindfulness to create more capable soldiers that can deploy more frequently feeds directly into the facile justification to fight more wars, almost always at the expense of soldiers. Having an isolated, professional, and highly capable fighting force that can be deployed frequently to combat missions due to the maximal optimization of each soldier's capability to give more of themselves for us, is a chilling and morally repugnant prospect. It also contravenes the medical and psychological professions' promise to do no harm. Military has long been a laboratory for medical and social testing despite such international prohibitions of testing without informed consent like the Nuremburg Code (Boyce, 2009). The costs of such experimentation, not to mention the killing and sacrifice required, may not be evident upfront, but what is not paid upfront, will manifest in the further disconnection of soldiers from themselves and society. Moral injury may be the least of the soldier's suffering and mindfulness may be at a loss to reconnect them.

Is There a Place for Mindfulness and the Military to Coexist?

If mindfulness is fundamentally at odds with military ethics and culture, in all but the most minimalist application of John Kabat-Zinn's widely accepted operational definition, can mindfulness find some place in the military and veteran community? Mindfulness measures "may be useful for identifying soldiers at risk and resilient for post-deployment psychological distress" (Call, Pitcock, & Pyne, 2015, p. 1304). Mindfulness has been employed in protocols to treat PTSD with at least one study demonstrating mindfulness' efficacy, at a biological level, in treating PTSD while other studies have shown the effectiveness of mindfulness in addressing pain and physiological stress that co-occurs with PTSD (Bergen-Cico, Possemato, & Pigeon,

2014). Mindfulness-Based Stress Reduction (MBSR) is employed by the United States Veterans Administration to assist veterans who are not necessarily suffering PTSD or any other psychological or physical ailment. Those who seek out MBSR are typically "older," in their forties, fifties, or sixties, with younger veterans dropping out at a higher rate (Kearney et al., 2015).

We can hypothesize that once the veteran has achieved distance and time from the powerful influences of military culture, then individual autonomy has an opportunity to emerge. Younger veterans still heavily influenced by military culture could be repelled by the contrary culture of mindfulness practice. Interestingly, "older Veterans also seem prepared to work with an acceptance-based approach" since they have "experienced firsthand the limitations of attempts to suppress or avoid chronic symptoms, coupled with the realization that personal growth and healing are often slow processes that require some effort." (Kearney et al., 2015, pp. 5–6).

The older veterans' realizations also correspond with broader intentions of mindfulness including "discernment, wise action, or wisdom" (Monteiro et al., 2015, p. 3). Kabat-Zinn (2003) emphasizes the "universal qualities of being human" as being "wakefulness, compassion, and wisdom" (p. 283). Older veterans who have faced chronic illness and endured much suffering perhaps have woken up sufficiently from the military indoctrinated sleep to be more accepting of themselves and the world. The question for many ethicists and a growing number of mindfulness teachers is how to wake up the military. Perhaps not so coincidentally, military ethical codes, however unsuccessful at having their virtues internalized, along with mindfulness seek similar goals: *phronesis*, a practical wisdom or discernment (Robinson, 2007a, 2008). Timothy Challans (2007), in his scathing dissection of the ethical hypocrisy and distortions of humanity in current military culture and practices, calls for the "Awakening Warrior" to become aware in a "fully reflective life." Van Gordon et al. (2015), in noting that current mindfulness practices in the military are "something other than mindfulness," also call for awakening:

> In such an uncertain and arguably hostile economic and political global climate, rather than refuse to introduce responsible military leaders to the principles of mindful awareness, we argue that a more rational solution is to deploy military personnel and leaders that are fully aware of the consequences of their thoughts, words, and actions and who carry out their role with wisdom and compassion. (p. 53)

Given what we know about military's intractable culture, which is highly resistant to change, along with the correspondingly resultant persistent and profound changes upon each and every soldier, such calls are optimistic at best. Nevertheless, such calls are necessary pressures that must be exerted to ensure that we do not segregate and marginalize one segment of our humanity to serve our purposes. We need something more than ethical codes or attempts to resurrect the quasi myths of the Samurai and chivalry (Farrell, 2007) or call upon such vague moral terms as "honor," which is "always morally impressive," but is only "sometimes successful" and may mean very little (Axinn, 2009, p. 49). We do not know if military culture's attempts to comprehensively suppress the wakefulness of fellow humans in the military continue to be necessary for them to carry out their work. We are all interconnected, mindfulness tells us, and mistreating or using others as tools for our own benefit is incongruous with a compassionate wisdom or a mindful ethic. Mindfulness, however, is all about helping others and alleviating suffering, suffering that hopefully was not caused or, aided and abetted by mindfulness.

Conclusion

For mindfulness teachers, being aware of the seismic forces engaged to manipulate soldiers to distance them from their humanity and connect exclusively with institutional goals certainly presents significant challenges to delivering mindfulness programs. This clash of cultures can alienate soldiers and veterans who are already profoundly alienated from both society and themselves. Employing mindfulness in a manner that allows soldiers to do more soldier-type things furthers, once again, institutional goals and not the long-term needs and limitations of the humanity in each and every human being wearing a military uniform. Such disconnection, institutionalized and socially legitimized, further isolates soldiers and veterans from themselves and society.

However, such large-scale deformation of humanity offers opportunity for, if not demands, the rest of humanity help soldiers reconnect with themselves, the society for which they sacrificed, and the life that surrounds all of us each day. Mindfulness offers such relational tools to re-establish connectedness, but also to develop discernment and wisdom. Mindfulness-based stress reduction is "grounded in a non-authoritarian, non-hierarchical perspective that allowed for clarity, understanding, and wisdom" (Kabat-Zinn, 2011, p. 292). That the deeper aspects of mindfulness clash with military culture may be self-evident. However, teaching and guiding veterans to shed their deeply inculcated deference to authority so they may live in equanimity with life around them while cultivating *clarity, understanding, and wisdom* offers them hope to awake from their military-induced sleep. For serving soldiers still heavily influenced by the forces of indoctrination and socialization on a daily basis, mindfulness goals should be perhaps more modest, seeking maybe to simply plant seeds of wisdom and compassion. There is always hope that societies will demand that their militaries become less *institutionalized* and more mindful of not just the missions they define, but how they can cultivate wisdom and compassion, the roots of mindfulness, in each and every soldier. This is a very large hope but learning to "communicate with honesty and candor, and at the same time with mutual respect" (Kabat-Zinn, 2013, p. 480) may help humanity find less costly and more beneficial solutions to our global conflicts. It would be a more compassionate act than sending our fellow humans into the fray to lose their humanity so that we may maintain the myth that we are preserving our own.

References

Amaro, A. (2015). A holistic mindfulness. *Mindfulness, 6*(1), 63–73.

American Psychological Association (APA). (2011). *Competency benchmarks in professional psychology.* Retrieved from https://www.apa.org/ed/graduate/revised-competency-benchmarks.doc

Axinn, S. (2009). *A moral military: Revised and expanded edition, with a new chapter on torture.* Philadelphia: Temple University Press.

Bacevich, A. (2005). *The new American militarism: How Americans are seduced by war.* Oxford: Oxford University Press.

Bacevich, A. (2013). *Breach of trust: How Americans failed their soldiers and their country.* New York: Metropolitan Books/Henry Holt and Company.

Baer, R. A. (2003). Mindfulness training as a clinical intervention: A conceptual and empirical review. *Clinical Psychology: Science and Practice, 10*(2), 125–143. https://doi.org/10.1093/clipsy.bpg015

Baer, R. A. (2015). Ethics, values, virtues, and character strengths in mindfulness-based interventions: A psychological science perspective. *Mindfulness, 6*(1), 956–969.

Bardenwerper, W. (2011, November 10). U.S. soldiers at war: The forgotten 1 percent. *The Washington Post.* Retrieved from https://www.washingtonpost.com/opinions/us-soldiers-at-war-the-forgotten-1-percent/2011/11/10/gIQAzn7s9M_story.html?utm_term=.4460364fb6ea

Baron, R. S. (2000). Arousal, capacity, and intense indoctrination. *Personality and Social Psychology Review, 4*(3), 238–254. https://doi.org/10.1207/S15327957PSPR0403_3

Benesch, O. (2016). Reconsidering Zen, Samurai, and the martial arts. *The Asia-Pacific Journal, 14*(17/7), 1–23. Retrieved from http://eprints.whiterose.ac.uk/108831/1/article_4921.pdf

Bergen-Cico, D., Possemato, K., & Pigeon, W. (2014). Reductions in cortisol associated with primary care brief mindfulness program for veterans with PTSD. *Medical Care, 52*(12), S25–S31. Retrieved from www.lww-medicalcare.com

Bishop, S. R., Lau, M., Shapiro, S., Carlson, L., Anderson, N., Carmody, J., & Devins, G. (2004). Mindfulness: A proposed operational definition. *Clinical Psychology: Science and Practice, 11*(3), 230–241.

Black, T. R. (2007, November 5). *Canada's vets face tough transition to civilian life.* Retrieved from http://communications.uvic.ca/releases/release.php?display=release&id=865

Boyce, R. M. (2009). Waiver of consent: The use of pyridostigmine bromide during the Persian Gulf War. *Journal of Military Ethics, 8*(1), 1–18.

Bruyea, S. (2011, November). *A challenging homecoming: How military culture, indoctrination as well as physical and psychological injury complicate a successful transition.* Paper presented at the Military and Veterans Health Review Forum, Kingston, Ontario, Canada.

Bruyea, S. (2016). *Remembrance forgotten: Seventy years of neglect and our obligation to Canadian Forces veterans.* Masters Dissertation-unpublished.

Bryan, C. J., & Morrow, C. E. (2011). Circumventing mental health stigma by embracing the warrior culture: Lessons learned from the Defender's Edge Program. *Professional Psychology: Research and Practice, 42*(1), 16–23.

Burk, J. (2008). Military culture. In L. Kurtz (Ed.), *Encyclopedia of violence, peace & conflict* (2nd ed., pp. 1242–1256). Oxford: Academic Press (Elsevier).

Call, D., Pitcock, J., & Pyne, J. (2015). Longitudinal evaluation of the relationship between mindfulness, general distress, anxiety, and PTSD in a recently deployed National Guard sample. *Mindfulness, 6*(1), 1303–1312.

Capstick, M. D. (2003, Spring). Defining the culture: The Canadian Army in the 21st century. *Canadian Military Journal, 47*–53. Retrieved from http://www.journal.forces.gc.ca/index-eng.asp

Challans, T. L. (2007). *Awakening warrior: Revolution in the ethics of warfare.* Albany, NY: State University of New York Press.

Christian, J. R., Stivers, J. R., & Sammons, M. T. (2009). Training to the warrior ethos: Implications for clinicians treating military members and their families. In M. Freeman, S. Moore, & B. A.

Freeman (Eds.), *Living and surviving in harm's way: A psychological treatment handbook for pre- and post-deployment of military personnel*. New York: Routledge. Retrieved from http://site.ebrary.com/lib/oculottawa/reader.action?docID=10308653

Coffey, K. A., Hartman, M., & Fredrickson, B. L. (2010). Deconstructing mindfulness and constructing mental health: Understanding mindfulness and its mechanisms of action. *Mindfulness*, *1*(4), 235–253.

Cook, M. L. (2008). Ethics education, ethics training, and character development: Who 'owns' ethics in the US Air Force Academy. In P. Robinson, N. De Lee, & D. Carrick (Eds.), *Ethics education in the military* (pp. 57–66). Aldershot: Ashgate.

Coronado-Montoya, S., Levis, A. W., Kwakkenbos, L., Steele, R. J., Turner, E. H., & Thombs, B. D. (2016). Reporting of positive results in randomized controlled trials of mindfulness-based mental health interventions. *PloS One*, *11*(4), e0153220.

Cotton, C. A. (1982/83). A Canadian military ethos. Canadian Defence Quarterly, 12(3), 10–18.

Deschamps, M. (2015). *External review into sexual misconduct and sexual harassment in the Canadian Forces*. Retrieved from http://www.forces.gc.ca/assets/FORCES_Internet/docs/en/caf-community-support-services-harassment/era-final-report-(april-20-2015)-eng.pdf

Donagan, A. (1977). *The theory of morality*. Chicago: University of Chicago Press.

Duty with honour. (2003). National defence.(hereafter cited in-text as *"Duty"*)

Dwyer, D. P. (2003, May–June). An engaged spirituality. *Health Progress*, 62–64. Retrieved from www.chausa.org

Eidelson, R. (2011, March 25). The dark side of "Comprehensive Soldier Fitness". *Psychology Today*. Retrieved from https://www.psychologytoday.com/blog/dangerous-ideas/201103/the-dark-side-comprehensive-soldier-fitness

Elwy, A. R., Johnston, J. M., Bormann, J. E., Hull, A., & Taylor, S. L. (2014). A systematic scoping review of complementary and alternative medicine mind and body practices to improve the health of veterans and military personnel. *Medical Care*, *52*(12, Suppl. 5), S70–S82.

English, A. D. (2004). *Understanding military culture*. Kingston, ON: McGill-Queen's University Press.

Farber, I. E., Harlow, H. F., & West, L. J. (1957). Brainwashing, conditioning and DDD (debility, dependency and dread). *Sociometry*, *20*(4), 271–285. Retrieved from http://www.jstor.org/stable/2785980

Farrell, S. (2007). *The road to Abu Ghraib. Chivalry, mercy and self-restraint*. Retrieved from http://chivalrytoday.com/road-abu-ghraib/

Fiala, A. (2010). *Public war, private conscience: The ethics of political violence*. London: Continuum.

Fields, R. (1991). *The code of the warrior: In history, myth, and everyday life*. New York: HarperPerrennial.

Fotion, N., & Elfstrom, G. (1986). *Military ethics: Guidelines for peace and war*. Boston: Routledge & Kegan Paul.

French, S. E. (2003). *The code of the warrior: The values and ideals of warrior cultures throughout history*. New York: Rowman & Littlefield.

Gigerenzer, G., & Gaissmaier, W. (2011). Heuristic decision making. *Annual Review of Psychology*, *62*, 451–482.

Gilbert, P., & Choden, K. (2014). *Mindful compassion: How the science of compassion can help you understand your emotions, live in the present, and connect deeply with others*. Oakland, CA: New Harbinger.

Giner-Sorolla, R., & Chaiken, S. (1997). Selective use of heuristic and systematic processing under defense motivation. *Personality and Social Psychology Bulletin*, *23*(1), 84–97.

Goffman, E. (1961). The characteristics of total institutions. In A. Etzioni (Ed.), *A sociological reader on complex organizations* (2nd ed., pp. 312–338). New York: Hold, Rinehart & Winston.

Gray, J. G. (1998). *The warriors: Reflections of men in battle*. Lincoln, NE: University of Nebraska Press (Bison Books). (Original work published 1959).

Greenberg, M. T., & Mitra, J. L. (2015). From mindfulness to right mindfulness: The intersection of awareness and ethics. *Mindfulness, 6*(1), 74–78.

Grossman, D. (2009). *On killing: The psychological cost of learning to kill in war and society.* New York: Back Bay/Little, Brown.

Grossman, P. (2015). Mindfulness: Awareness informed by an embodied ethic. *Mindfulness, 6*(1), 17–22.

Gunaratana, B. H. (2015). *Mindfulness in plain English.* Somerville, MA: Wisdom Publications.

Hackett, J. W. (1983). *The profession of arms.* New York: Macmillan.

Hanh, T. N. (1976). *The miracle of mindfulness: An introduction to the practice of meditation.* Boston, MA: Beacon Press.

Hare, J. (2014, Winter). Religion and morality. In E. N. Zalta (Ed.), *The Stanford encyclopedia of philosophy.* Retrieved from http://plato.stanford.edu/entries/religion-morality/.

Harrison, D., & Laliberté, L. (1994). *No life like it: Military wives in Canada.* Toronto: James Lorimer.

Haynie, J. M., & Shepherd, D. (2011). Toward a theory of discontinuous career transition: Investigating career transitions necessitated by traumatic life events. *Journal of Applied Psychology, 96*(3), 501–524.

Hedges, C. (2003). *War is a force that gives us meaning.* New York: Anchor Books.

Janowitz, M. (1959). *Sociology and the military establishment.* New York: Russel Sage.

Janowitz, M. (1960). *The professional soldier* (1964, paperback ed.). New York: The Free Press.

Jha, A. P., Morrison, A. B., Dainer-Best, J. D., Parker, S., Rostrup, N., & Stanley, E. A. (2015). Minds "At Attention": Mindfulness training curbs attentional lapses in military cohorts. *PloS One, 10*(2).

Jha, A. P., Morrison, A. B., Parker, S., & Stanley, E. A. (2017). Practice is protective: Mindfulness training promotes cognitive resilience in high-stress cohorts. *Mindfulness, 8*(1), 46–58.

Kabat-Zinn, J. (1990). Full catastrophe living: Using the wisdom of your body and mind to face stress, pain and illness. New York: Delacorte

Kabat-Zinn, J. (2003). Mindfulness-based interventions in context: Past, present, and future. *Clinical Psychology: Science and Practice, 10*(2), 144–156.

Kabat-Zinn, J. (2005). *Coming to our senses.* New York: Hyperion.

Kabat-Zinn, J. (2011). Some reflections on the origins of MBSR, skillful means, and the trouble with maps. *Contemporary Buddhism, 12*(1), 281–306.

Kabat-Zinn, J. (2013). *Full catastrophe living: Using the wisdom of your body and mind to face stress, pain, and illness (Revised and updated edition).* New York: Bantam Books.

Kasher, A. (2008). Teaching and training military ethics: An Israeli experience. In P. Robinson, N. De Lee, & D. Carrick (Eds.), *Ethics education in the military* (pp. 133–146). Aldershot: Ashgate.

Kearney, D. J., Martinez, M., Felleman, B. I., Bernardi, N., Sayre, G., & Simpson, T. L. (2015). *Teaching mindfulness to veterans: A resource.* Seattle, WA: VA Puget Sound Health Care System.

Kraft, H. S. (2007). *Rule number two: Lessons I learned in a combat hospital.* New York: Little, Brown and Company.

Lester, P. B., McBride, S., Bliese, P. D., & Adler, A. B. (2011). Bringing science to bear: An empirical assessment of the Comprehensive Soldier Fitness program. *American Psychologist, 66*(1), 77–81.

Lindahl, J. R. (2015). Why right mindfulness might not be right for mindfulness. *Mindfulness, 6*(1), 57–62.

Litz, B. T., Stein, N., Delaney, E., Lebowitz, L., Nash, W. P., Silva, C., & Maguen, S. (2009). Moral injury and moral repair in war veterans: A preliminary modal and intervention strategy. *Clinical Psychology Review, 29*(8), 695–706.

Loomis, D. C., & Lightburn, D. T. (1980). Taking into account the distinctness of the military from the mainstream of society. *Canadian Defence Quarterly, 10*(2), 16–22.

Mader, H. M. (2002). Riterlichkeit. Eine Basis de humanitären Völkerrechts un ein Weg zu seiner Durchsetzung. *Truppendienst, 2*, 122–126.

Magrid, M., & Poirier, M. R. (2016). The three shaky pillars of Western Buddhism: Deracination, secularization, and instrumentalization. In R. M. Rosenbaum & B. Magrid (Eds.), *What's wrong with mindfulness (and what isn't): Zen perspectives* (pp. 39–52). Somerville, MA: Wisdom Publications.

McGurk, D., Cotting, D. I., Britt, T. W., & Adler, A. B. (2006). Joining the Ranks: The role of indoctrination in transforming civilians into service members. In A. B. Adler, C. A. Castro, & T. W. Britt (Eds.), *Military Life: The psychology of serving in peace and combat, Volume 2: Operational stress* (pp. 13–31). Westport, CT: Praeger Security International.

Mileham, P. (2010). Unlimited liability and the military covenant. *Journal of Military Ethics, 9*(1), 23–40. https://doi.org/10.1080/15027570903353836

Moelker, R., & Kümmel, G. (2007). Chivalry and codes of conduct: Can the virtue of chivalry epitomize guidelines for interpersonal conduct? *Journal of Military Ethics, 6*(4), 292–302.

Monteiro, L., & Musten, F. (2013). *Mindfulness starts here: An eight-week guide to skillful living.* Victoria, BC: FriesenPress.

Monteiro, L. M., Musten, R. F., & Compson, J. (2015). Traditional and contemporary mindfulness: Finding the middle path in the tangle of concerns. *Mindfulness, 6*(1), 1–13.

Moore, B. A., Hopewell, C. A., & Grossman, D. (2009). After the battle: Violence and the warrior. In S. Morgillo Freeman, B. A. Moore, & A. Freeman (Eds.), *Living and surviving in harm's way: A psychological treatment handbook for pre- and post-deployment of military personnel.* New York: Routledge: Taylor & Francis Group.

Moskos, C. C., Williams, J. A., & Segal, D. R. (Eds.). (2000). *The postmodern military: Armed forces after the cold war.* New York: Oxford University Press.

Nuciari, N. (2007). National differences in military values and civilian values: Is the gap culture-free or culture-bound. In G. Caforio (Ed.), *Cultural difference between the military and parent society in democratic countries* (Vol. 4, pp. 225–237). Bingley: Emerald Group. https://doi.org/10.1016/S1572-8323(07)04010-6

Ohnishi, S. T., & Ohnishi, T. (2009). Philosophy, psychology, physics and practice of ki. *Evidence-based Complementary and Alternative Medicine: Ecam, 6*(2), 175–183. https://doi.org/10.1093/ecam/nen005

Olsthoorn, P. (2007). Courage in the military: Physical and moral. Journal of Military Ethics, 6(4), 270–279. Retrieved from https://doi.org/10.1080/15027570701755471.

Ota, F. (2008). Ethics training for the Samurai warrior. In P. Robinson, N. De Lee, & D. Carrick (Eds.), *Ethics education in the military* (pp. 147–160). Aldershot: Ashgate.

Pew Research Center. (2011). *The military-civilian gap: War and sacrifice in the post-9/11 era.* Retrieved from October 5, http://www.pewsocialtrends.org/2011/10/05/war-and-sacrifice-in-the-post-911-era/

Poirier, M. R. (2016). Mischief in the marketplace for mindfulness. In R. M. Rosenbaum & B. Magrid (Eds.), *What's wrong with mindfulness (and what isn't): Zen perspectives* (pp. 13–27). Somerville, MA: Wisdom Publications.

Purser, R. (2014, Spring). The militarization of mindfulness. *Inquiring mind, 30*(2). Retrieved from http://www.inquiringmind.com/Articles/MilitarizationOfMindfulness.html

Purser, R. E. (2015). Clearing the muddled path of traditional and contemporary mindfulness: A response to Monteiro, Musten, and Compson. *Mindfulness, 6*(1), 23–45.

Purser, R., & Loy, D. (2013, July 1). Beyond McMindfulness. *Huffington Post.* Retrieved from http://www.huffingtonpost.com/ron-purser/beyondmcmindfulness_b_3519289.html.

Reber, C. A. S., Boden, T., Mitragotri, N., Alverez, J., Gross, J. J., & Bonn-Miller, M. O. (2013). A prospective investigation of mindfulness skills and changes in emotion regulation among military veterans in posttraumatic stress disorder treatment. *Mindfulness, 4*(4), 311–317.

Rees, B. (2011). Overview of outcome data of potential meditation training for soldier resilience. *Military Medicine, 176*(11), 1232–1242.

Rendtorff, T. (1986). *Ethics Volume 1: Basic elements and methodology in an ethical theology* (K. Crim, Trans.). Philadelphia: Fortress Press.

Robinson, P. (2007a, Spring). Ethics training and development in the military. *Parameters, 22*–36. Retrieved from http://cape.army.mil/cgsc-ethics/repository/Ethics-Training-and-Development-in-the-Military_Robinson_Parameters_Spring%202007_pages%2023-36.pdf

Robinson, P. (2007b). Magnanimity and integrity as military virtues. *Journal of Military Ethics, 6*(4), 259–269.

Robinson, P. (2008). Introduction: Ethics education in the military. In P. Robinson, N. De Lee, & D. Carrick (Eds.), *Ethics education in the military* (pp. 1–12). Aldershot: Ashgate.

Robinson, P., De Lee, N., & Carrick, D. (Eds.). (2008). *Ethics education in the military*. Aldershot: Ashgate.

Rochman, B. (2009, September 26). Samurai mind training for modern American warriors. *Time*. Retrieved from http://content.time.com/time/nation/article/0,8599,1920753,00.html

Rock, E. R. (2009, September 10). Meditation and the military – an oxymoron? Or is meditation going mainstream? Retrieved from http://searchwarp.com/swa546457-Is-Meditation-Going-Mainstream-Meditation-And-The-Military.htm

Rose, S. (2015). Applying Durkheim's theory of suicide: A study of altruism and anomie among Canadian veterans of Afghanistan. Doctoral dissertation. Retrieved from https://qspace.library.queensu.ca/handle/1974/13511

Rothschild, S., Kaplan, G., Golan, T., & Barak, Y. (2017). Mindfulness meditation in the Israel Defense Forces: Effect on cognition and satisfaction with life—A randomized controlled trial. *European Journal of Integrative Medicine, 9*(1). https://doi.org/10.1016/j.eujim.2017.01.010

Schein, E. H. (1992). *Organizational culture and leadership* (2nd ed.). San Francisco: Jossey-Bass.

Segsworth, W. (1920). *Retraining Canada's disabled soldiers*. Ottawa: King's Printer.

Senauke, H. A. (2016). One body, whole life: Mindfulness and Zen. In R. M. Rosenbaum & B. Magrid (Eds.), *What's wrong with mindfulness (and what isn't): Zen perspectives* (pp. 69–79). Somerville, MA: Wisdom Publications.

Shapiro, S. L., Carlson, L. E., Astin, J. A., & Freedman, B. (2006). Mechanisms of mindfulness. *Journal of Clinical Psychology, 62*(3), 373–386.

Shapiro, S. L., & Schwartz, G. E. (2000). The role of intention in self-regulation: Toward intentional systemic mindfulness. In M. Boekaerts, P. R. Pintrich, & M. Zeidner (Eds.), *Handbook of self-regulation* (pp. 253–273). San Diego, CA: Academic Press.

Shay, J. (2002). *Odysseus in America: Combat trauma and the trials of homecoming*. New York: Scribner.

Sherman, N. (2015). *Afterwar: Healing the moral wounds of our soldiers*. Oxford: Oxford University Press.

Smith, R. T., & True, G. (2014). Warring identities: Identity conflict and the mental distress of American veterans of the wars in Iraq and Afghanistan. *Society and Mental Health, 4*(2), 147–161.

Snider, D. (1999). The future of American military culture: An uninformed debate on military culture. *Orbis, 43*(1), 11–26.

Soeters, J. L., Poponete, C. R., & Page, J. T. (2006). Culture's consequence in the military. In A. B. Adler, T. W. Britt, & C. A. Castro (Eds.), *Military culture-military life: The psychology of serving in peace and combat* (Vol. 4, pp. 13–34). Westport, CT: Praeger Security International.

Stanley, E. A. & Jha, A. P. (2009, October 30). Mind fitness: Improving operational effectiveness and building warrior resilience. *Army*. Retrieved from http://www.army.mil/mobile/article/?p=29549

Stanley, E. A., Schaldach, J. M., Kiyonaga, A., & Jha, A. P. (2011). Mindfulness-based mind fitness training: A case study of a high-stress predeployment military cohort. *Cognitive and Behavioral Practice, 18*(4), 566–576. https://doi.org/10.1016/j.cbpra.2010.08.002

Sue, D. W. (1981). *Counselling the culturally different: Theory and practice*. New York: Wiley.

Teasdale, J. D., Segal, Z. V., & Williams, J. M. G. (2003). Mindfulness training and problem formulation. *Clinical Psychology, 10*(2), 157–160.

Thompson, M. (2011, November 21). The other 1%. *Time*, 34–39.

Tick, E. (2014). *Warriors return: Restoring the soul after war*. Boulder, CO: Sounds True.

Tisdale, S. J. (2016). The buffet: Adventures in the New Age. In R. M. Rosenbaum & B. Magrid (Eds.), *What's wrong with mindfulness (and what isn't): Zen perspectives* (pp. 80–90). Somerville, MA: Wisdom Publications.

Tracey, I., & Flower, R. (2014). The warrior in the machine: Neuroscience goes to war. *Science and Society*, *15*(12), 825–834.

Turchik, J. A., & Wilson, S. M. (2010). Sexual assault in the U.S. military: A review of the literature and recommendations for the future. *Aggression and Violent Behavior*, *15*(4), 267–277. https://doi.org/10.1016/j.avb.2010.01.005

Van Gordon, W., Shonin, E., Griffiths, M. D., & Singh, N. N. (2015). There is only one mindfulness: Why science and Buddhism need to work together. *Mindfulness*, *6*(1), 49–56.

Verweij, D. (2007). Comrades or friends? On friendship in the armed forces. *Journal of Military Ethics*, *6*(4), 280–291.

Wadell, P. (1989). *Friendship and the moral life*. Notre Dame, IN: University of Notre Dame Press.

Waller, W. (1944). *The Veteran comes back*. New York: The Dryden Press.

Index

© Springer International Publishing AG 2017
L.M. Monteiro et al. (eds.), *Practitioner's Guide to Ethics and Mindfulness-Based Interventions*, Mindfulness in Behavioral Health,
DOI 10.1007/978-3-319-64924-5